First Steps

Exploring Arizona's Back Country

A Word of Caution

While the author has made every effort to insure the aaccuracy of the information in this book, changes do occur in weather, geography or roads and trails. It is the responsibility of each hiker to use good judgement and make wise decisions regarding their activities. The author and all associated with this book, directly or indirectly, disclaim any liability for accidents, injuries, damages or losses which may occur when using this book. The responsibility for safety while hiking these trails remains with the individual hiker. We wish you the very best experience while enjoying Arizona outdoors!

Mileage

Mileage may vary from that listed as odometers may be slightly different for each vehicle. We have attempted to describe routes so that hikers may arrive at their destination even with the mechanical vagarities of odometers.

Maps

Most of the hikes in this book can be found using a Forest Service map or by checking an internet browser online. In the more remote areas, a topographical map may also be useful. If in question, check with your local governing agency, whether federal, state or private, for further information on any trail.

Cover Photo: Bog Springs

First Steps: Exploring Arizona's Back Country / Eileen Moore
Published by Morten Moore Publishing, LLC
        415 E. Mohawk, Flagstaff, AZ 86005
Copyright 2022 Kenneth & Ruth Mortenson
ISBN 978-0-9991108-9-8

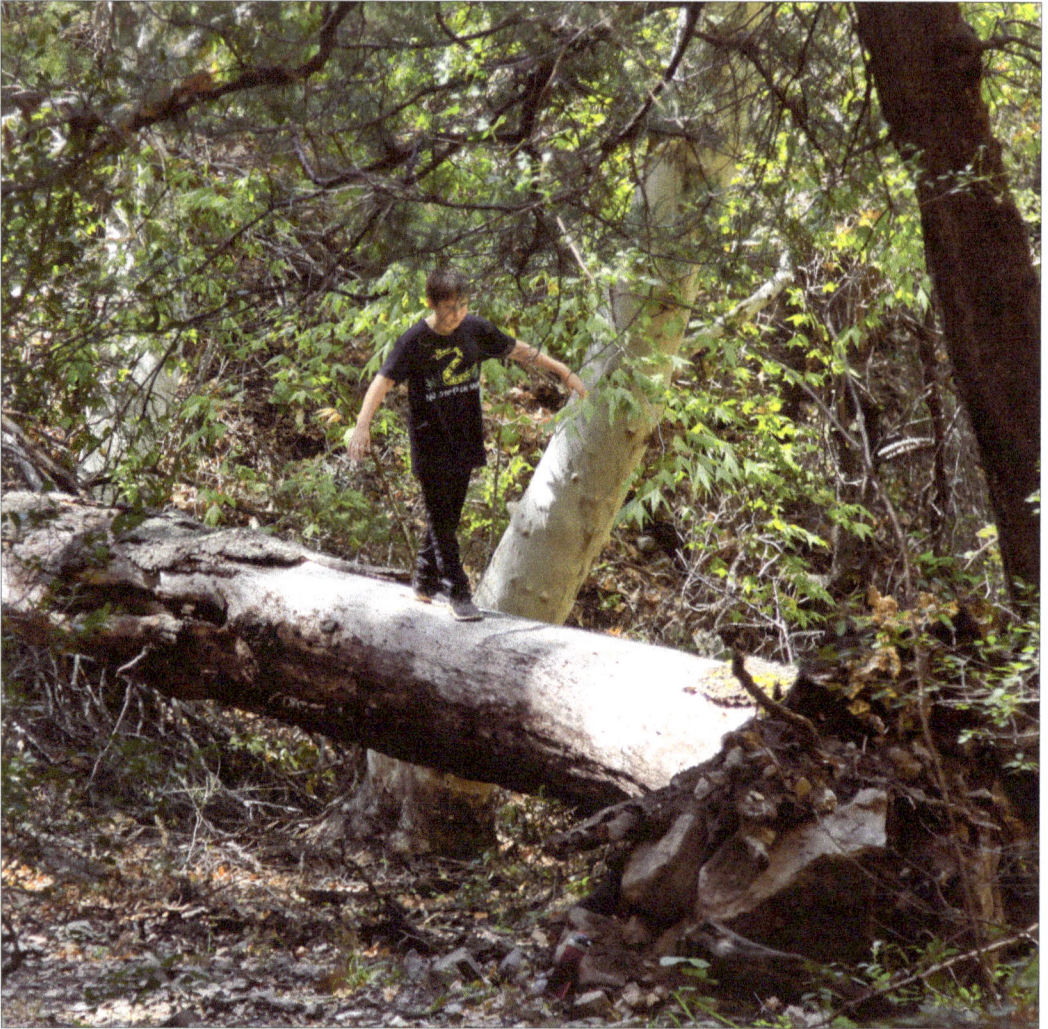

Oh, the places you'll go,
the things you'll see . . .

First Steps

Exploring Arizona's Back Country

Each adventure begins with those first steps from our home into new territory. We step out of our comfort zone to accept new challenges and find previous experience give us confidence to accept the challenge of the unknown. Those first steps lead to places we would not experience unless we take that first step and keep moving.

You may be an experienced hiker looking for a new area or a novice wishing to explore beyond your doorstep. This book is an introduction to family friendly trails that lead through territory close to your home base, hopefully sparking your curiosity to explore more of Arizona. Most of the trails are relatively short, not too demanding and have a specific destination other than a 'nice view.'

We've picked out several trails for each region that families will enjoy. If you search the internet for these trails, other routes will most likely pop up, expanding your options. Once you become familiar with a region, you'll want to start checking other locations for new trails to explore.

Let's first think about being prepared to hike in the back country.

1) Pick a hike, find a map. That little map on your phone is helpful but a paper map of the area you're

hiking in gives you an overall view of what surrounds you. Much of the back country has no cell service and it is important to be familiar with the terrain.

2) Place the appropriate supplies in your backpack, including sufficient water. Arizona is an ARID state. See the list of items to pack on the next page.

3) Don't exceed your physical abilities. Whether the distance or the endurance demanded, know your limitations and avoid a call to medics.

4) VERY IMPORTANT - Call a responsible person and let them know where you are hiking and when you expect to return. Request that if they don't hear from you, they check back to ensure you have returned. If you don't show up within a reasonable amount of time they alert the authorities.

5) If you're with a group, don't get separated. That means the more fit hikers wait for the slower members. On only one occasion have I willingly sent my partner away and that was in an emergency. We are stronger together.

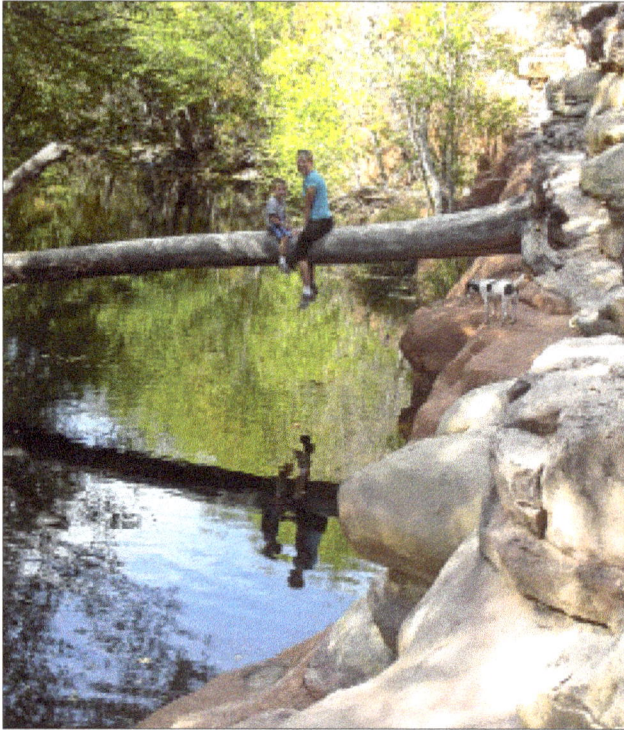

eyes, we renew our sense of wonder at the world around us.

First tip: Slow down. See the wonder in your child's mind. Live within that moment. The longer hikes will come later.

Second tip: Your child will alternate between the minute and the grand discoveries. Live in the moment, drawing their attention to what they don't see.

Third tip: Your child's legs are shorter than your legs. They take two, maybe three steps, for every one of your steps. It may seem like your child has more energy than you as they bound around the house but they are short on endurance. Don't push your child beyond what they are capable of doing.

Fourth tip: Those who are very young and those who are very old share a vulnerability to the climate in which they live. Both children and the elderly have a hard time adjusting and maintaining their core body

Hiking with a Child's Perspective

Before we set out into the back country, let's look at the world from a child's point of view. There is so much to discover from shiny rocks in a clear stream to the challenge of climbing a huge boulder. Too often we lay out a route and forget that a child may want to slow down and explore the natural world. Maybe they want to make tracks through squishy mud or examining the water bugs skating on a creek surface.

When hiking with a child we should respect their age and abilities, their level of endurance, their experience in being outdoors and plan appropriately. If we plan realistically, our expectations are less likely to crash. And through their

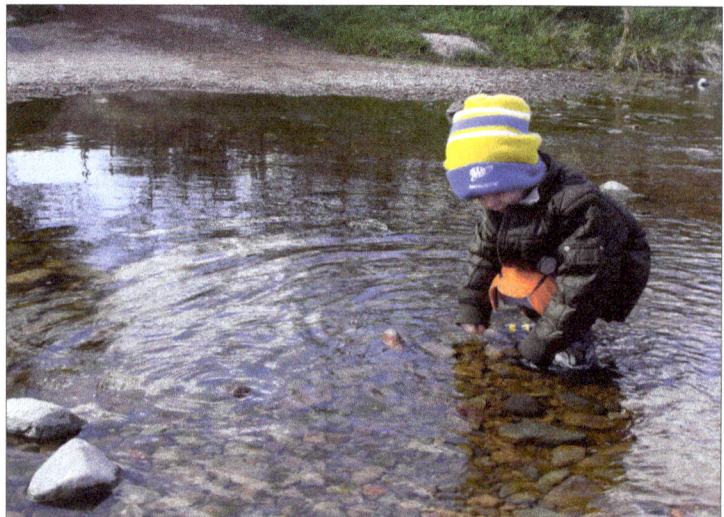

temperature to the current conditions. Think ahead and protect your child from extreme conditions, whether cold or hot, rainy or dry.

In cold weather, you child may need one more layer than you're wearing. With overheated temperatures, their bodies will overheat more quickly. It is far better to retreat than to push onward for the sake of completing a hike.

Fifth Tip: The time you spend outdoors is not about the distance you cover but about the character you are developing in that child. Your child will not forget the time you've spent with him and if it is done well, it will become a treasured memory. This is something more valuable than anything we can buy them. Make the time worthwhile.

And finally, the last tip: I have no problem with resorting to bribery to urge my child to take a few more steps.

Being Prepared

Experienced hikers load their packs with a few supplies. You just never know what might be useful when unexpected things happen. They also know the value of a good pair of hiking boots. We've drawn up a list of items that may come in handy when you're far from home and need the tools for survival.

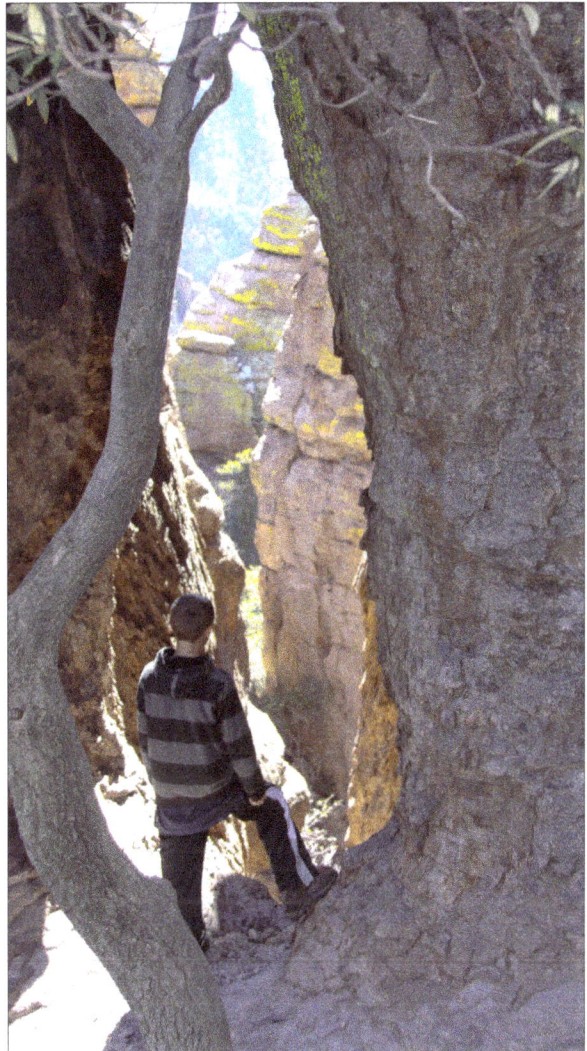

Echo Canyon trail, Chiricahua Mountains

Basic Supplies	
Water! Lots of water!	Pocket Knife and/or Leatherman tool
Snacks	Compass (know how to use it)
First aid kit	A foil survival blanket
A windbreaker or jacket.	Toilet paper & plastic bag
Flashlight	Whistles
Water-proof matches or a lighter	Water filtration device or iodine tablets

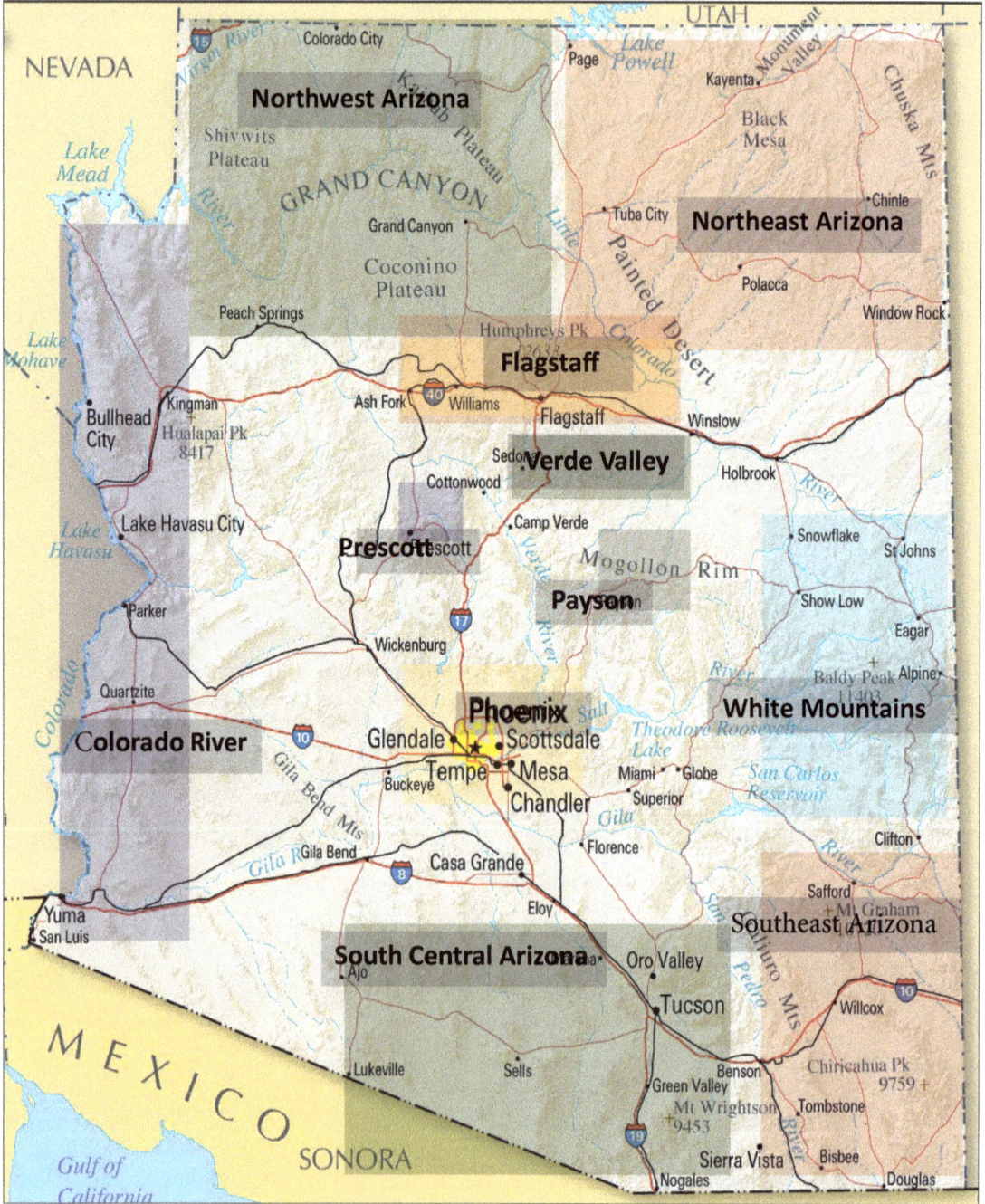

NEVADA

UTAH

Colorado City

Lake Powell

Page

Kayenta

Monument Valley

Northwest Arizona

Shivwits Plateau

Chuska Mts

Black Mesa

Chinle

GRAND CANYON

Lake Mead

Virgin River

Kaibab Plateau

Little

Tuba City

Northeast Arizona

Grand Canyon

Coconino Plateau

Polacca

Lake Mohave

Painted Desert

Window Rock

Peach Springs

Humphreys Pk

Colorado

Flagstaff

Ash Fork

Williams

Flagstaff

Winslow

Kingman

Hualapai Pk
8417

Sedona

Verde Valley

Holbrook

River

Bullhead City

Cottonwood

Camp Verde

Snowflake

St Johns

Lake Havasu City

Prescott Prescott

Verde

Mogollon Rim

Show Low

Lake Havasu

Parker

Payson

Eagar

Colorado

Wickenburg

River

Baldy Peak
11403

Alpine

Quartzite

Phoenix

Salt

White Mountains

Colorado River

Glendale

Scottsdale

Theodore Roosevelt Lake

Tempe

Mesa

Miami

Globe

San Carlos Reservoir

Buckeye

Chandler

Superior

Gila Bend Mts

Gila

Clifton

Gila R

Gila Bend

Florence

Casa Grande

River

Yuma

Eloy

Safford

Mt Graham

Southeast Arizona

San Luis

South Central Arizona

Oro Valley

Willcox

MEXICO

Ajo

Tucson

Chiricahua Pk
9759

Lukeville

Sells

Benson

Green Valley

Mt Wrightson
9453

Tombstone

Bisbee

SONORA

Nogales

Sierra Vista

Douglas

Gulf of California

The Ups and Downs of Arizona

Arizona is such a diverse state, from deserts to snow-capped mountains, from pine trees and fir down to saguaro cactus. If you don't like one ecological zone, just drive a couple of hours to a different one. Arizona residents do just that. Urban dwellers crowd the towns in the high country during warm weekends while those in the snow zone escape to a warmer climate during the winter.

Let's take a moment to look at the geography of Arizona. The basin and range region around Phoenix is pure desert with arid grit and sand supporting a wide range of cactus and succulents.

An eclipse of mountain ranges, known as the transitional zone, stretches from the southeast corner of the state, around Phoenix, and up to the Northwest corner. In the north, it is possible to chart a course from Flagstaff to the east border and south to the sky islands without dipping into the lowest elevations. In the south the mountain ranges are called sky islands and tend to be isolated, one range from another.

Moving northeast from Flagstaff across the central highlands, travelers traverse a high desert that once supported wild grasses. Today this zone is mostly covered with arid brush till we reach the pine forests along the eastern border.

Arizona's diverse landscape presents some unique challenges to those who enjoy the outdoors. Recreational visitors can dress for summer temperatures. Then, summer monsoonal rains move in and hikers find they are drenched and shivering in the cooler air. It is important to know the weather conditions, how they can change and to be prepared before we set out to enjoy a hike and time exploring the back country.

There are six to seven life zones spread over these three regions. Eash zone has unique flora and fauna, making Arizona a great place to explore. The desert zone is found below 6,000 feet in the central and southeastern parts of the state. The pinon pine and juniper zone, known as woodlands, is found between 6,000 to 7,000 feet. The ponderosa pine dominates the zone between 7,000-8,000 feet. The fir zone is up to 9,200 feet followed by the spruce zone up to 11,000 feet. Timberline is around 11,500 with the Alpine zone at the very top of the highest peaks.

Why is this important? If we pay attention to what grows in each zone, we have a better idea of what challenges the climate may throw at us as we prepare to be outdoors. We generally would not expect a snowstorm in the desert but we sure want to be prepared above 6,000 feet in the spring and fall.

I've divided the state into 11 regions. Each section features trails for hikers that are looking for something comfortable, usually under five miles, not too strenuous with something interesting to catch their attention along the route. Once you've grown comfortable with the trails we've suggested, you can find a whole lot more listed online. Head over to Alltrails with your internet browser and enter a trail you know in the search bar. That trail should pop-up with other options in the same area for you to consider.

We wish you the best in exploring Arizona. Stay safe!

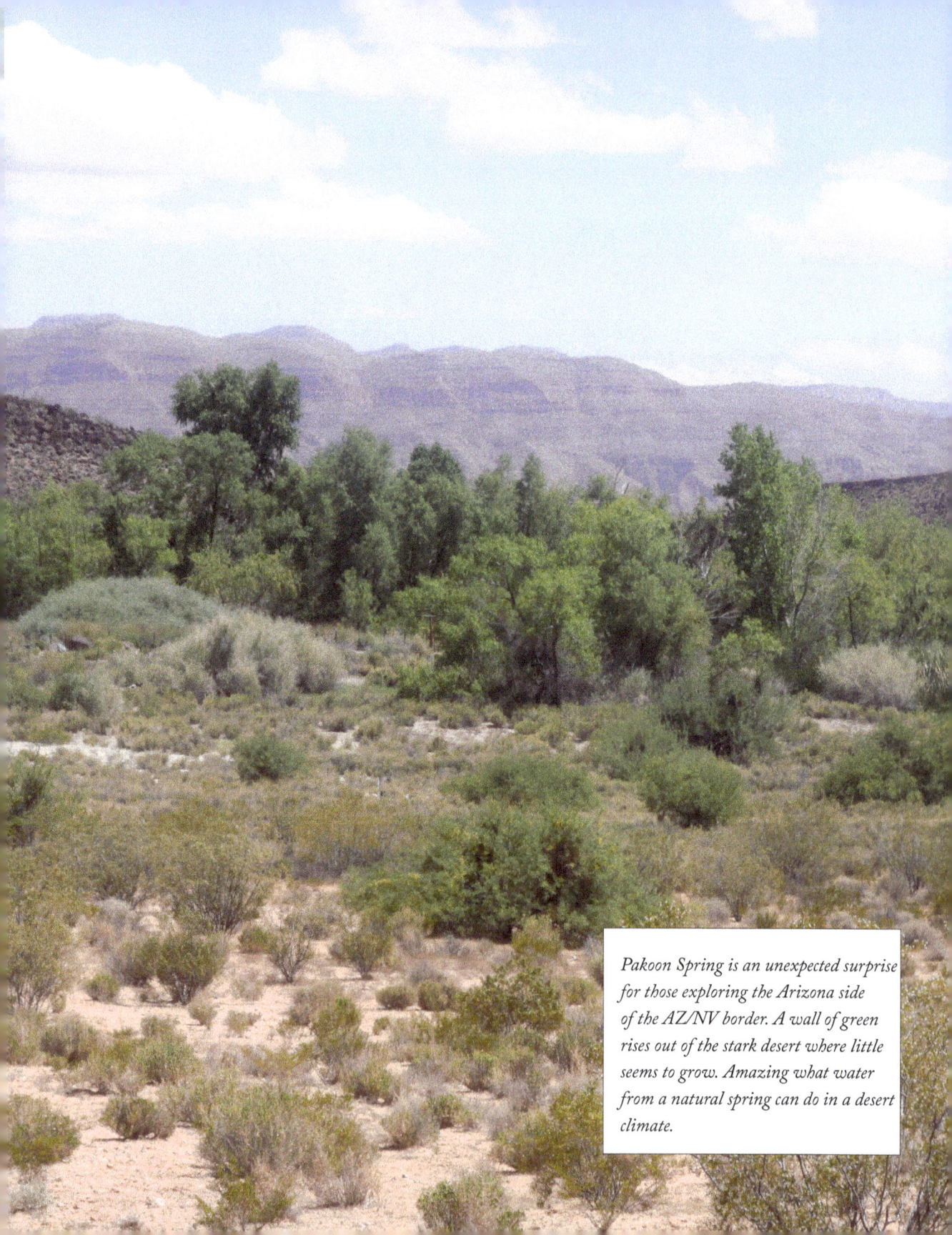

Pakoon Spring is an unexpected surprise for those exploring the Arizona side of the AZ/NV border. A wall of green rises out of the stark desert where little seems to grow. Amazing what water from a natural spring can do in a desert climate.

The Arizona Strip refers to the land north of the Grand Canyon and south of Utah, between Nevada on the west and US Highway 89A on the east. The terrain, west to east, forms a series of steps that rises from desert to a pine-shrouded plateau, 8,000 feet in elevation. The snow and rain that fall on the mountains around Jacob Lake. Don't be surprised to see buffalo and herds of deer north of the Grand Canyon.

Families wishing to explore further would be well advised to seek out those with experience in the forests and high desert of the Arizona Strip.

The Arizona Strip and Northwestern Arizona

plateau, drain through sharply cut canyons into the Grand Canyon and the Colorado River. Human settlements are far and few between, leaving a lot of land to explore, providing you are properly prepared for harsh conditions.

We've featured a few short hikes that will introduce hikers to the region. Two of our favorite historic sites are located in the strip and well worth checking out. Expect to find a wide range of conditions from high summer temperatures along the western border to heavy winter snow in the

Despite a number of trips into the area, in 2018, we found ourselves in trouble deep in a canyon on the North Rim. We should have heeded the old saying, 'An ounce of prevention is worth a pound of cure."

We recommend traveling with two vehicles when you go off the main highways as more than one flat tire is common. Be sure to take plenty of supplies and water. Always let someone know when you will return and where you will be! Go slow and easy, learn as you go!

1 Whitney Pockets
2 Pipe Springs
3 Big Springs /
   Brow Monument
4 Lees Ferry &
   Lonely Dell
5 Mt Trumbull &
   Toroweap
6 Angels Window &
   Cliff Spring
7 Bright Angel Point
8 Grand Canyon
   Village
9 East Rim
10 Roaring Springs
11 Red Butte
12 Grand Canyon
   Caverns
13 Havasupai

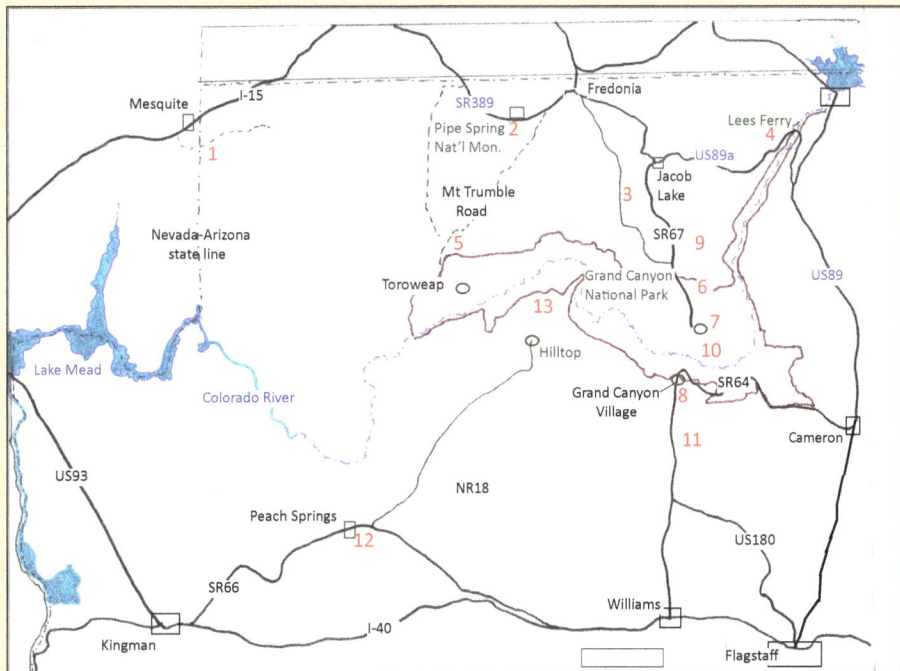

Pipe Springs National Monument

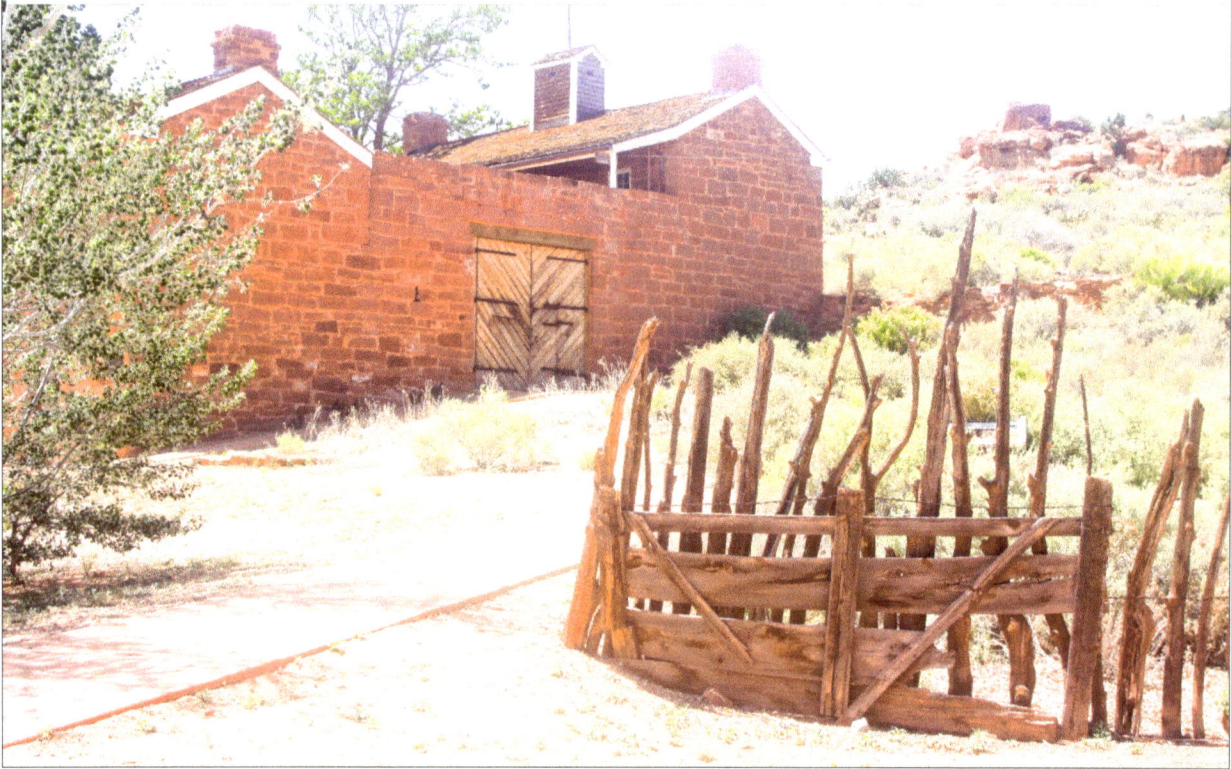

Pipe Springs National Monument is one of my favorite historic parks in the state. There is so much history to learn. Not just the history of the early LDS settlers but the history of how settlers survived, abuse to the land and the cost to be paid when we fail to understand our environment. As a family, you can tour the old fort and hike up the low ridge overlooking the site.

The springs were an important stop on the Old Spanish Trail between Santa Fe, New Mexico and the Spanish town of Los Angeles in the 1700s. In the late 1800's LDS settlers settled at the springs, moving down from Utah into Arizona. They established a ranch and brought thousands of head of cattle and sheep to graze the plains around the springs. They did not suspect that they were permanently damaging the grasslands.

Today, the US National Park Services manages the monument, giving us a taste of living history. The spring supports life, an oasis in the harsh dry land. The ponds provide water for gardens and a orchard. The water provides a cool respite to visitors.

Windsor Castle was a fortified home with large gates at either end of the structure, allowing easy, fast access for a wagon team if under attack. The rooms are built on either side of the courtyard and are filled with antiques from the descendants of Mormon settlers in the area.

Most intriguing is the room where milk was processed into cheese. Early settlers recognized the role of clean water in daily life and channeled the water from Main Spring that emerges under the fort to flow through a long trough in a room next

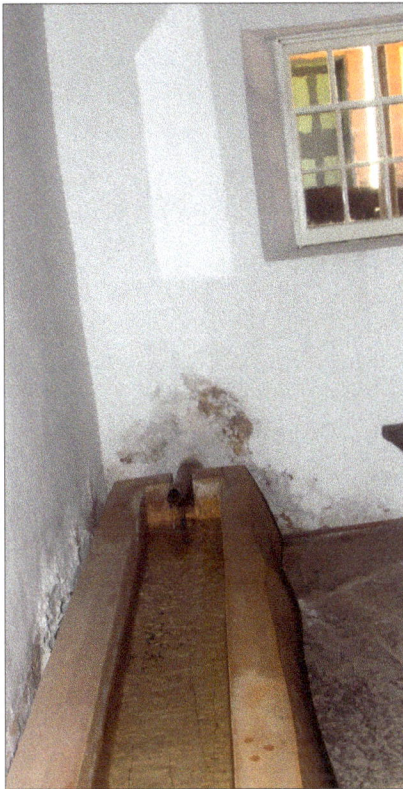

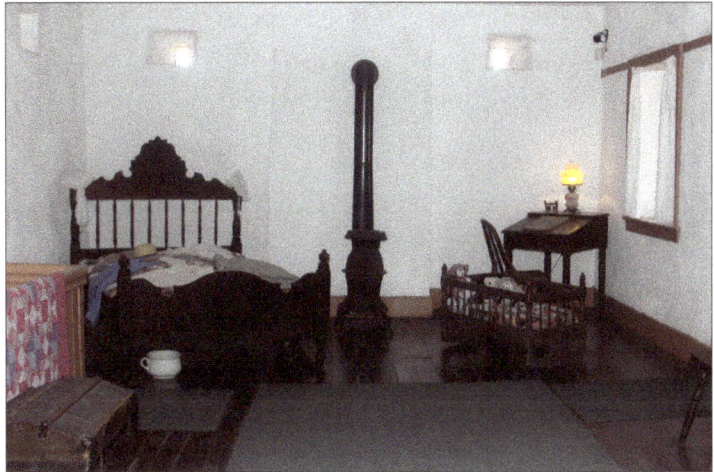

to the kitchen. Not only was a clean supply of water guaranteed but it helped to cool a room that must have been very warm on hot summer days.

A half-mile nature trail runs up the side of the mesa rising over the monument. The trail offers a wonderful view out over the valley and a chance to visualize how the grassland appeared before settlers moved in.

Pipe Spring is located between Fredonia and Colorado City, just south of the Utah border. From Fredonia, turn west from US 89A onto SR 389 and drive 15 miles. The Monument is clearly visible on the north side of the road.

Photo, left: Winsor Castle
Photo above: Spring water channeled through the 'cheese room'.
Photo, top right: the Sitting Room

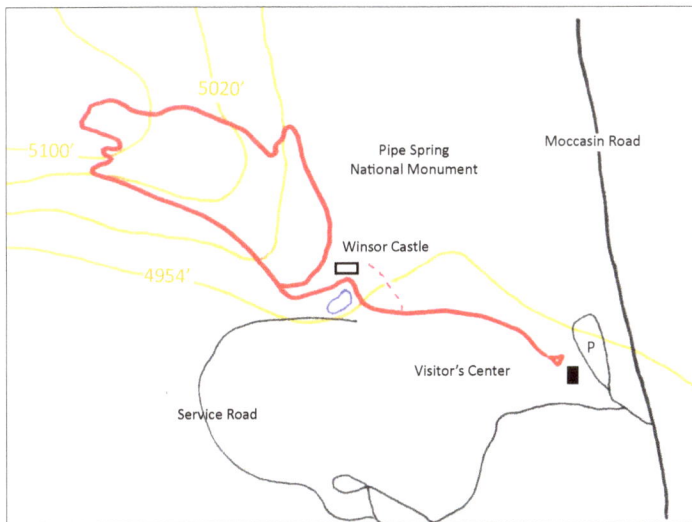

Driving Distance: 14 miles from Fredonia
Hiking Distance: .65 mile
Rating: Easy
Elevation: 5000'
Best Seasons: Spring & fall
Special Features: Historic site with unique   pioneer museum.
Precautions: Dry, warm climate and few services. Tourism is a large factor in local economy.
Maps: Arizona Highways map
Information:
Pipe Spring National Monument
(928) 643-7105

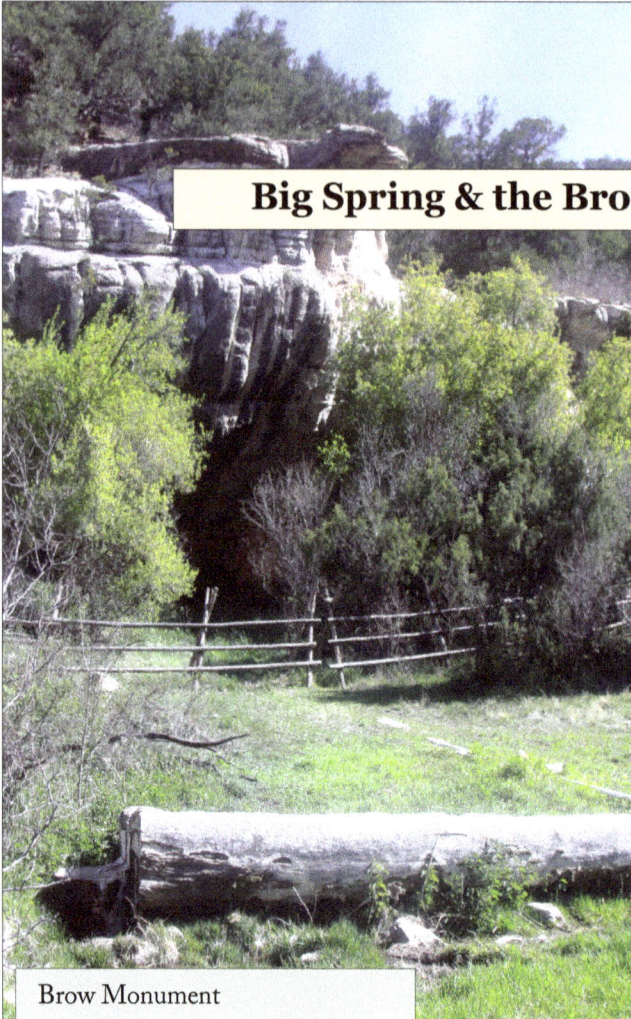

Big Spring & the Brow Monument Trail

Natural springs drew settlers to live in Nail Canyon, north of the Grand Canyon. **Big Spring** is the largest in a line of springs that emerge from the canyon walls with thousands of gallons of water flowing down a limestone cliff to a small pond.

The Forest Service established a camp on the site of an old ranch at Big Spring. They built small cabins for their personnel that are rented to summer visitors. A cookhouse and bathhouse complete the lay- out on one end of the camp while the Forest Service maintains a work site and houses for fire crews at the other end of the camp.

On the south end of the camp, a trail switchbacks up the cliff to top out on the plateau. The trail winds through the meadows and forest to a 100-foot tall fire tower with a view beyond the neighboring pines. During warm months, a lookout stands watch, scanning the terrain for the first signs of smoke. Most lookouts will permit visitors to climb the tower, providing they are respectful of tower personnel.

If the trail seems a bit long, there is road access along a circuitous route south and east of the camp. This route passes Castle Spring, a good place to stop and explore the natural spring that seeps from an overhanging ledge of limestone.

To reach Big Springs, drive south from Kanab, UT along FR 22 for just over 36 miles.

Brow Monument
Driving Distance: 15 miles from
   Jacobs Lake
Hiking Distance: 2 miles one way
Rating: Easy   Elevation: 7405'
Best Season: Spring - fall
Special Features: Historic site
Precautions: No services, isolated.
Maps: North Kaibab US Forest
   Service Map.
Information: Kaibab Plateau
   Visitor's Center
   928-643-7298

Brow Monument--

Imagine what it must have been like to be the first white man to explore the Grand Canyon.

John Wesley Powell lost an arm during a battle in the Civil War but this did not stop him from exploring uncharted territory across the western states. Powell is best known for leading the expedition that floated down the Colorado River, through the Grand Canyon.

Powell also led an expedition to chart the country north of the Grand Canyon. We can hike to a point overlooking the Arizona strip, toward the rim of the Grand Canyon and a monument commemorating Powell's expedition on the Brow Monument Trail.

From Big Springs Camp on Forest Road 422, drive south to FR 447. Turn right and drive a half mile to FR 252. Just under a mile further, turn left on FR252C which can be poorly marked. Follow FR252C to a parking area. Trail #108 follows an old road out to the brow of the mesa where you'll find the monument marker.

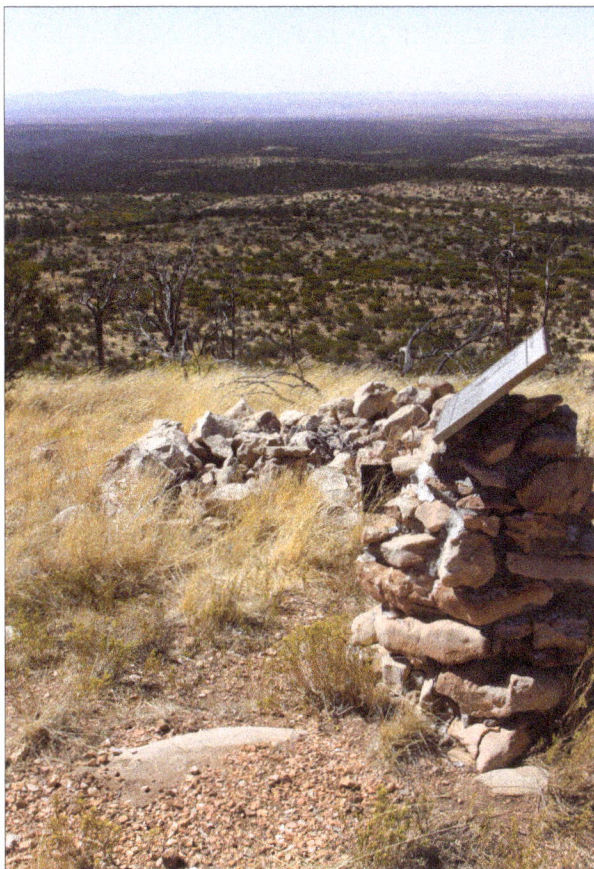

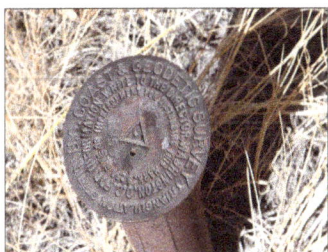

I love the views on either side of the ridgeline walked out to the monument. And to think we are walking in the footsteps of early explorers!

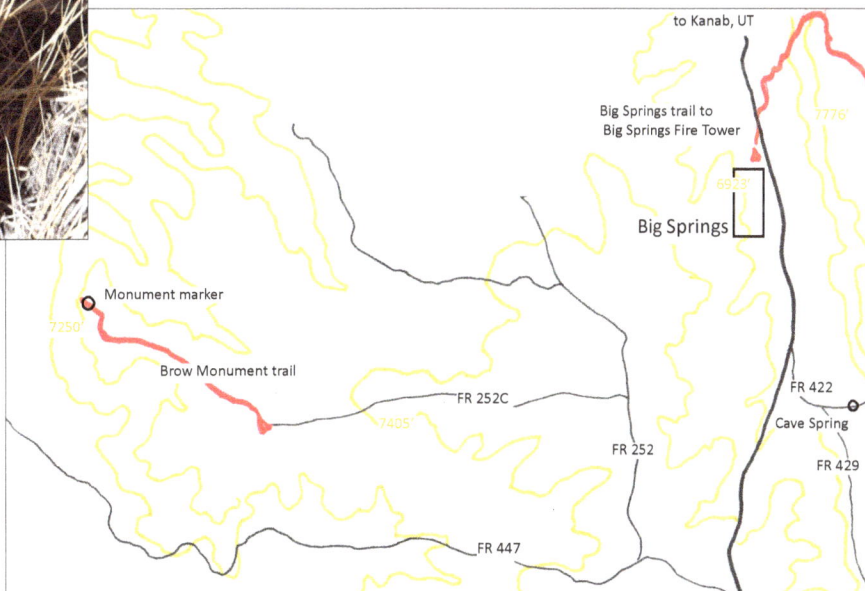

to Kanab, UT

Big Springs trail to
Big Springs Fire Tower

7776'

6883'

Big Springs

Monument marker

7250'

Brow Monument trail

FR 252C

7405'

FR 422

Cave Spring

FR 252

FR 429

FR 447

11

Lees Ferry, Riverside and the Sterling Trail

The Grand Canyon presented a mighty challenge to settlers moving south into Arizona from Utah. At best, those who lived around the canyon followed game trails to the river in this crack in the earth's surface.

Brigham Young, the leader of the LDS church, sought to expand his influence across the western states by sending out followers to operate ferries crossing the major rivers. John D. Lee was assigned to a hazardous crossing above what we now call Marble Canyon.

Lee began to operate a ferry at the crossing in 1870. The ferry became a key stop along the 'Honeymoon Trail,' named for the couples who followed the track to the LDS Temple in Saint George to have their unions blessed by the LDS leadership.

The ferry service ended in 1928 and the Navajo Bridge was completed in 1929. The site became the northern terminus for the Glen Canyon National Recreation Area, established in 1972.

Lonely Dell, the former home of Emma Lee, one of John's wives, is a short walk from Lees Ferry. This is a great place for visitors to stretch their legs while en route to the North Rim of the Grand Canyon. Visitors have an opportunity to explore and touch part of Arizona's history.

John W. Powell, one of the first white men to take a boat through the inner gorge spent several months at the site.

Several old buildings at Lees Ferry date back to a mining venture. Charles Spencer was convinced there was gold in the canyon walls

For outdoor enthusiasts, Lees Ferry is known for fishing and as the launch point for those rafting down the Colorado River. This is point zero on the river maps.

An aerial cable marks the site as the dividing line between the upper and lower basins of the Colorado River, an important demarcation point when it comes to distributing the water between the western states.

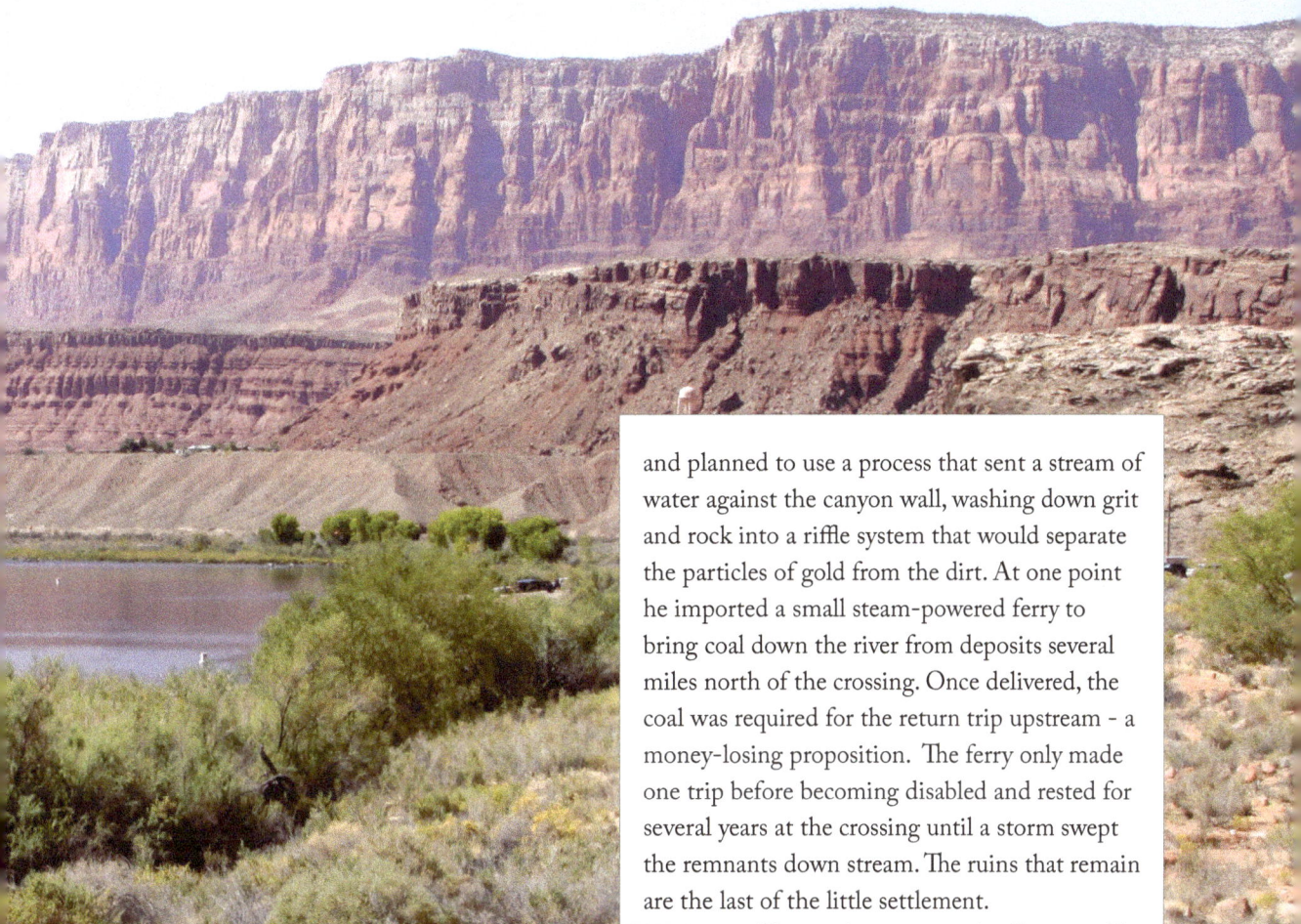

and planned to use a process that sent a stream of water against the canyon wall, washing down grit and rock into a riffle system that would separate the particles of gold from the dirt. At one point he imported a small steam-powered ferry to bring coal down the river from deposits several miles north of the crossing. Once delivered, the coal was required for the return trip upstream - a money-losing proposition. The ferry only made one trip before becoming disabled and rested for several years at the crossing until a storm swept the remnants down stream. The ruins that remain are the last of the little settlement.

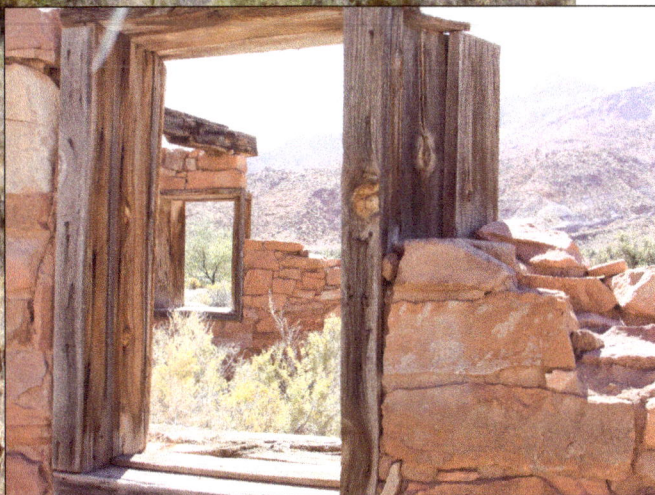

Two trails remain at the Crossing. The river trail follows the river's western bank upstream for about a mile, climbing and descending with the rocky terrain.

The **Spencer trail** climbs the western wall to the rim. It was carved out of the rock by Charles Spencer as a mule trail. He hoped to freight the coal to the site. We don't recommend climbing this trail as the fractured rock is unstable. Instead, enjoy some time along the river. For those who wish to wade, be aware that the river currents are dangerous.

Lonely Dell at Lees Ferry

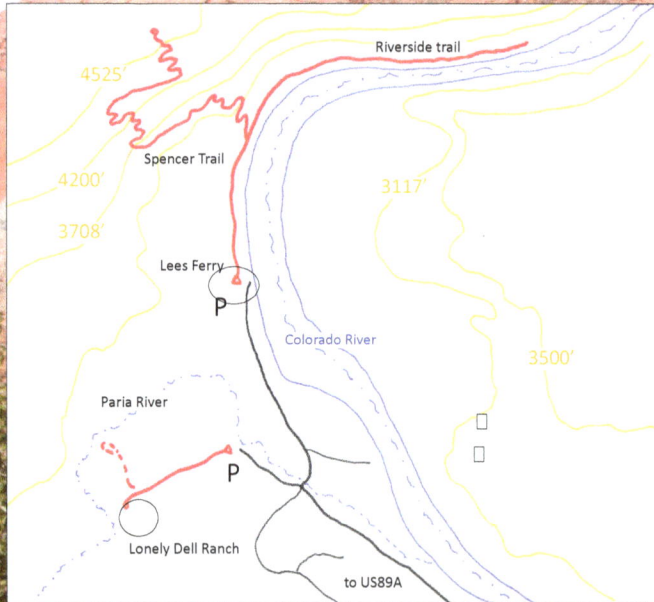

- 4525'
- Riverside trail
- Spencer Trail
- 4200'
- 3708'
- 3117'
- Lees Ferry
- P
- Colorado River
- 3500'
- Paria River
- P
- Lonely Dell Ranch
- to US89A

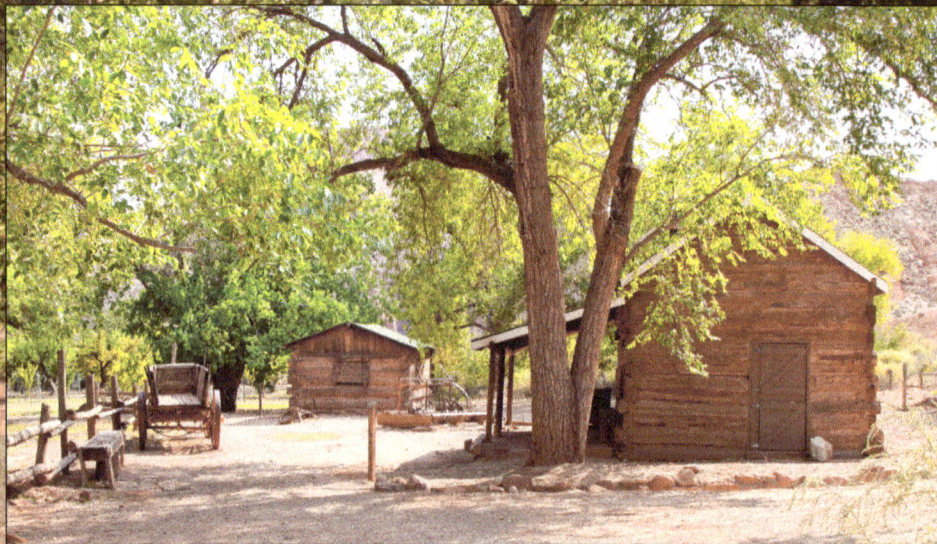

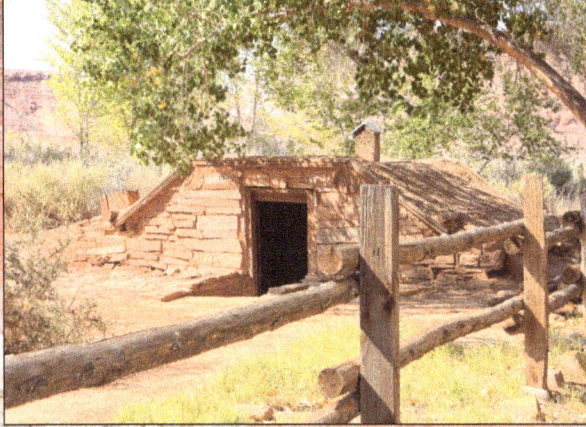

When Emma Lee, one of John Lee's wives, arrived at the junction of the Paria and Colorado Rivers, she exclaimed, "What a lonely dell."

What choice did she have in following her husband who had been banished to the site to operate a small ferry? Following the work ethic of the Latter Day Saints, they built a home and root cellar and planted a large garden and orchard. This all remains at the site along with a more modern building that was once part of a cattle ranch with headquarters at the site.

The Paria is a fickle river, at times awash in run-off from storms on the Kaibab Plateau before receding to a shallow stream thick with silt from the sandstone cliffs. The floods frequently washed out Emma's labor. When crops were lean, the family imported food from St. George to stave off starvation.

Today, hikers drop down through Buckskin Canyon, just off US89 between Page and Kanab, following the watercourse through narrow slots to emerge after a couple of days just north of Lonely Dell.

Parking is off the Lees Ferry Road above the Paria River. Cross the access road to follow a dirt track southwest a half mile to Lonely Dell. If arriving in early summer, you may find fruit on the trees and yes, you may pick what you can use.

Hiking Distance; .75 mile
Rating: Easy
Best Season: Spring & fall
Elevation: 3,160'
Special Feature: Historic site, old orchard
Maps: Arizona Highways

Branching Out on the Arizona Strip

Here are three other areas we like for exploring the Arizona Strip. They are a bit challenging but each offers a great opportunity to explore a part of Arizona that is not visited by crowds of people.

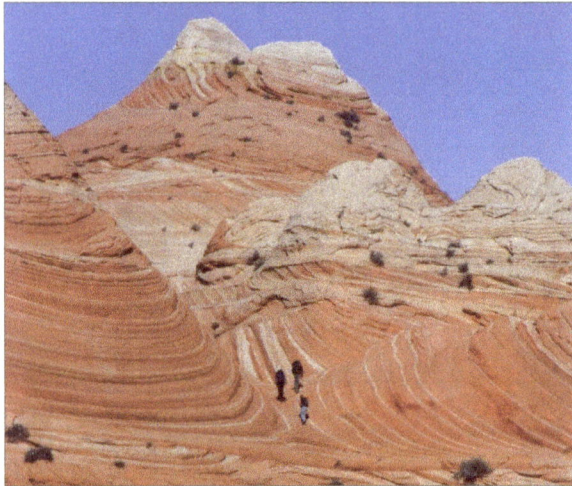

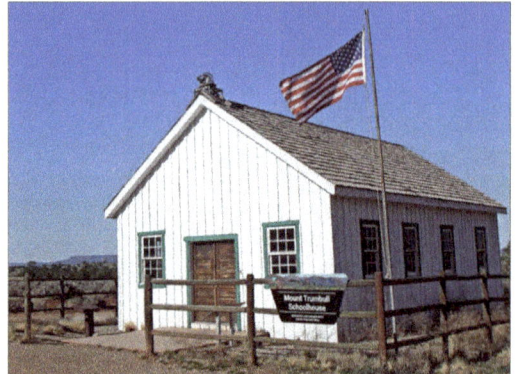

The loneliest schoolhouse in Arizona
Courtesy of the Bureau of Land Management

The Wave & Buckskin Canyon

The **Wave** has become enormously popular over the last two decades but access is restricted. To apply for a pass, either enter the lottery for a permit or check with the office for a daily walk-in pass. Either way, obtaining a hiking permit to venture into this back-country site can be difficult

The trailhead is located off House Rock Valley Road/FR1065 in a narrow canyon between Page and Saint George, Utah. The footpath ascends out of the canyon to cross two miles of rock flats. You will receive a packet of instructions with photos of landmarks along the route. Follow these instructions, using the photos as a guide, or you may not find the Wave.

Hikers can make a side trip into the narrow confines of Buckskin Canyon, a slot. This trailhead has become popular with hikers as a route to follow the Paria River down to the Colorado and Lees Ferry, a multi-day hike that requires careful planning.

Whitney Pockets

Whitney Pockets is a cluster of sandstone formations in the far northwestern corner of Arizona. To get there, drivers cross into Nevada. The easiest route to this region is from exit 120 off Interstate 15. After turning south from I-15, cross the Virgin River and turn right following the river along the Gold Butte Back Country Byway. The first 15 miles are paved, mostly. As the Byway approaches the state line, red and white rock formations rise on either side of the road - This is an other worldly landscape of rocky pockets, arches and spires. No official trail, just a great place to explore.

If you find a desert tortoise, they are a protected species.

Just beyond Whitney Pockets, the road divides with the right side descending through Nevada toward the Colorado while the left side ascends a mountain pass to drop toward Pakoon Spring in Arizona. This is not an area that drivers should take lightly. There are no services - only the kindness of those who pass in a whirl of dust.

Mt. Trumbull &
Toroweap

Caution: We aren't joking about the tire-eating road. Two vehicles are a good idea as services don't exist on the Arizona Strip beyond the small towns. For those who wish to get away from the crowds, these rolling hills covered with tall grass and scrub may be a national treasure!

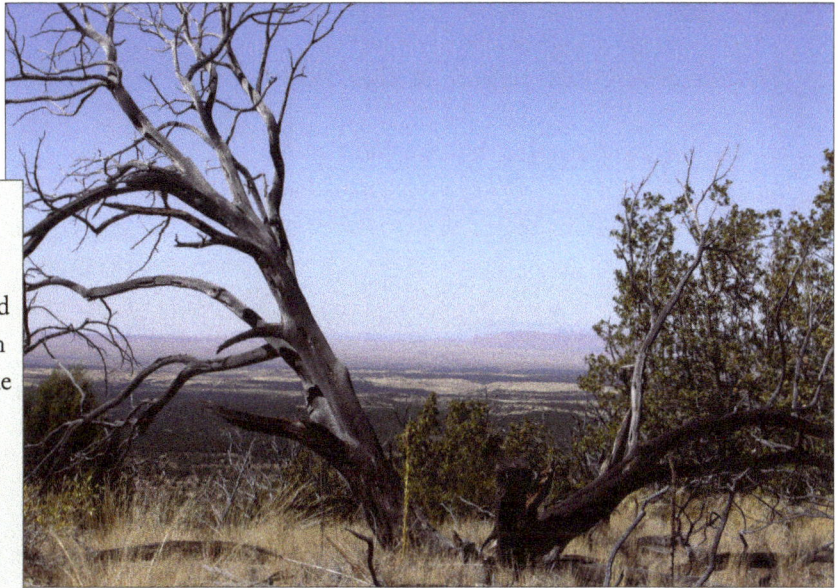

Along the Brow Monument trail

Toroweap Point stands atop vertical cliffs above the Colorado River in the western Grand Canyon. The Tuweep National Park station is a long way from anywhere on this tire-eating road. (Hint: tire repair kit and two vehicles a plus!)

A precipitous trail descends the cliffs to the river below - we don't recommend this trail for families. Instead, after getting an eyeful of the canyon, turn back and follow the route around **Mount**

Trumbull to the Nixon Administrative Site. A logging town with a one-room school house once stood here for children from neighboring ranches. A sawmill produced timber for construction in Saint George, Utah.

A rough un-maintained trail ascends the northeast side of Mt. Trumbull, from the water tank to the summit. Toward the top, route-finding skills become essential.

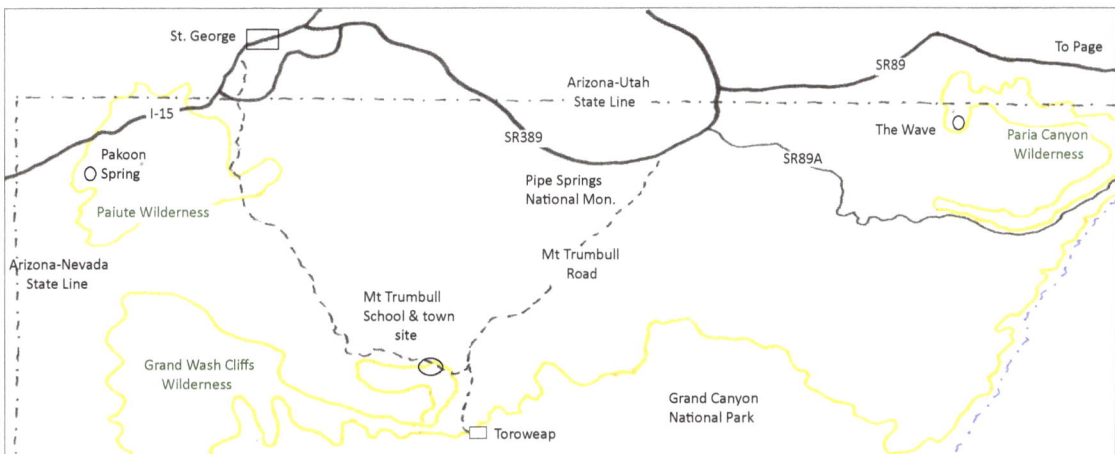

The **Grand Canyon**

The **Grand Canyon**, north or south? Visitors ponder this question as they plan to visit this grand national park.

While the south rim offers expansive view of monuments and totems, the north rim offers the grandeur of Point Sublime and hidden niches along a rim bathed in isolation. I like both rims but the lush forests of the north rim leave me feeling as if I'm home.

If you're up to hiking a distance, the river is just seven miles below the south rim. That's 14 miles round trip. If that is a bit lengthy, there are trails of shorter distances that will leave you feeling as if you have become acquainted with this grand rift in the earth's surface.

Photo: Point Imperial, North Rim

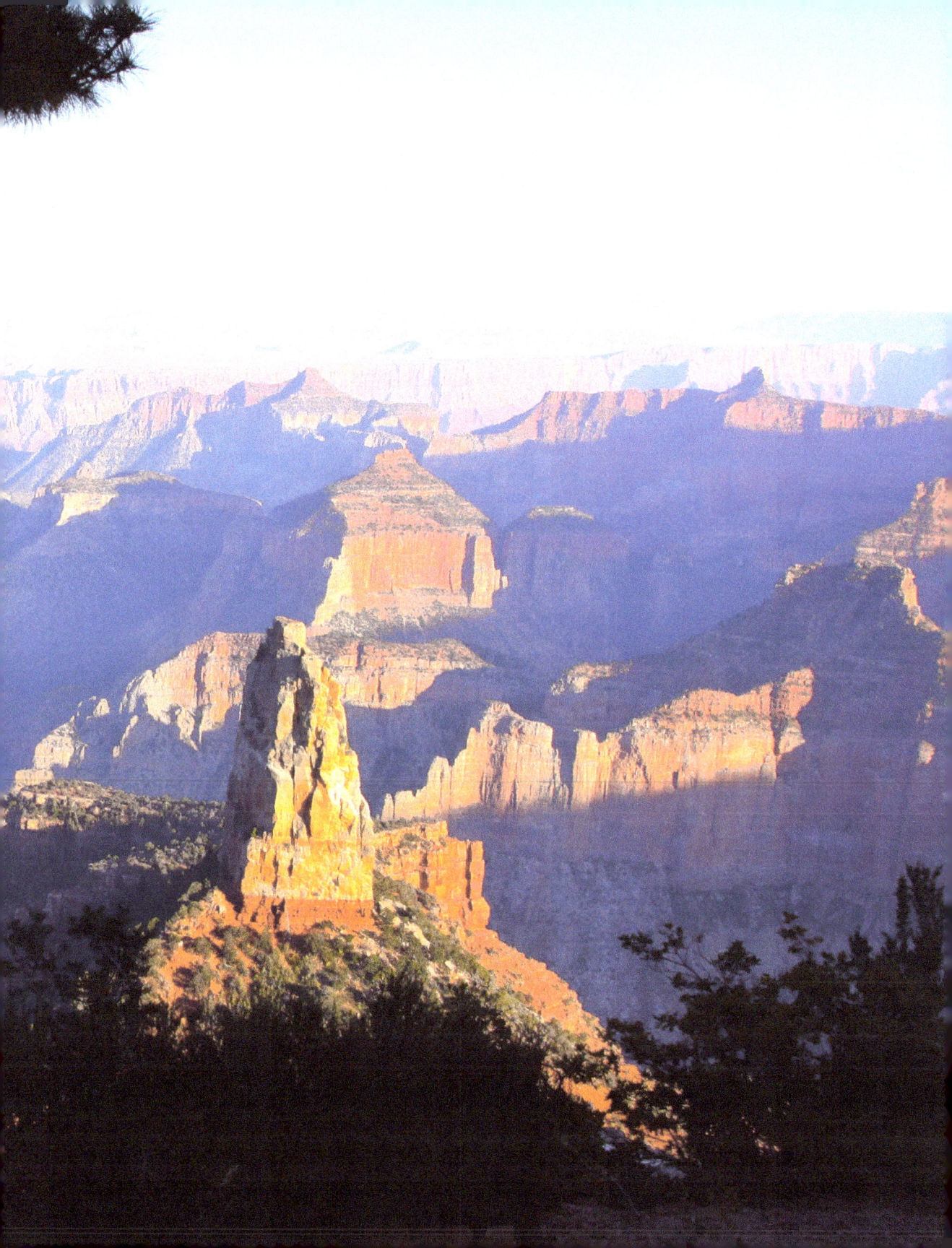

Grand Canyon North Rim

Visitors from all over the world come to hike the Grand Canyon. The trails dropping into the Inner Gorge are long and hard but there are several options that are easier for novice hikers.

Angel's Window & Cliff Springs

One of Arizona's best known arches invites visitors to cross an open span for a view of the monuments below the north rim. Imagine soaring as a bird through **Angel's Window**, sliding along warm air thermals over the canyon.

To visiting the arch drivers turn off SR64 to drive 21 miles across the Wallahalla Plateau. Just before arriving at the parking area, visitors catch a glimpse of the arch east of the road. From the large parking lot, a half-mile trail leads visitors out to Point Royal.

After a visit to the arch, drive back .3 mile to a wide bend in the road. Parallel park along the road. On the west side of the road, a well-marked trail drops steeply into a side canyon of the Grand. Enroute to **Cliff Spring**, hikers pass a prehistoric structure hidden under a rocky ledge that may have served as storage for native people.

Cliff Spring is classified as a dripping spring with water percolating through the rock ledge above the trail to drip into a muddy pool below. Dripping springs like this one are very important to the wildlife of the Grand Canyon. Take a moment to search the muddy surface for the prints of animals that may have visited this perennial water source during the evening hours. If we sit quietly, small birds fly in to grasp the moss clinging to the walls as they sip the water.

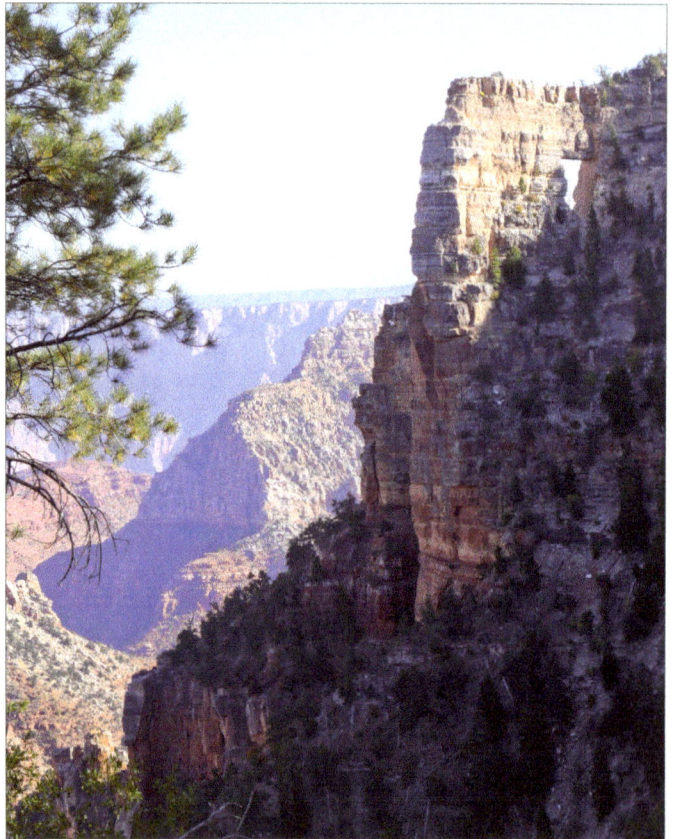

Driving Distance: 61 miles from Jacobs Lake, 25 miles from the Grand Canyon Lodge.
Hiking Distance: 1.25 mile one way.
Rating: Easy
Elevation: 7875'
Best Season: Summer, early fall.
Special Features: Hidden spring, Indian ruin.
Precautions: Steep drop-offs toward the end of trail.
Maps: GCN Park map
Information: Grand Canyon National Park
(928) 638-7888

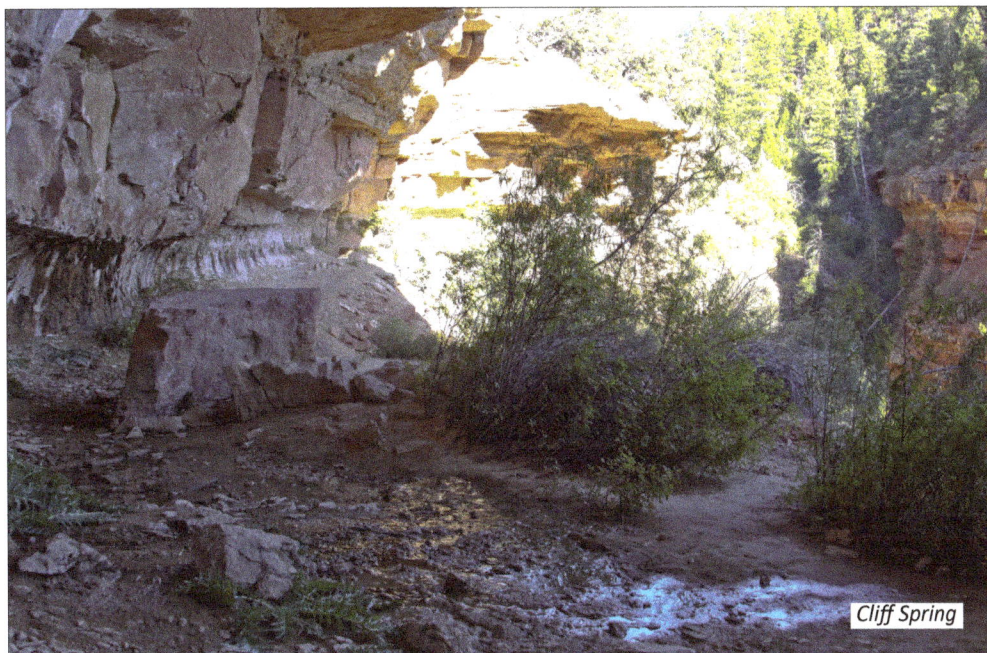
Cliff Spring

Bright Angel Point

At the North Rim Lodge, a footpath extends almost a mile out to **Bright Angel Point**. Some parents find this trail unnerving as the finger ridge has steep dropoffs on either side. The view from Bright Angel Point is stunning and a favorite place to catch the sun sinking below the horizon.

Back at the North Rim lodge, take a moment to visit the statue of the mule known as Brighty. The little mule led prospectors down the steep trails of the canyon and inspired visitors to explore beyond the rim.

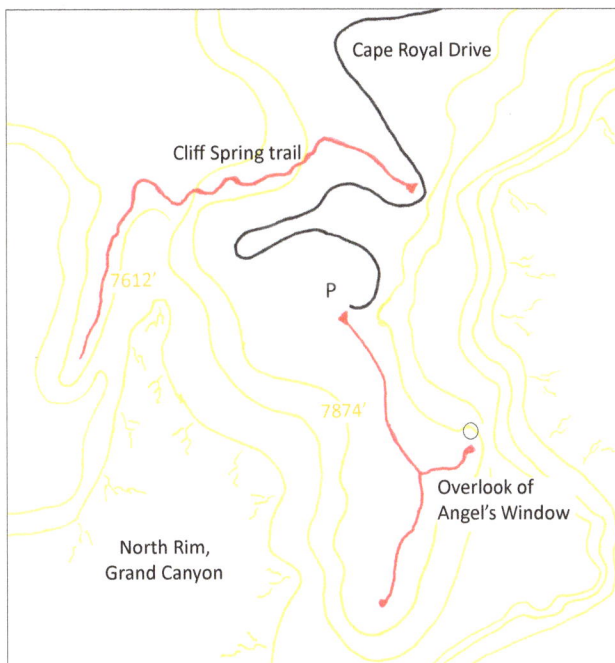
Cape Royal Drive

Cliff Spring trail

7612'

P

7874'

Overlook of Angel's Window

North Rim, Grand Canyon

Fans of Edward Abby, an environmental writer, can still visit his cabin and a small fire tower just east of the Park's North Rim entrance station. Imagine being a ranger in this isolated locale back in the 1950's.

Grand Canyon South Rim

Four trails drop into the canyon, from the South Rim to the Colorado River. **Bright Angel trail** begins just below the Village. The **South Kaibab trail** begins from a viewpoint east of the Village and is accessed by shuttle. The **Grandview trail** begins at Grandview Point, east of the Village. The **Hermit trail** begins at Hermit Rest, seven miles west of the Village. Do not expect to hike the trails to the river without adequate preparation, a lot of water and snacks. These are not trails to be taken lightly as the ascent back to the trailhead is difficult!

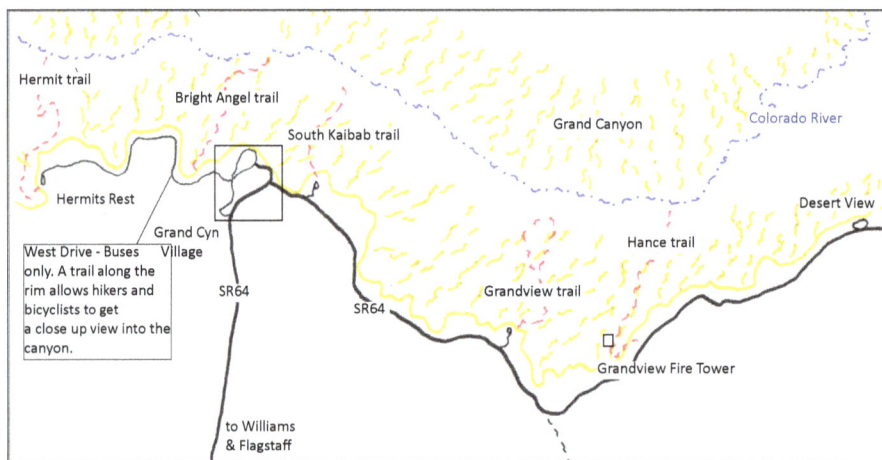

Map labels: Hermit trail, Bright Angel trail, South Kaibab trail, Grand Canyon, Colorado River, Hermits Rest, Desert View, Grand Cyn Village, Hance trail, West Drive - Buses only. A trail along the rim allows hikers and bicyclists to get a close up view into the canyon., SR64, SR64, Grandview trail, Grandview Fire Tower, to Williams & Flagstaff

Most visitors to the Grand Canyon arrive at Grand Canyon Village and walk the paved trail along the canyon rim. During the warmer months, the trail is crowded. Some visitors drop down the Bright Angel trail to a tunnel a quarter mile south of the rim and take a few photos. The trail that seemed so easy with the descent, proves to be more challenging coming out.

A footpath leads west from the village along the rim to **Hermit's Rest.** During the warmer months, the road to Hermit's Rest is closed to passenger vehicles but shuttles have designated stops for visitors who wish to ride all or part of the seven miles. Village bike rentals are also popular.

Turning east, novice hikers might also consider the rim trail that passes between viewpoints. The trail is mostly level and fairly easy for young hikers.

We love to take visitors to the Desert View Watch Tower and encourage them to climb the three flights of stairs to the top for a bird's-eye view of the canyon.

For those who want to try a short hike into the canyon, we could suggest **OohAhh Point**. This is along the South Kaibab trail with OohAhh Point .9 mile below the rim. Skeleton Point is another 1.5 miles beyond OohAhh. Both viewpoints give spectacular views of the canyon and a demanding climb back to the rim.

Arizona Trail & Grandview Fire Tower
Many visitors turn south off SR64 to visit the Grandview Fire tower. At 80 feet high, the historical structure towers above the ponderosa pines. The tower stands along the **Arizona Trail,** which follows crosses Arizona from from Utah to Mexico.

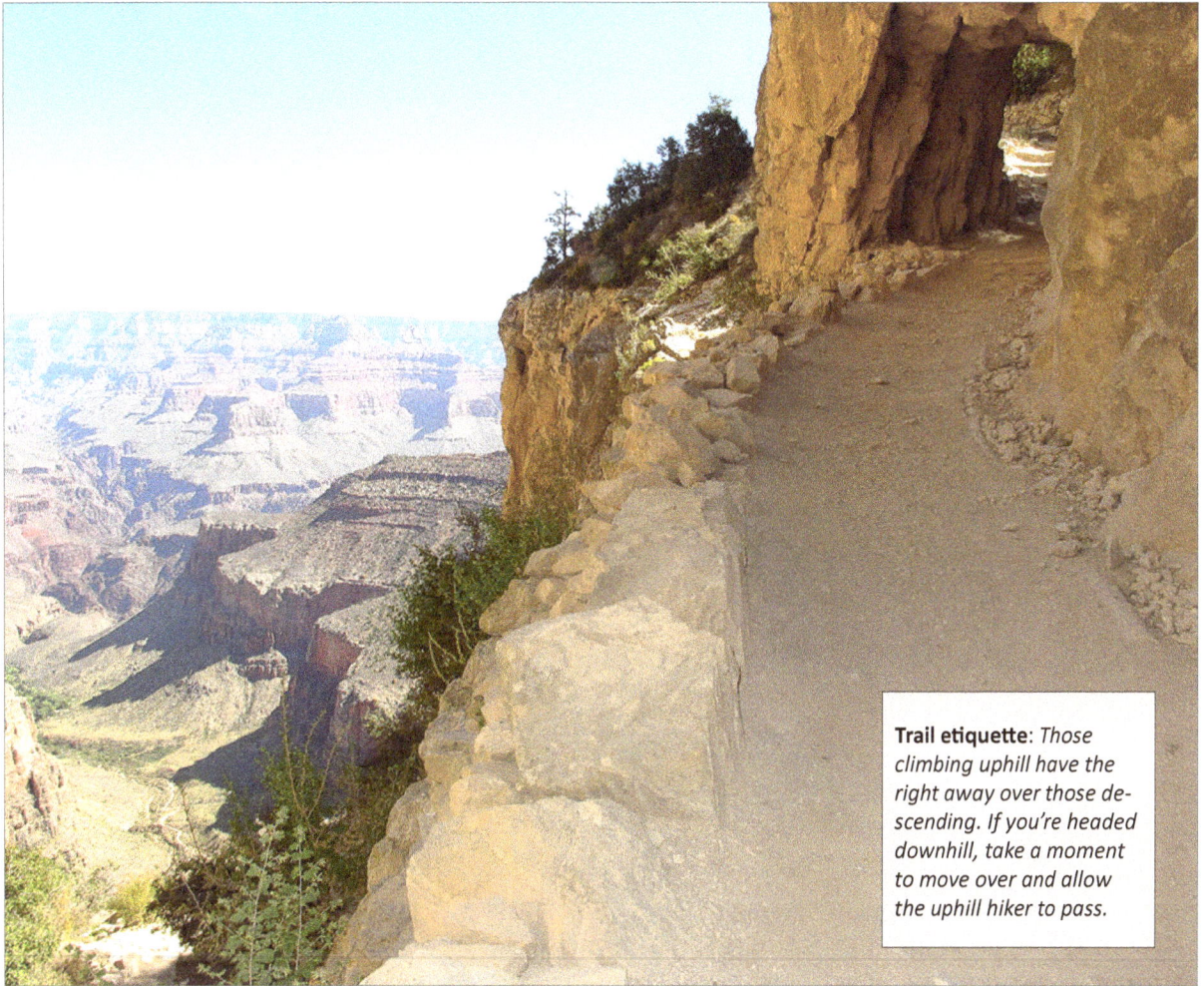

Bright Angel Trail with Indian Gardens far below.

Indian Gardens / South Rim

To visitors standing on the south rim of the Canyon, **Indian Gardens** below the rim seems like a short hike, easily accomplished. Down the trail they come in sandals without water, seemingly unaware of the effort to return to the rim.

The round trip is eight miles and not to be taken lightly, especially during the summer months. There are two rest stops along the route at 3-mile and 1.5-mile, providing water and restrooms. Watch out for the mule trains as they do not give way to hapless visitors who fail to move to the side of the trail.

Indian Gardens is lovely with mature trees and the sound of running water from a small spring-fed stream. Just above the campground, a spur trail take visitors an additional 1.5 miles out to Plateau Point and a view of the Inner Gorge.

Beyond Indian Gardens, Bright Angel Trail drops through a section known as the Devils Corkscrew to Pipe Creek and the river.

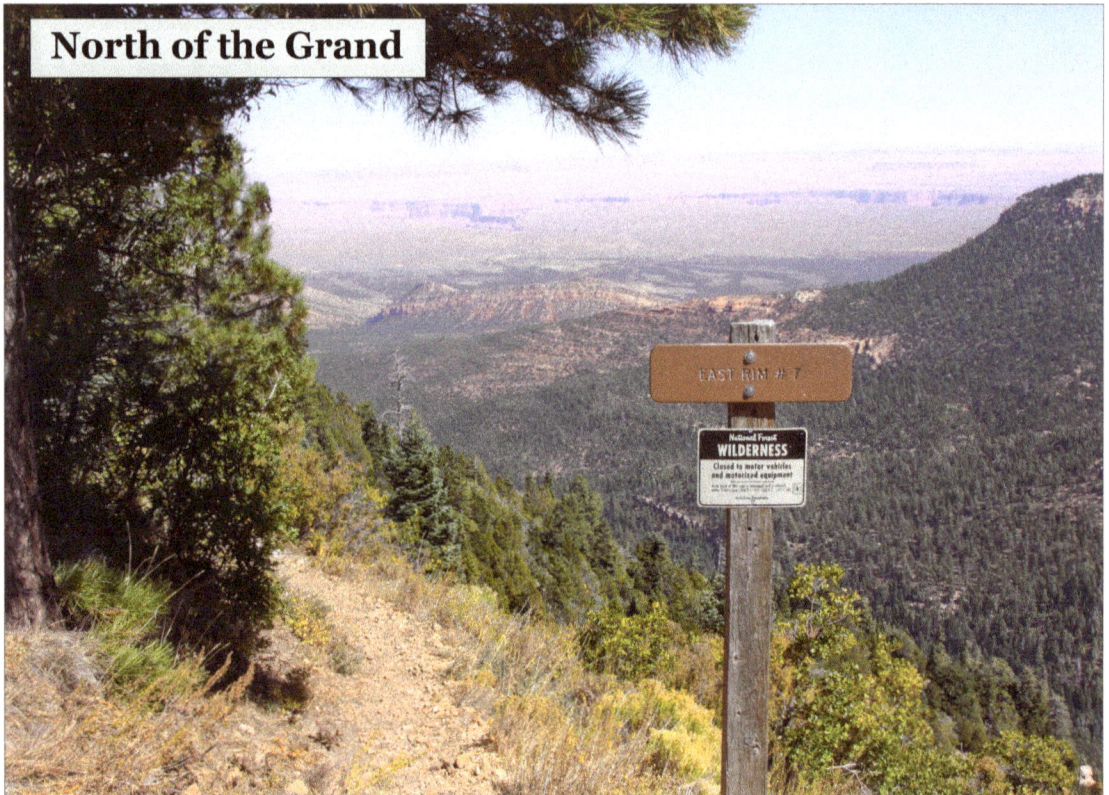
North of the Grand

East Rim & North Canyon

I love the lush fir and spruce forest of the north rim and the descent into North Canyon does not disappoint as visitors pass through lush forest and red sandstone monuments. However, the climb out of North Canyon is tough due to the steep terrain. The canyon floor is narrow with only a few hours of sunlight lighting the shallow stream.

For novice hikers, following the trail along the East Rim may be a better choice though it requires caution to keep from tripping over roots and protruding rock.

The trailhead is south of Jacob Lake off SR67. After passing Kaibab Lodge in Demotte Park, turn left (east) on FR611 and follow it to the clearly marked trailhead for the East Rim trail in a large parking lot on the east side of the road. A wide path leads east a quarter mile to the edge of the canyon where it intersects the Arizona trail. Turn left and follow the rim trail to the trailhead. The East Rim trail drops into the canyon while the rim trail turns away from the canyon.

Driving Distance: 30 miles from Jacob Lake
Hiking Distance: 1.5 miles one way
Rating: Moderate
Elevation: 7200' - 8800'
Best Season: Summer & fall.
Special Features: Access into one of the side canyons of the Grand Canyon, native fish in the stream.
Maps: North Kaibab NFS map
Information: North Kaibab Ranger Station
(928) 643-7395

Roaring Springs / North Rim

The **North Rim** trail into the Grand Canyon is not as crowded as the Bright Angel but it does see a lot of traffic from day trippers and cross-canyon hikers. The 11-mile round hike to Roaring Spring is demanding and the ascent is steep. However, the trail allows hikers to visit a spring pumping hundreds of thousands of gallons out of the aquifer, providing water through a pipeline to Grand Canyon village on the South Rim. The trail is a witness to the heroic effort of crews that blasted a route along sheer rock cliffs. Those who wish to do this as a day hike would be wise to start early in the morning.

Below the spring, the trail descends to Cottonwood Campground. Beyond the campground the trail is a gentle grade over six miles to Phanton Ranch, passing Ribbon Falls and through the 'box', a narrow passage with vertical rock walls.

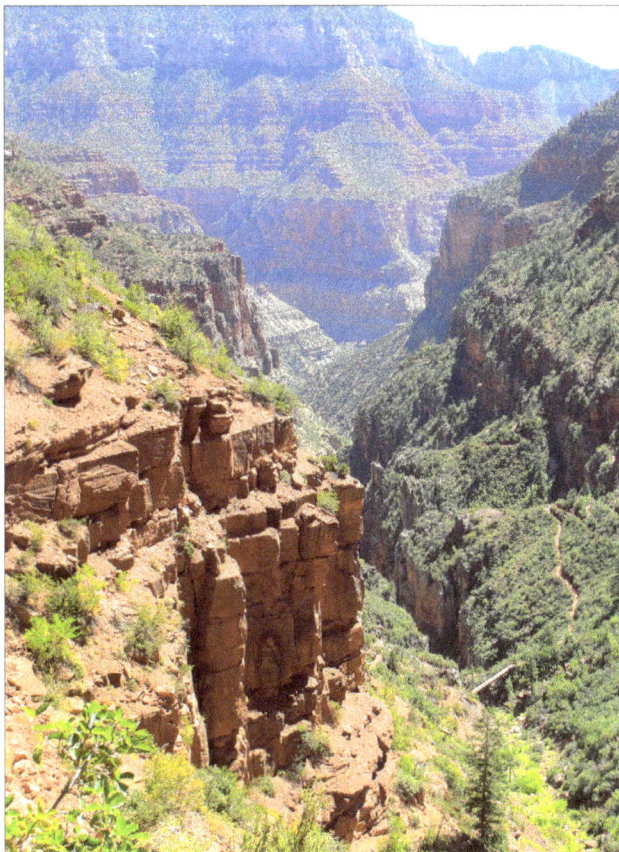

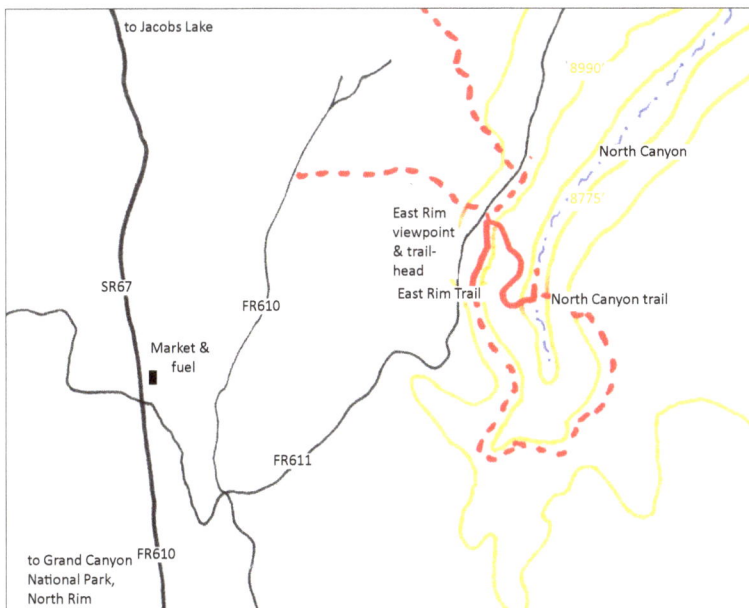

Driving Distance: 30 miles
 from Jacob Lake
Hiking Distance: 5.5 miles
 one way.
Rating: Moderately difficult
Elevation: 8,235 - 4,718'
Best Season: Summer & fall.
Special Features: Access to
 one of Az's largest springs
Maps: North Kaibab NFS
 map
Information:
 Grand Canyon Nat'l Park
 928-638-7888

Red Butte

Many visitors leaving Flagstaff, drive north, their windshield filled with dreams of the Grand Canyon. Just north of Valle, a small community at the junction of US180 and SR64, a red sandstone butte rises above the forest of pinyon and juniper. **Red Butte** is a remnant of the rock layers that once covered this region. The summit is protected by a lava cap. The butte certainly does not see the crowds visiting the South Rim. In fact, hikers may not see anyone until reaching the summit.

At the summit, is a fire tower, only 16 feet in height with one flight of stairs to a balcony surrounding the one-room cab. For those with a fear of heights, the tower is reasonable. It is a bit disappointing to find a poor view north of the Canyon rim but the perspective looking out over the plain gives a whole new understanding of the forces of nature and how they work on the landscape. During the summer the tower is manned and sees only a few visitors unlike towers closer to population centers. There is a road up the back side of the butte but it is closed off with a gate to all but Forest Service personnel.

From Flagstaff, drive north, along US 180. Forty-eight miles north of Flagstaff, US 180 joins SR 64 at Valle, continue north on SR 64, 10.5 miles to the sign for Red Butte at mp 224. Turn right on to FR 320 and travel 1.4 miles, turn left on to FR 340. At just under a mile, turn right again and park at the foot of Red Butte. The trailhead is well-marked.

Driving Distance: 41 miles from Williams, 64 miles from Flagstaff by US 180, 23 miles from South Rim.
Hiking Distance: 1.5 miles one way.
Rating: Moderate
Elevation: 6400' - 7300'
Best Season: Spring, summer & fall.
Special Features: Fire tower, good geology lesson is layers of rock.
Precautions: Watch footing to avoid nasty fall where the trail has eroded.
Maps: Kaibab NFS map
Information: Chandler Ranger District

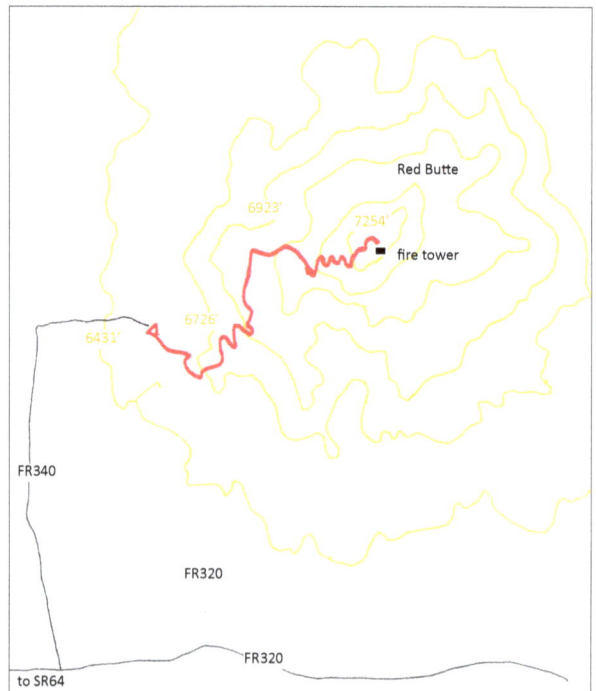

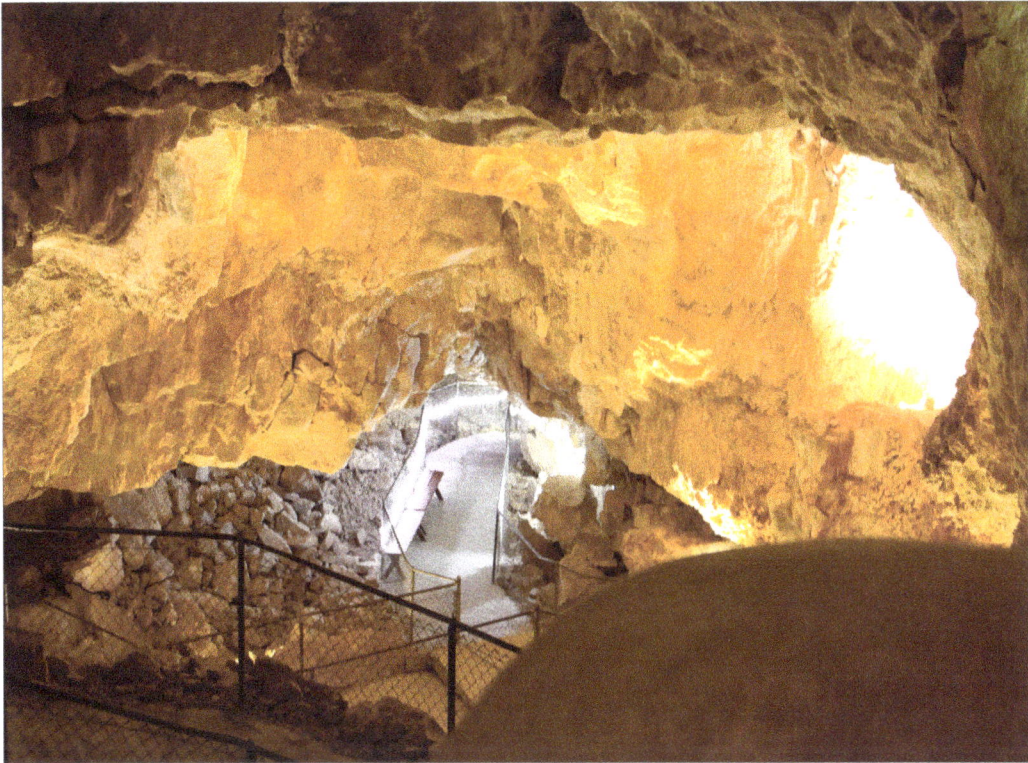

Grand Canyon Caverns

Many visitors are awed by the grandeur of Karchner Caverns southeast of Tucson, but Arizona has other caves not as well known that get their share of attention. The **Grand Canyon Caverns** are a series of 'rooms' with a walking tour introducing visitors to the unique features of this landmark. The caverns are locationed on Old Highway 66 a few miles east of Peach Springs, and the headquarters for the Hualapai Tribe.

The forty-five minute tour cover three-quarters of a mile. The guide points out stalactites, stalagmites and draperies, all rock formations created by water passing through the limestone that is the primary rock in this part of Arizona. In the largest room, visitors pass by a deposit of emergency supplies stored in the cool chamber for times of national emergencies.

Despite the well lit chambers and stairs, it is a relief to emerge from the elevator that ascends from the cavern and breathe air above ground once again. The exit is strategically placed so that visitors pass through the gift shop.

Driving Distance: 101 miles east of Flagstaff
Hiking Distance: .75 mile loop.
Rating: Easy
Elevation: 5,310'
Best Season: Year round.
Special Features: Large cave with easy access.
Maps: Arizona Highways map
Information: Grand Canyon Caverns (928) 422-3223

Cataract Canyon and Havasupai

Despite the distance to **Havasupai**, I can not fail to mention this hike as it remains a favorite for so many interested in the Grand Canyon. This is the canyon of the blue-green waters with tremendous waterfalls and travertine pools that lure hikers from all over the world.

The trailhead is located at Hilltop, north of Peach Springs, a community located on Route 66. The parking area is crowded with vehicles, a snack shop, helipad and scores of people, dogs and horses all in a narrow corridor at the top of a cliff. Reservations are required, whether hiking or riding the eight miles to the village. Many hikers complain about how difficult it can be to reach the tribe to make a reservation.

The first 1.5 miles drop along switchbacks into **Cataract Canyon**. This is followed by 6.5 miles in the dry creek bed through gravel and river rock. This passage is fascinating as the walls rise higher, the trail steadily dropping.

As hikers emerge from the canyon, the air is cooled by the irrigation ditches that brings water to the village. Hikers pass through the village, covering another mile before descending the last two miles into the campground. The campground stretches a mile along Cataract Creek.

Hikers encounter the first of the falls between the village and the campground. As hikers descend deeper into the canyon, the iconic Havasupai Falls drop over a cliff on the right side of the trail. The campground has porta-potties at the entrance. The campsites are located between a cliff on the left and the stream on the right. No reserved spots, look for an open table.

Just below the campground, the trail descends through a tunnel and down a ladder to the foot of Mooney Falls - an adventure as hikers trust the ladder to be solid and sturdy.

Those who follow the creek an additional three miles come to Beaver Falls. Much, much further, the creek enters the Colorado River, tinting the river a shade of aquamarine.

Reservations?

Making reservations with the Havasupai tribe is challenging. However, visitors should be persistent as it is a long hike back to Hilltop if the tribe refuses to accomodate visitors who arrive without a without a permit to stay overnight.

The Village has a small lodge. There are no motels where one can walk in and obtain a room.

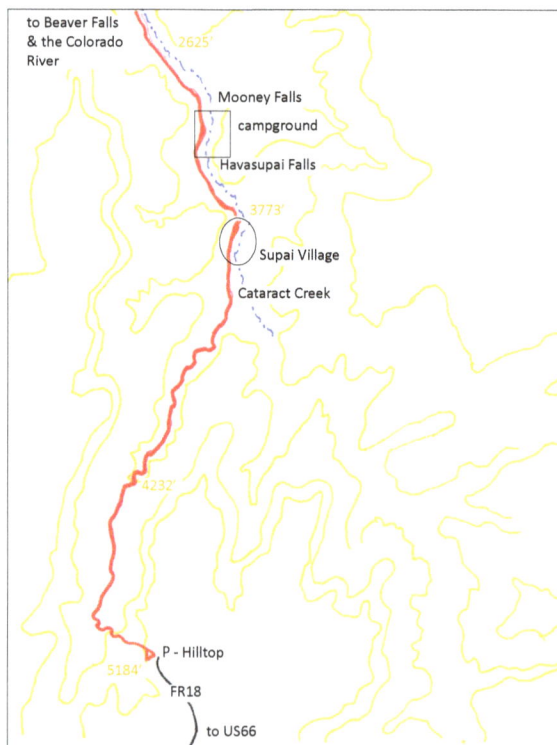

to Beaver Falls & the Colorado River
2625'
Mooney Falls
campground
Havasupai Falls
3773'
Supai Village
Cataract Creek
4232'
P - Hilltop
5184'
FR18
to US66

Driving Distance: 90 or 127 miles
from I-40 exits onto
Route 66
Hiking Distance: 8 miles to village,
10 miles to Havasupai Falls,
11 miles to Mooney Falls
Rating: Strenuous due to length and
gravel.
Elevation: 5900' - 3200'
Best Season: Spring or Fall
Special Features: Scenic falls and pools
to play in.
Precautions: Carry enough water! Long
hike in and out. Watch out for
nasty spills on travertine rock
around the creek. Stay out of
the way of the horses on the trail.
Maps: Arizona Highways map
Information:
Havasupai Tourist Enterprises
Supai, AZ 86435
(928) 448-2180

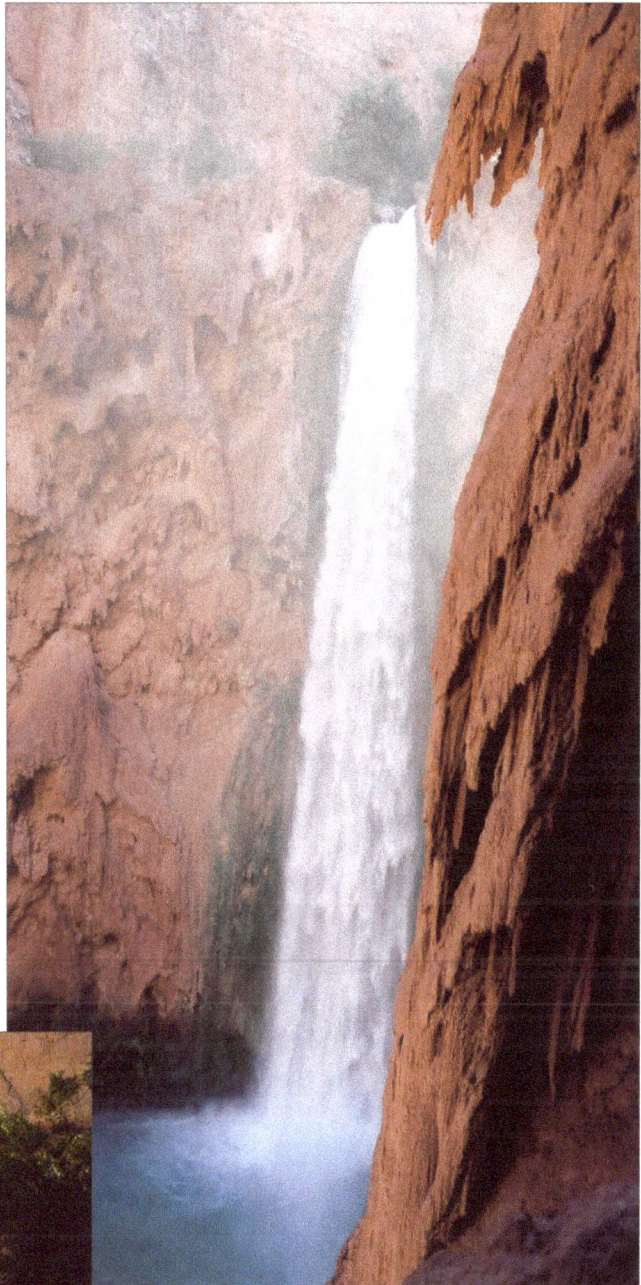

Mooney Falls

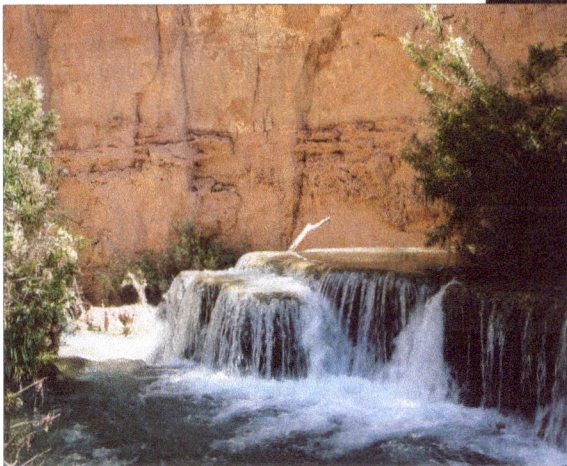

We no longer recommend **Antelope Canyon**
or the overlook above **Horseshoe Bend** as great hikes.

The Navajo Nation is now charging an exorbitant fee for hikers to be led through **Antelope Canyon** with tours running every 15 minutes. No time to sit and absorb the the quiet and solumn beauty of this slot.

Unfortunately, **Waterhole Canyon**, a second slot nearby seems to be headed in the same direction. There are other slots on Navajo land but access is limited to tribal members.

Off Limits

White Mesa Arch was another location we loved to recommend. A Navajo family's residence sits along the route to the base of the arch. They have grown tired of the traffic passing through their 'front yard'. We've recently heard that they are no longer allowing visitors to the arch. The only access is a cross country hike with miles of scrambling through steep side washes and a pinyon-juniper forest.

At one time we recommended climbing to the arch at **Windowrock** as well. The tribe considers the arch sacred and you could be fined for trespassing if you attempt to climb the ridge above tribal headquarters. There are social trails around the monument at the foot of the arch for those who visit the capital of the Navajo Nation.

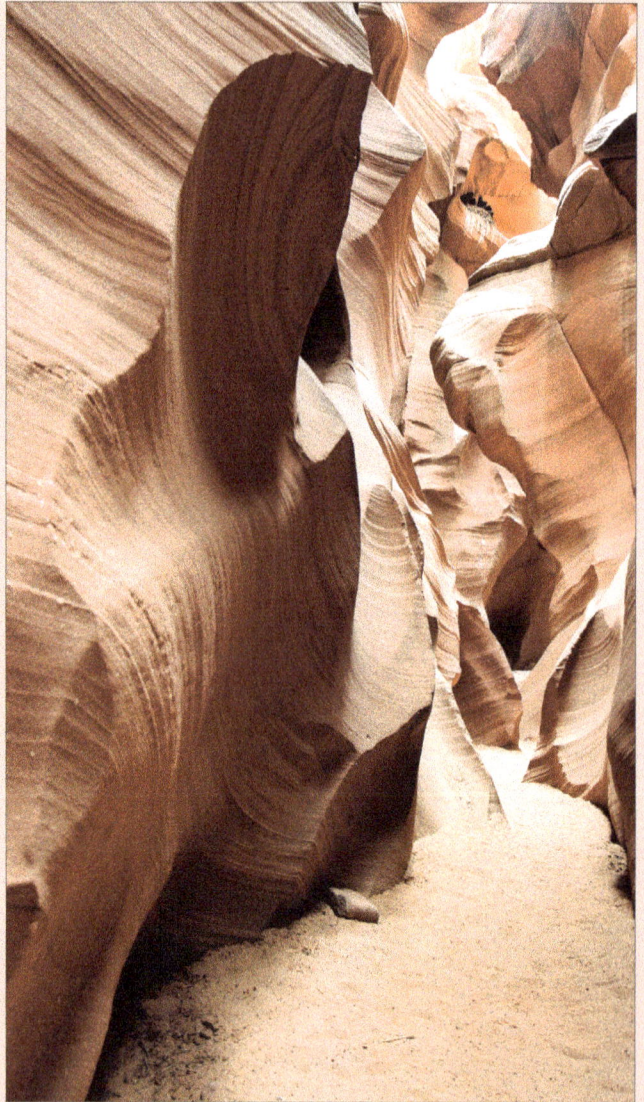

Antelope Canyon

As settlers poured into the western half of the continent in the late 1800's, a great conflict arose with the native tribes that roamed these wild lands. Ultimately, the federal government would set aside land for many of the tribes.

purchase a hiking permit at either the headquarters in Windowrock or at the governmental center for the western reservation in Cameron.

On Hopi ancestral lands, please remember that some of the villages are considered traditional and

The Navajo Nation and Northeastern Arizona

When we consider hiking on the ancestral lands alloted to the Hopi and Navajo Nations, we must remember we are under Navajo tribal law. Along with consideration of the tribal laws, is the request to be respectful of the residents and their rural homesteads.

The Navajo Nation does expect hikers to

tourists are not welcome.

If you should come across a remote hogan, please do not approach the dwelling as if this was a tourist site. If you should encounter a Navajo who requests that you leave his location, please do so. This request applies to all of the 22 reservation across Arizona.

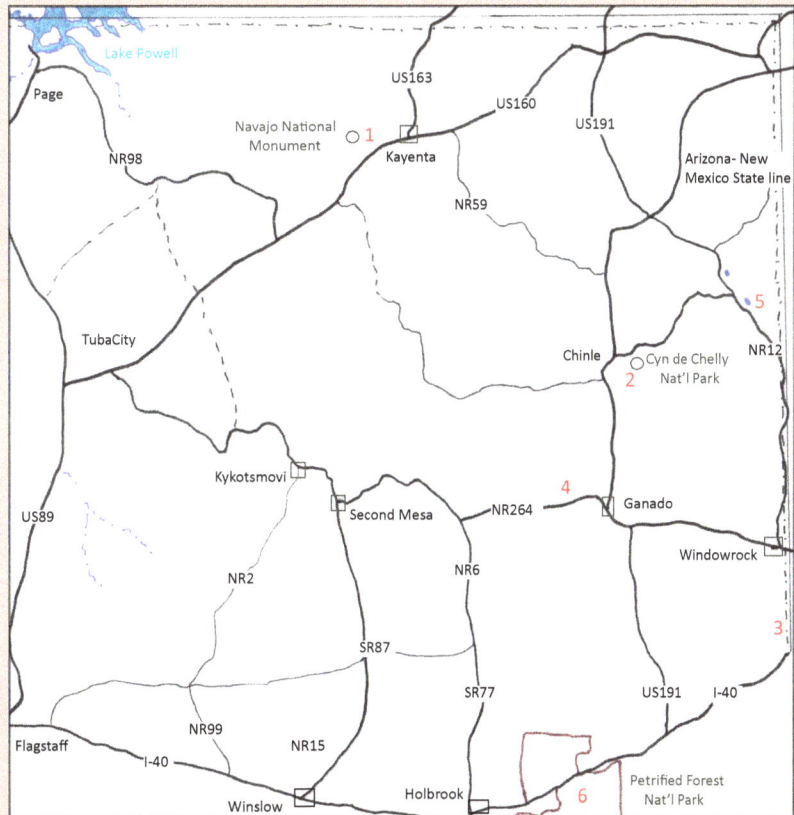

1 Betatakin & Navajo National
      Monument
2 Canyon De Chelly
3 Route 12 Ampitheatre
4 Kinlichee
5 Wheatfields & Black Pinnacle
6 Petrified Forest

Betatakin & Navajo National Monument

Betatakin is one of the most visited ancient ruins in Arizona. Once inhabited by the Ancestral Puebloan people, the cliff-side pueblo was built into the sandstone cliffs overlooking Tsegi Canyon.

The Sandal Trail from the Visitors Center takes visitors along the canyon rim to an overlook of the massive alcove and the ruin under the sheltering rim. The Aspen trail descends into the canyon to the edge of the ruin. Visitors are no longer allowed to climb into the ruin.

If you are reasonably fit, I recommend the three to four hour guided tour along the Aspen trail into the canyon. Call ahead to reserve a place on the tour.

Visitors are led to a small parking area. The trail descends through a locked gate to a set of steep stairs cut into the sandstone. At the foot of the steps, visitors walk along a rocky shelf above a narrow canyon up to an alcove sheltering the ruin. Returning to the trailhead is a steep climb.

Aspen and pine trees fill the narrow valley below the ruin, making it a green oasis. Those who once lived in the pueblo would have burned the available wood in cooking fires and for warmth during the winter months. Since the ruins were abandoned, the forest has been restored.

The floor of Tsegi Canyon is still farmed by Navajo families, as their ancestors have done for centuries. From the trail it is possible to look down the canyon along the route to the Keet Seel ruin. Keet Seel is a large multi-dwelling ruin, accessible by permit only, with visitors either hiking or riding horses eight miles along the canyon floor. The Visitors Center can put visitors in touch with local guides. Traditional Navajos will not remain at the ruins overnight.

Betatkin and the Navajo National Monument are located 18 miles south of Kayenta, north of US 160. A small sign marks the turnoff onto NR 564. Follow the two-lane paved road 10 miles north into the Navajo National Monument, stopping at the Visitor's Center. The inner canyon trail may not be suitable for very young children but is certainly a great place for older kids to learn history first hand.

At one time visitors were allowed to enter parts of the ruin. This is no longer allowed. Instead, visitors descend into the canyon for a view of the alcove and forest that has filled the drainage.

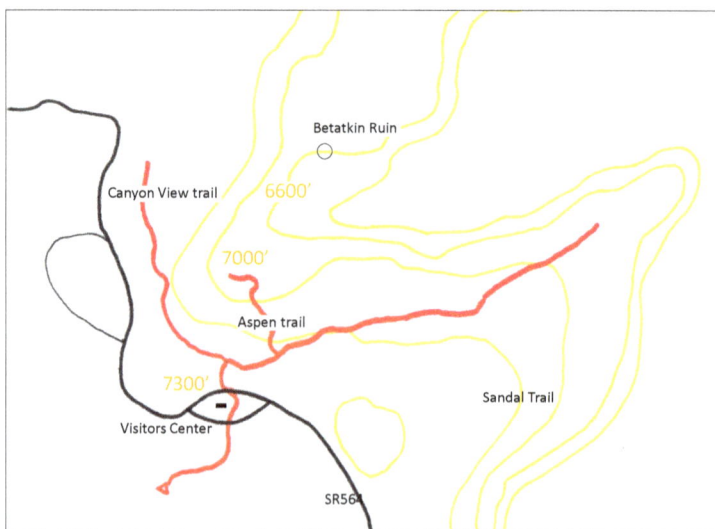

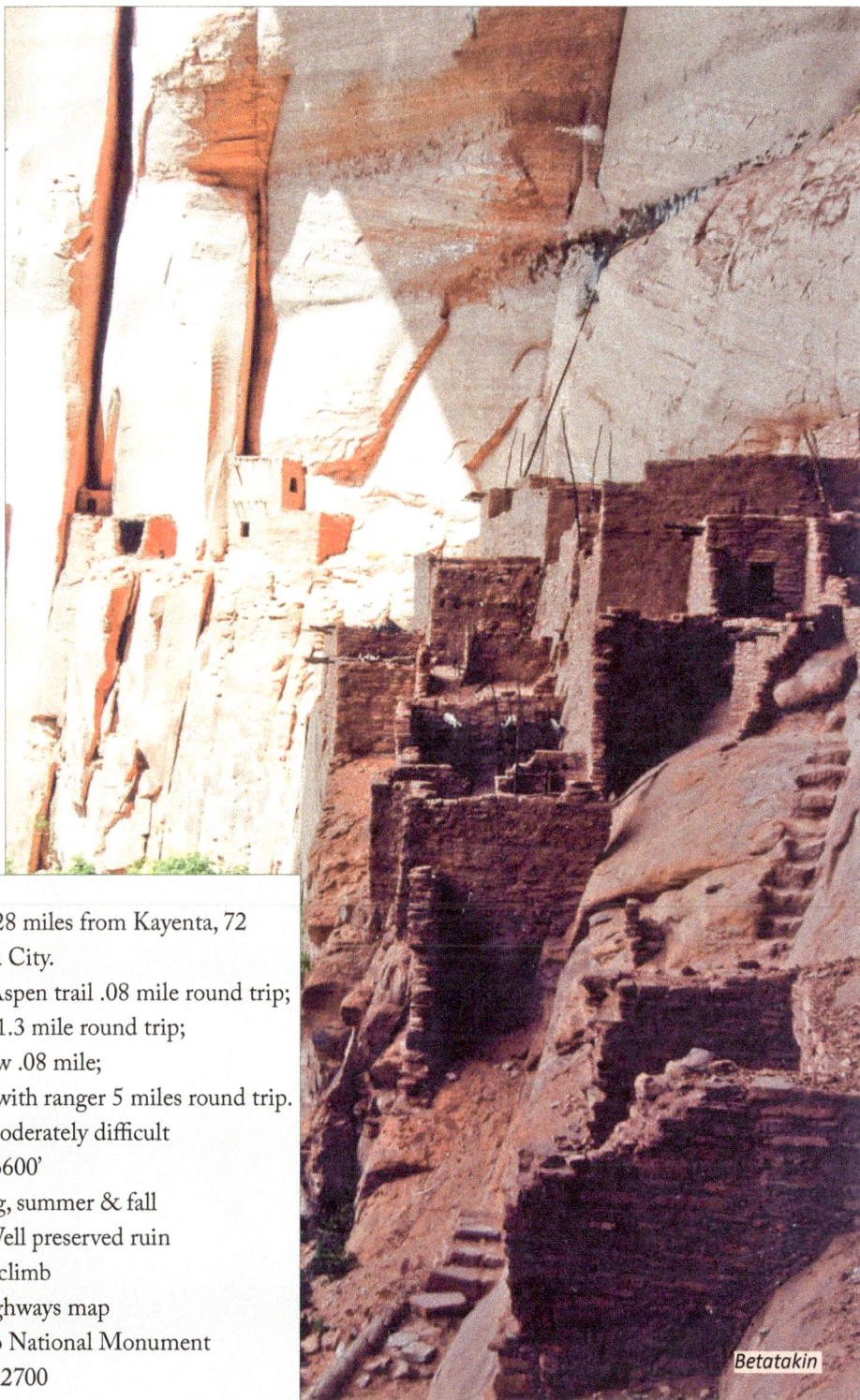
Betatakin

Driving Distance: 28 miles from Kayenta, 72
    miles from Tuba City.
Hiking Distance: Aspen trail .08 mile round trip;
        Sandal trail 1.3 mile round trip;
        Canyon View .08 mile;
        Tsegi Point with ranger 5 miles round trip.
Rating: Pueblo - moderately difficult
Elevation: 7300' - 6600'
Best Season: Spring, summer & fall
Special Features: Well preserved ruin
Precautions: Steep climb
Maps: Arizona Highways map
Infomation: Navajo National Monument
        (928) 672-2700

Canyon de Chelly & White House Ruin

Canyon de Chelly has long sheltered the Diné people. They've built their homes at the base of the sheer cliffs, grazed their flocks of sheep and raised crops in the bottom land of Cibique Creek. Much of Navajo storytelling revolves around Canyon de Chelly, including the tale of Spiderwoman holding Navajo children captive on her rock.

The vertical red sandstone walls of the canyon are stained with desert varnish from water seeping over the edges, adding to the aura of mystery that pervades the canyon. For those who wish to hike, one trail into the canyon is available without a Navajo guide. To reach the trailhead, turn east off NR 64, to follow the road behind the Visitor's Center. The South Rim Road winds past the campground, then climbs along the rim to different viewpoints. The turnoff to White House Ruins viewpoint is 4.9 miles from the Visitors Center with another .6 mile to the parking lot.

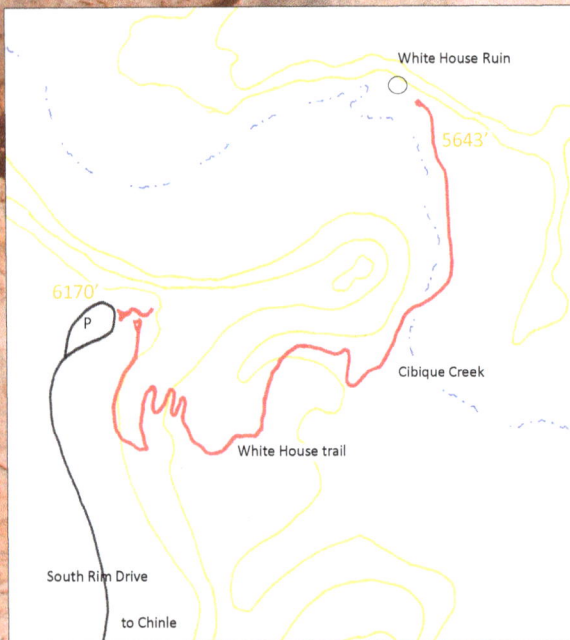

White House Ruin

5643'

6170'

P

Cibique Creek

White House trail

South Rim Drive

to Chinle

From the overlook, the trail crosses the rocky plain to the right to descend through a tunnel cut in the rim. Emerging from the tunnel, the canyon floor spreads below visitors feet, framed by sandstone monuments. The trail switchbacks along sheer cliffs to the canyon floor!

Once hikers have reached the canyon floor, the trail turns sharply left and crosses the creek toward White House Ruin. At times, heavy spring runoff has swept the bridge downstream. If the creek is too high, don't risk crossing.

The ruins are fenced off. A small plaque explains the origin of the ruins and the meaning of the "White House in the middle." During peak visitor season, Navajo people sell jewelry near the ruins.

Visitors follows SR 191 to Chinle in the northeastern corner of Arizona. Turn east on SR64 and drive 2.8 miles to the turnoff for the Park. The Visitors Center displays exhibits on the history and culture of the area; it includes a replica of a hogan and a small brush shelter.

Driving Distance: 8.3 miles from Chinle stop light.
Hiking Distance: 1.5 miles one way
Rating: Moderately easy
Best Season: Late Spring, summer & fall.
Special features: Rich native history and well preserved ruins in depth of beautiful canyon. Unique trail construction.
Precautions: Due to cliffs, hold onto small children along the trail approaching trail head. Please grant residents their privacy.
Maps: Arizona Highways
Infomation: Canyon de Chelly Visitors Center

During several trips along Navajo Route 12, I had been intrigued by the sculpted sandstone cliffs that tower over this narrow strip of asphalt. As part of the ridge, **Coffee Pot Rock** overlooks a natural amphitheater located off NR 12. The access into the ampitheater is through a break in a low ridge on the east side of the road, exactly three miles north of I-40. The shoulder does not provide parking and visitors should not block a dirt track leading off the road.

From the highway, walk downhill along the dirt track toward a depression filled with water and follow a wash running east-west. Find a safe place to climb down and follow the wash eastward till it intersects a larger wash rising toward the sandstone cliffs.

Upon reaching the cliffs, find a route up the side of the wash and climb the rim into the ampitheater. This requires route finding. The sculptured walls leave visitors feeling insignificant, dwarfed by the rosy glow with shafts of sunlight and green ponderosa. Some visitors sing or bounce echoes off the walls of the ampitheater. I preferred to referentially soak in the silence.

The area is not well visited making discretion while exploring the better part of valor. Don't go beyond what you can safely descend! The walls of the wash can collapse with little warning - don't trust them. And don't get caught in a flash flood coming down the wash - you cannot out run it!

If there is any sign of rain to the north, do not enter the wash or attempt this hike. Flash flood carved this wash and can catch hikers unaware of the danger of being swept downstream.

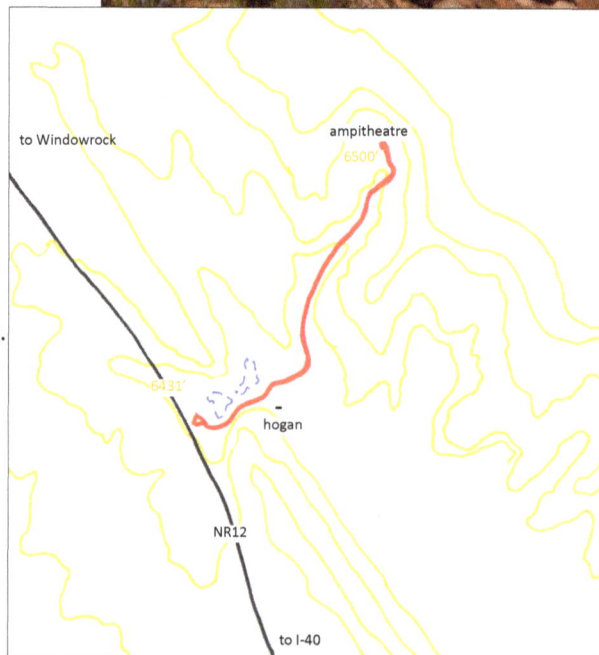

The Route 12 Natural Ampitheatre

Please heed the precaution about hiking on native land at the beginning of this chapter!

Distance: .5 mile one way
Driving Distance: 3 miles north of
    Lupton/I-40, 25 miles south from
    Windowrock.
Rating: Moderately easy
Best Season: Summer, fall
Special features: Beautiful red rock amphi-
    theater and a sandstone spire shaped
    like a coffee pot.
Precautions: Flash floods, poisonous in
    sects & reptiles. Do not attempt
    to descend or climb the steep dirt
    walls of the wash as they may col
    lapse. Do not enter the wash if there
    is any sign of rain upstream. If the
    wash floods, wait for the water to
    pass downstream!

More Exploring on the Navajo Nation

Hubbell Trading Post

The Hubbell Trading Post is located a half mile west of the intersection of US 191 and State Route 264 near Ganado on the eastern half of the Navajo Nation. The earliest white settlers arrived on the ancestral lands in the late 1800s and established posts to trade with the Navajo People. In operation for 150 years, the trading post, grants a glimpse into the history of the old west and the Navajo people.

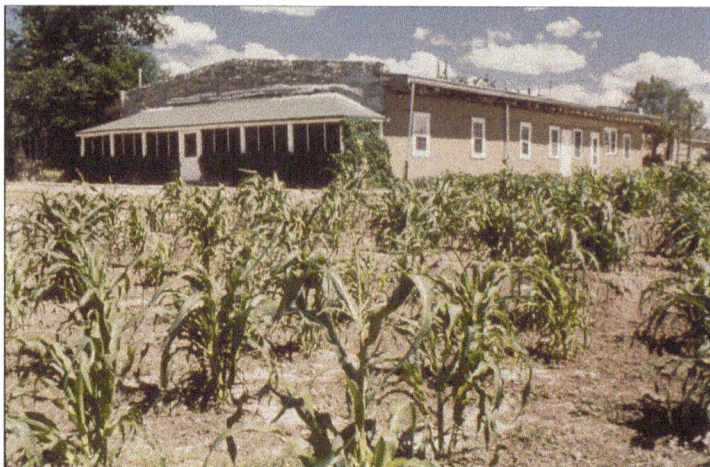

Hubbell Trading Post / NPS photo

Kinlichee

This site is an old pueblo ruin believed to date back to the ancient Anasazi, possibly built around 1100 AD. The pueblo is repidly disintegrating under the onslaught of winter and summer rains. A rickety ladder descends into a shallow kiva - do not attempt to climb down.

Look around! Why has this site been occupied for centuries, first by primitive people and now with modern Navajo homes nearby?

While exploring watch for rattlesnakes and please, do not enter the ruins.

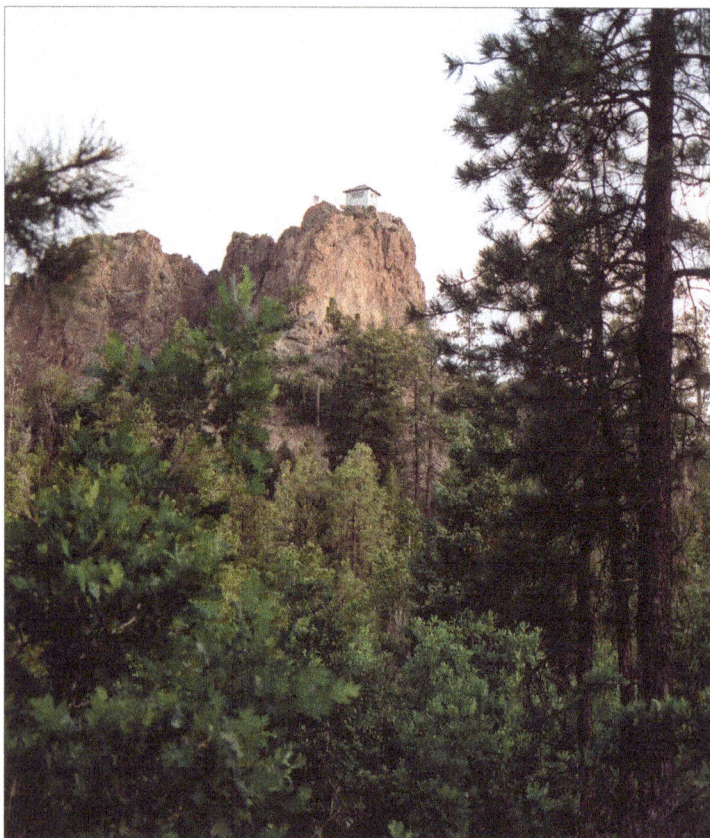

Black Pinnacle Fire Lookout - A metal stairway on the backside of Black Pinnacle allows access to the peak.

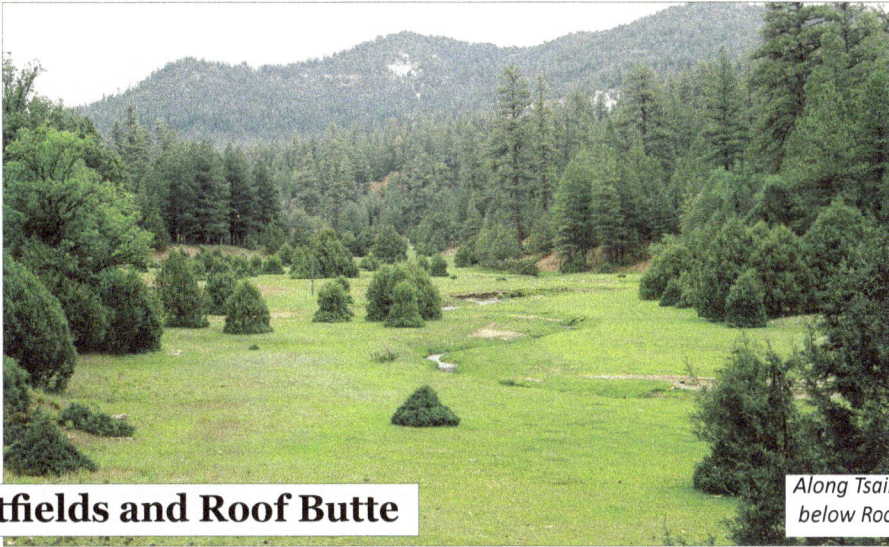

Along Tsaile Creek, below Roof Butte.

Wheatfields and Roof Butte

While many visitors are drawn to the dramatic vistas of Canyon de Chelly, a select few are drawn to the eastern end of the canyon along Navajo Route 12. A small primitive campground and boat launch for rowboats draws fishermen to try their luck on **Wheatfields Lake**. The canyon below the dam presents an invitation to explore further.

I am drawn to the eatern lands along Navajo Route 12 and to the Lukachukai Mountains as shown in the photo. Others would recommend Canyon de Chelly or other locations that are part of the Navajo National Monuments.

Driving north, note the small sign for **Black Pinnacle Fire Lookout**. Turning down the dirt track, park in a small lot on the backside of the rock cliffs and walk to a metal stairway that climbs to the lookout. It is manned during the warmer months.

Further north, just beyond Tsegi, visitors pass a dirt road that turns up Tsegi Canyon. I followed the dirt track to the summit of Roof Butte, finding pleasant meadows and beautiful groves of aspen along the road. It is easy to get lost in the Lukachikai Mountains. If you choose to explore, create a road map that you can use to return to Route 12 - don't rely on your memory. Establish your GPS settings before leaving home.

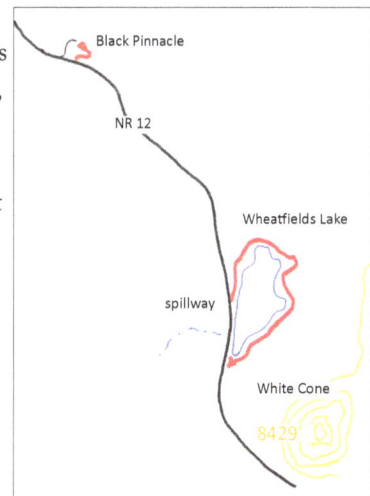

Taking a wrong turn at one junction, I emerged into a high meadow with several sheep camps around the perimeter. These are occupied during the summer by families who return to their homes in the winter months.

At the summit, a collection of radio towers and a fire lookout crowd a narrow ridge. Looking west, the landscape is one of rock and deeply incized canyons. Turn and look east, the ridges of fir and spruce covered mountains remind one of Colorado. In the summer, the lookout cabin is manned. I followed a communication service truck to the summit. For his part, he thought I might be lost, searching for the route to Shiprock on the other side of the Lukachukai Mountains. He was a gracious guide!

Petrified Forest National Forest & the Petrified Log Bridge

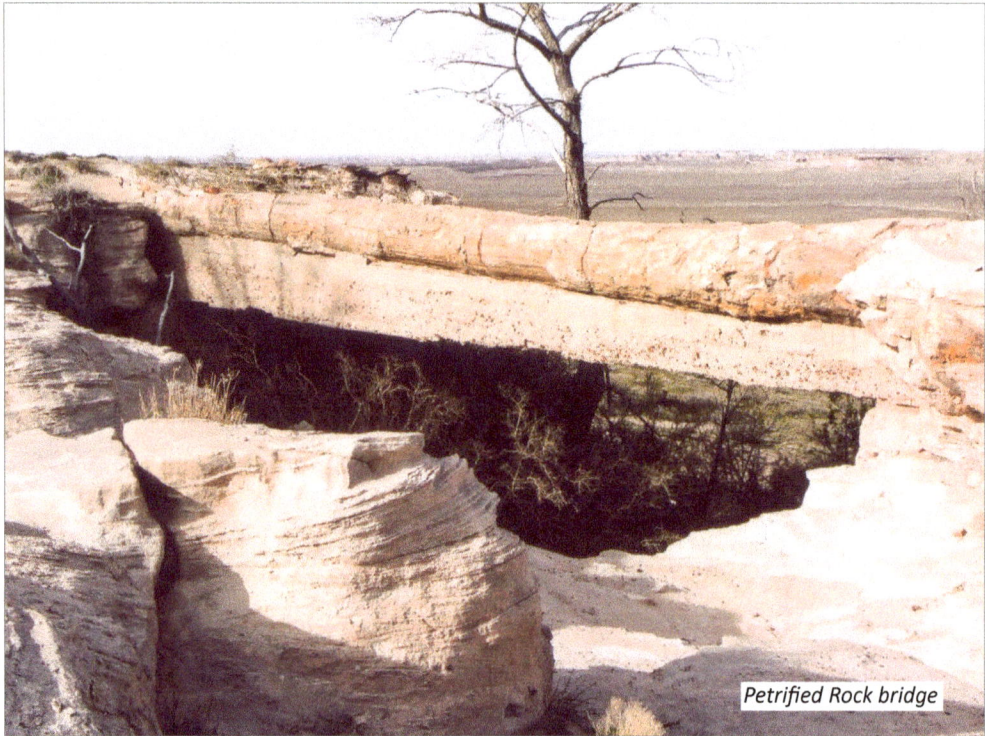

Petrified Rock bridge

The high desert around Holbrook wasn't always so dry. Vast wetlands once covered this area. Giant trees grew in the highlands around the marshy plain. As the trees fell, some scientists believe that a flood swept some of the trees down onto the plain where they were covered with layers of sediment.

Over the centuries, through the petrification process, the trees became hardened rock, now called petrified wood. As the softer rock around the logs eroded, the petrified wood was exposed. The federal government designated a select area as the **Petrified National Monument** to preserve the petrified wood. Trails lead through the giant logs, allowing us to examine the rock formations.

There are two entrances to the Petrified Forest, one off I-40, east of Holbrook. The other is off US 180, south of Holbrook. Each entrance leads

to one of two Visitor's Centers with a cluster of trails. Along with educational displays, the Visitors Center displays letters from people who have taken rocks illegally and later returned them. Some swear the rock has brought them bad luck and the only way to right this misfortune was to return the rocks.

At the southern entrance one trail takes hikers through a display of giant logs for .4 mile. Another trail visits the Agate House, a structure built from petrified wood. My favorite may be the petrified log bridge over a small wash. A cement foundation now supports the bridge.

The northern entrance offers hikers the Crystal Forest trail and the Blue Mesa trail. There are a number of pullouts for viewpoints along the main road overlooking the Painted Desert.

Along the Colorado River
and Just Beyond

Arizona residents love water! The Colorado River is sometimes referred to as the 'West Coast of Arizona', honoring the water sports along the Colorado River.

Along the Arizona/California state line, the Colorado River, passes through two of the driest deserts in North America. The land along the river would be chalky-dry but residents have channeled water into fields and urban landscapes. Beyond the urban areas, we find such a contrast between the dark green water of the Colorado and the dry landscape carpeted with desert scrub and cactus.

We've featured several trails with interesting destinations. But if you love hiking in the desert, you're sure to find more trails with a search on the internet. Please be careful when hiking or driving through flooded washes as only a a foot or so of water can wash a vehicle downstream. Better to wait till the water drops to a safe level. When hiking through a wash, if you hear a low roar behind you, get out! A flash flood may be coming your way or it may be a Marine Corps pilot out of Yuma testing his skills.

The Black Mountains and Mohave Mountains north of I-40 and the Kofa and Castle Dome Mountains to the south are a defining barrier between the Colorado and inland deserts. These mountain ranges are home to some of Arizona's big horn sheep though it is unlikely that visitors will encounter the animals along the perimeters of the mountain ranges.

The mountain are riddled with two-track dirt roads and abandoned mining shafts. Some of those shafts are still worked from time to time - pay attention to the No Trespassing signs!

Long before giant walls of cement blockaded this water course, the river ran red with silt. Today, the water emerging from the dams along the Colorado is cold and clear with the silt captured behind the dams.

1 Hualapai Mountain Park
2 Crack In the Mountain / SARA Park
3 Whytes Retreat / Cattail Cove
4 Buckskin State park
5 Burro Creek
6 Palm Canyon
7 Yuma Crossing & East Wetlands

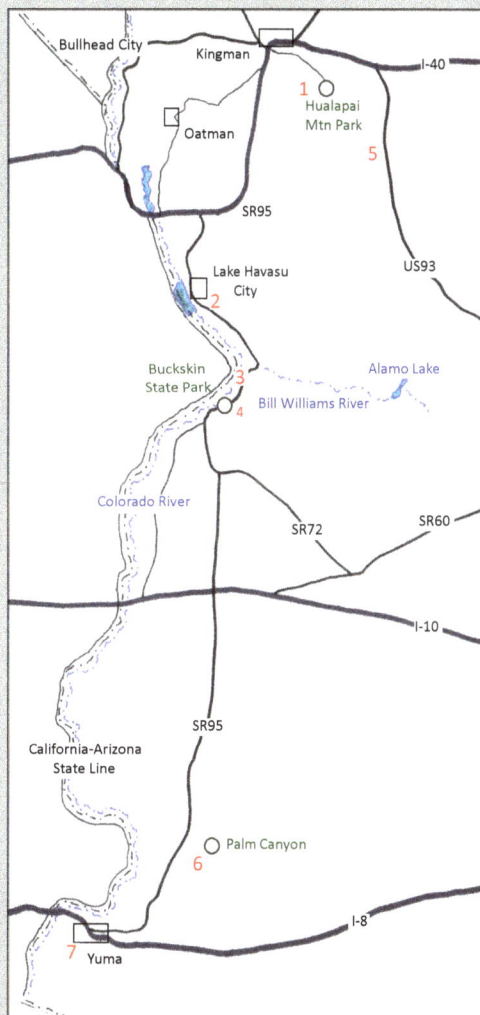

Hualapai Mountain Park

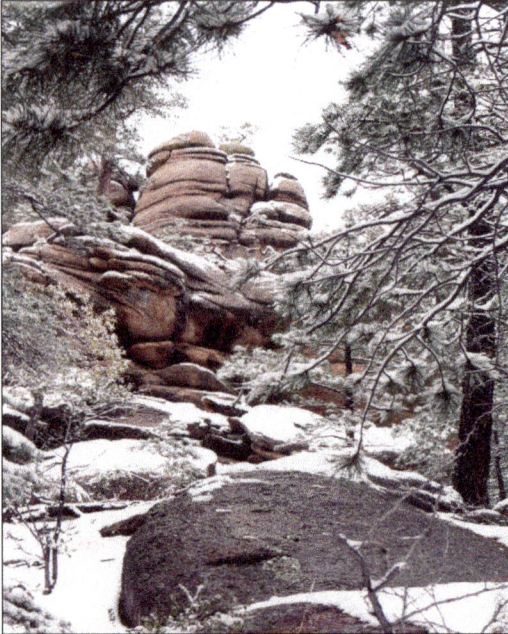

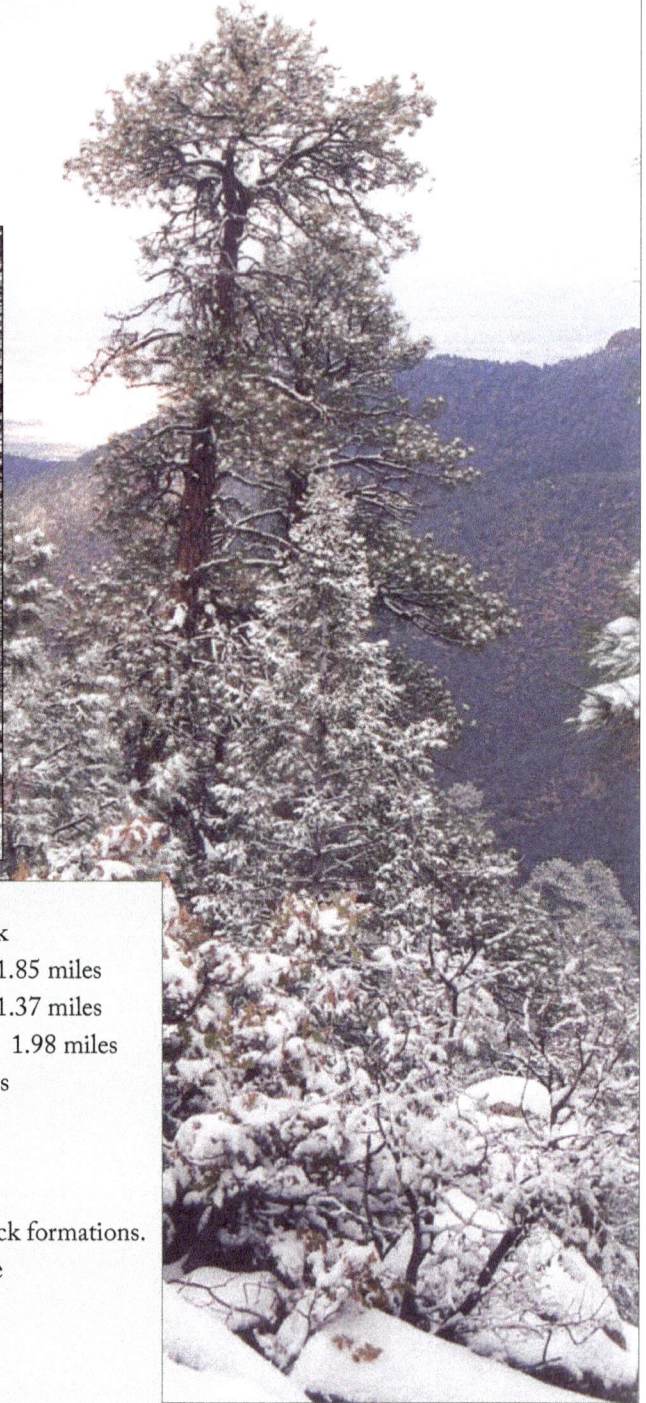

Driving Distance: 10 miles Kingman to Park
Hiking Distance: trailhead to CCC Camp 1.85 miles
                CCC camp to Aspen Peak   1.37 miles
                CCC camp to Hayden Peak   1.98 miles
                Potato Patch Loop   4.5 miles
Rating: Moderate
Elevation: 6800' - 8300'
Best Season: Spring, summer & fall.
Special Features: Historic area with great rock formations.
Precautions: Watch footing in rock scramble
Maps: Hualapai Mountain Park map
Infomation: Hualapai Mountain Park.
        (928) 757-3859

One of the most delightful areas for hiking in the western region of Arizona is hidden just outside of Kingman in the Hualapai Mountains. A network of pine-shaded trails wind through the peaks of the Hualapai Range.

From the junction of Andy Devine Street and Stockton Hill Street, Hualapai Mountain Road turns south for 10 miles into the **Hualapai Mountain Park**. During office hours, visitors can pick up a trail map at the entrance to the park. From the entrance, turn right and follow the main road to the trailhead. The road passes through campgrounds and cabins - those wishing to stay overnight, can make cabin reservations in advance.

From the trailhead, the first quarter mile is a steep climb through switchbacks before settling into a reasonable grade. Along the trail, are signs for some of the rock formations. My favorite was The Gossips, resembling three

slouching figures of pink Hualapai granite huddled on the side of the mountain.

En route to an old CCC camp, hikers pass a side trail to Stonestep lookout, an excellent lookout point. The CCC camp dates back to the 1940's, housing work crews that built roads and retaining walls. The site has been well maintained, offering tables and barbeque pits for a picnic lunch under the aspen and tall pines.

At a trail junction in the day-use area the left branch takes hikers up a steep ascent to Aspen Peak. Hikers scrambling over the last boulder, enter a small clearing with the remains of two old cabins. One last scramble over a rock formation reveals a great view of the plain below.

Back at the recreation area, those taking the right branch at the trail junction hike onward to Hayden Peaks, West and South.

Opposite page:
High in the Hualapai Mountains
after a spring snow.
Inset: The Gossips Rock Formation

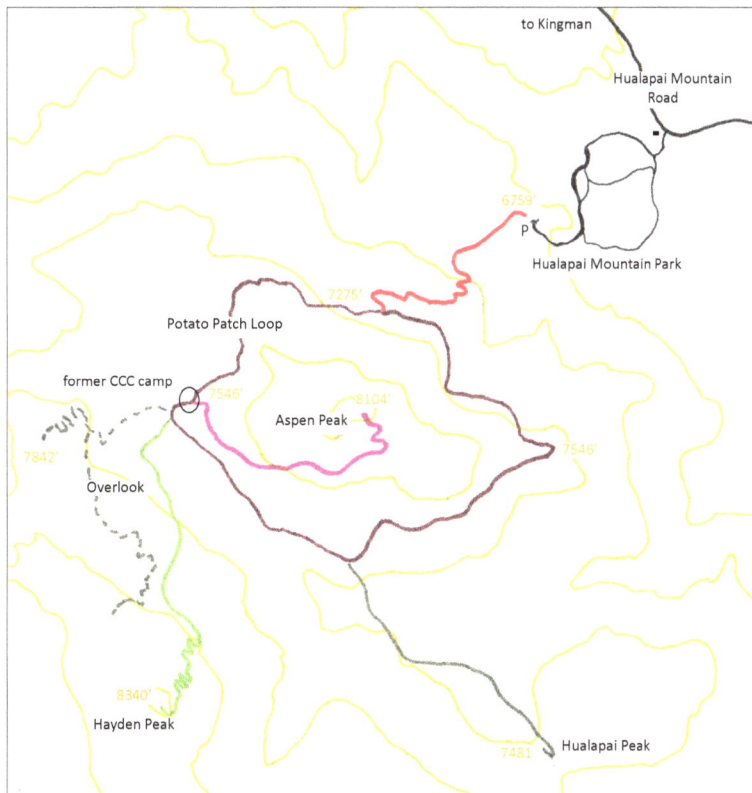

to Kingman

Hualapai Mountain Road

6759'

P

Hualapai Mountain Park

7275'

Potato Patch Loop

former CCC camp

7546'

8104'

Aspen Peak

7842'

7546'

Overlook

8340'

Hayden Peak

7481'

Hualapai Peak

The Crack in the Mountain

In 1967, Robert P. McCullough, Sr, purchased a stone bridge in London, England for $1.2 million dollars with the intention of shipping the bridge to a desert town that few people knew or visited. Shipping doubled the cost and then, there was the cost of reassembling the numbered blocks over a section of dry desert. Arizona residents thought the man was crazy. Turns out McCullough was a visionary and today Lake Havasu City is a bustling town with a laidback vibe. The bridge extends over a narrow channel aside from river's main channel.

The Lake Havasu City Council set aside property at the southern end of town for **SARA Park** and within its bounds is the trail known as the **Crack in the Mountain**. From the roadside parking area, hikers descend into a wash and follow the yellow trail markers toward a narrow slot between two hills.

Two other trails cross and recross the yellow route. As hikers follow the wash, the canyon walls developed. The wash is transformed into a slot a mile from the trailhead, the canyon walls become vertical and large red boulders emerge out of the gravel in the wash. The highlight of the slot is an eight-foot rock slide with a rope anchored to a boulder near the top. Hikers either slide down the rock face or turn back to take a route high on the hill above the slot to reach the river. On the return, hikers follow the blue trail markers to avoid climbing the slide.

On our return, we chose to follow the wash, not noting the yellow markers. Somehow, we managed to divert to a secondary wash and ended up a half mile from the parking area. Pay attention to your route as you return!

Follow the yellow triangles. If you miss your turn, just stay in the bottom of the wash and head downhill. This doesn't work so well on the return. A good sense of direction is helpful or you may end up at the wrong trailhead.

Driving Distance: Within Lake
    Havasu City Limits
Hiking Distance: 1.75 miles one way
    to the pour-over
Rating: Moderate
Elevation: 855 - 558'
Best Season: Winter, maybe spring,
    or fall.
Special Features: A natural pour-over
    creating a rock slide.
Precautions: Slick rock, poisonous
    vipers.
Maps: Trail map at site

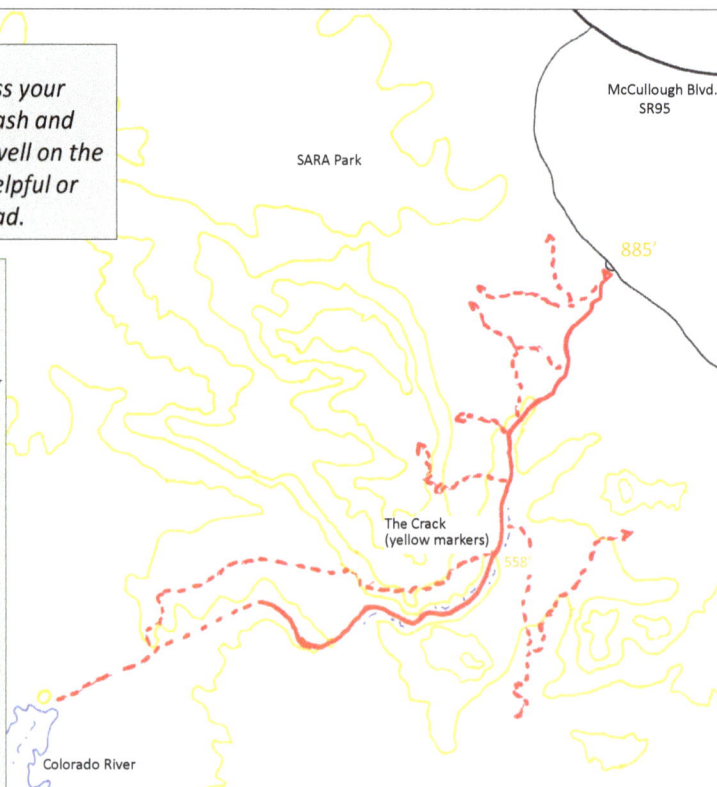

McCullough Blvd.
SR95

SARA Park

885'

The Crack
(yellow markers)

558'

Colorado River

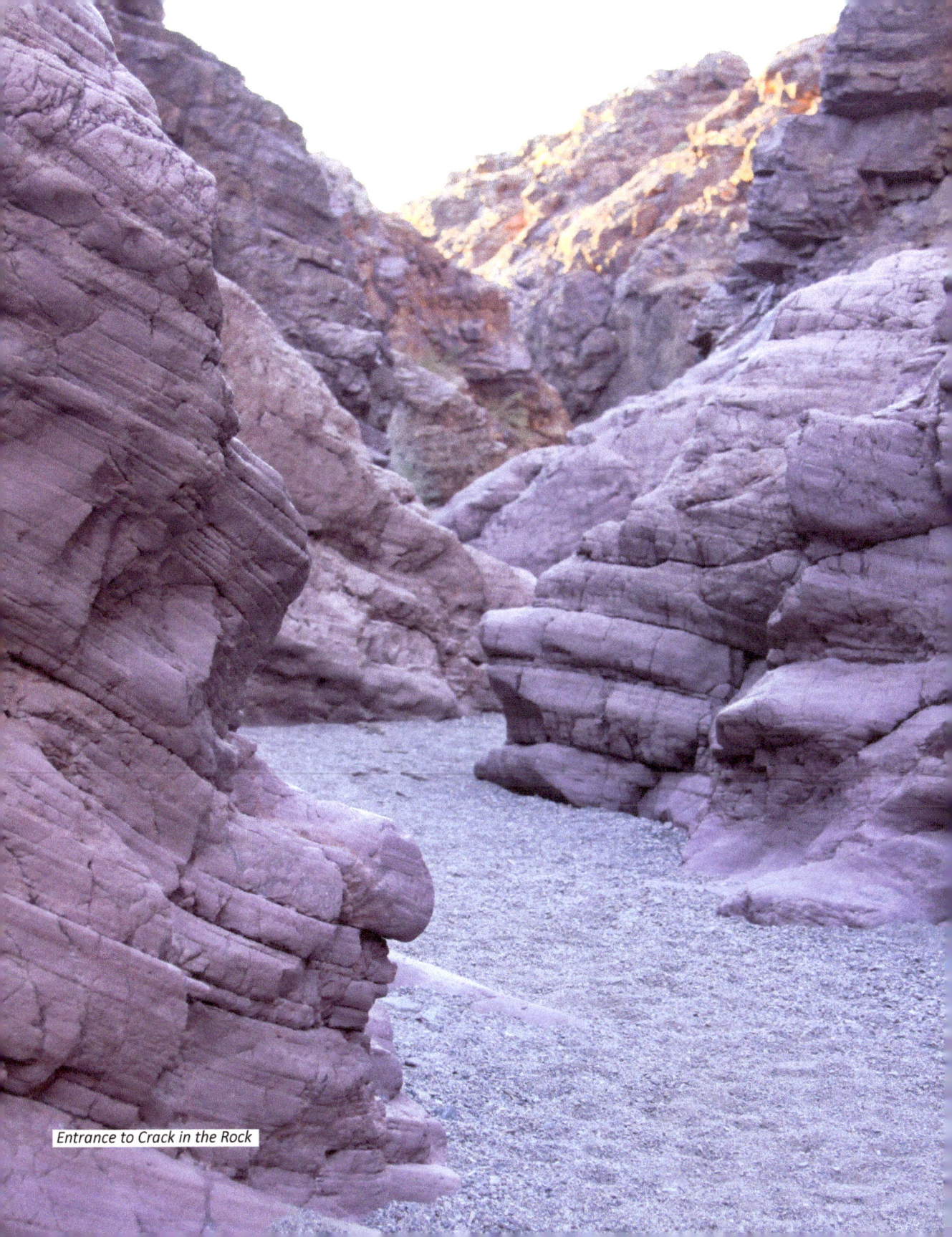

Entrance to Crack in the Rock

Cattail Cove / Colorado River

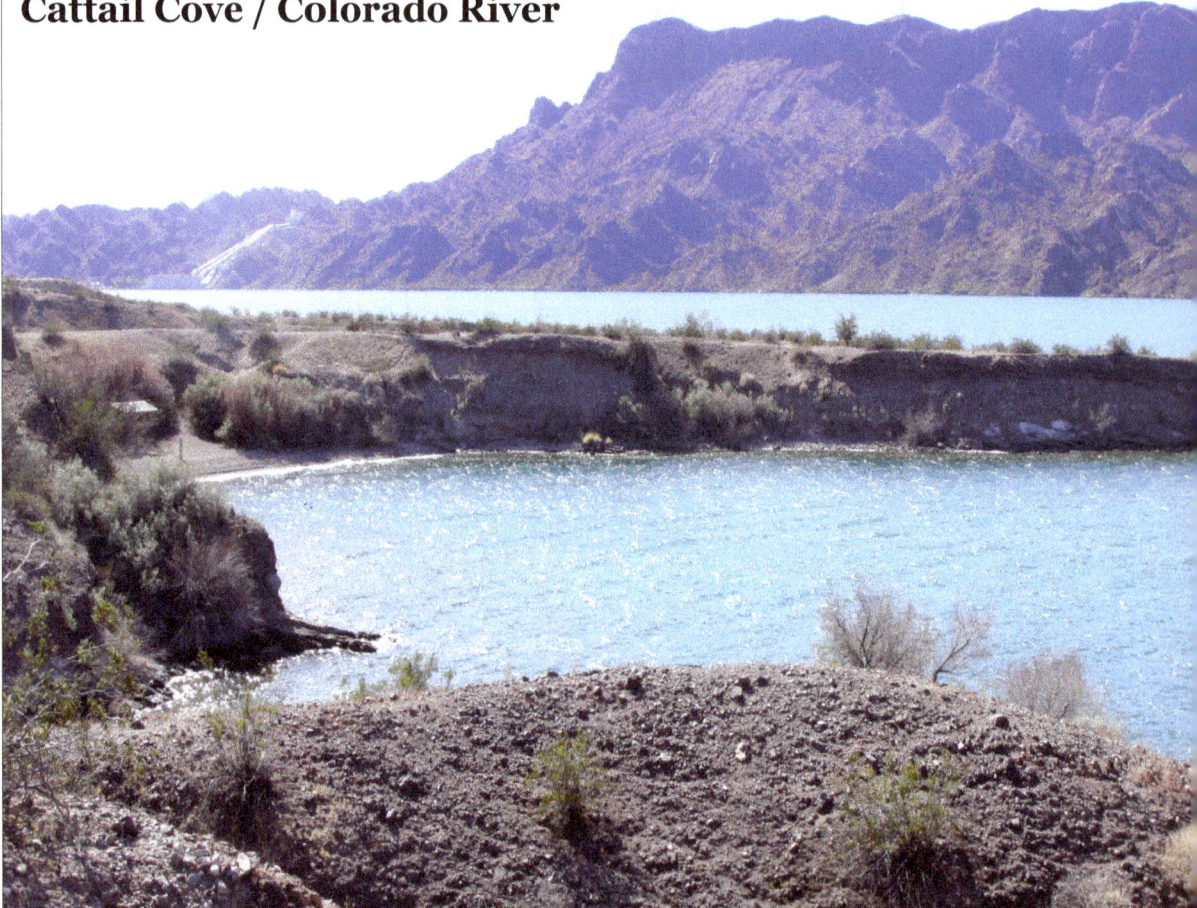

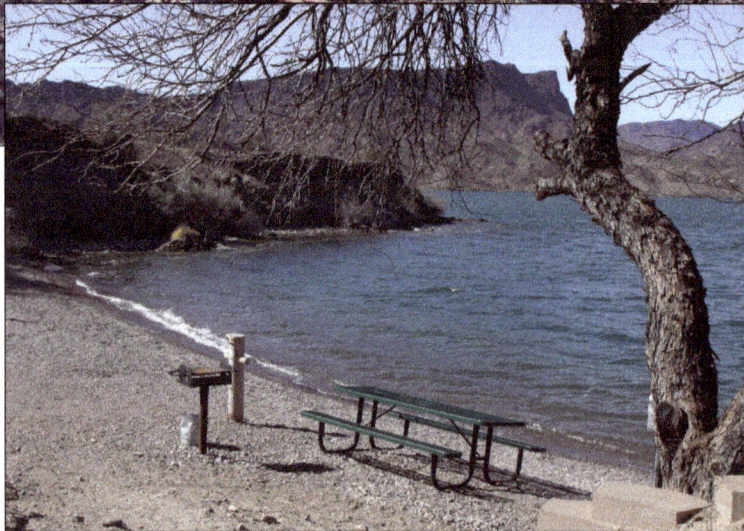

Driving Distance: 15 miles from
    Lake Havasu City

Rating: Easy

Elevation: 450'

Best Season: Winter, maybe
    early spring, or fall.

Special Features: Water! Lakeside
    hiking

Precautions: Crumbly edges
    along lakeside trail,
    poisonous snakes.

Info: Vis. Center 928-855-1223

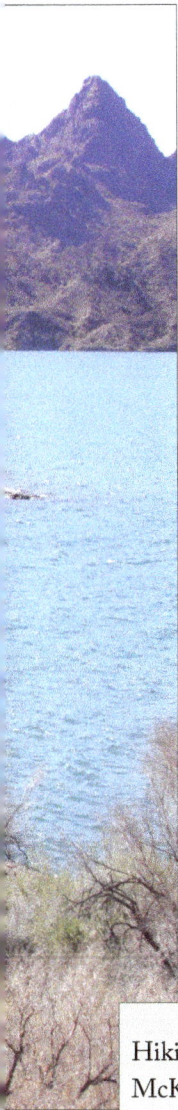

Cattail Cove State Park, with a marina and campground, is located 10 miles south of Lake Havasu City at mp 168. There is a fee to enter this park with designated day use parking. A network of trails is located west of the marina. The southern trailhead is at the end of the west parking lot.

The northern trailhead sits behind a chain link fence at the loading ramp, along the river's edge. This leads to a footpath carved out of a sloping hillside, with a steep drop to the water below. The view is beautiful but the trail requires attention as tripping could result in a sudden skid down to the water.

At the far end of the loop, the trail turns southwest toward a small cove called Whytes Retreat. Hikers may choose to stay left at the junction and return to the marina. Whytes Retreat has a beach of fine river rock with a small ramada and vault toilet.

Ted's Trail takes hikers from Whytes Retreat along a direct route to Wayne's Way. Ripley's Run takes a longer route inland to Wayne's Way with all trails returning to the parking lot. All trails give hikers a good look at the Mohave desert and desert shrubs. During the winter months, the parking lots are not crowded and temperatures perfect for hiking.

Photos:
Whytes Retreat

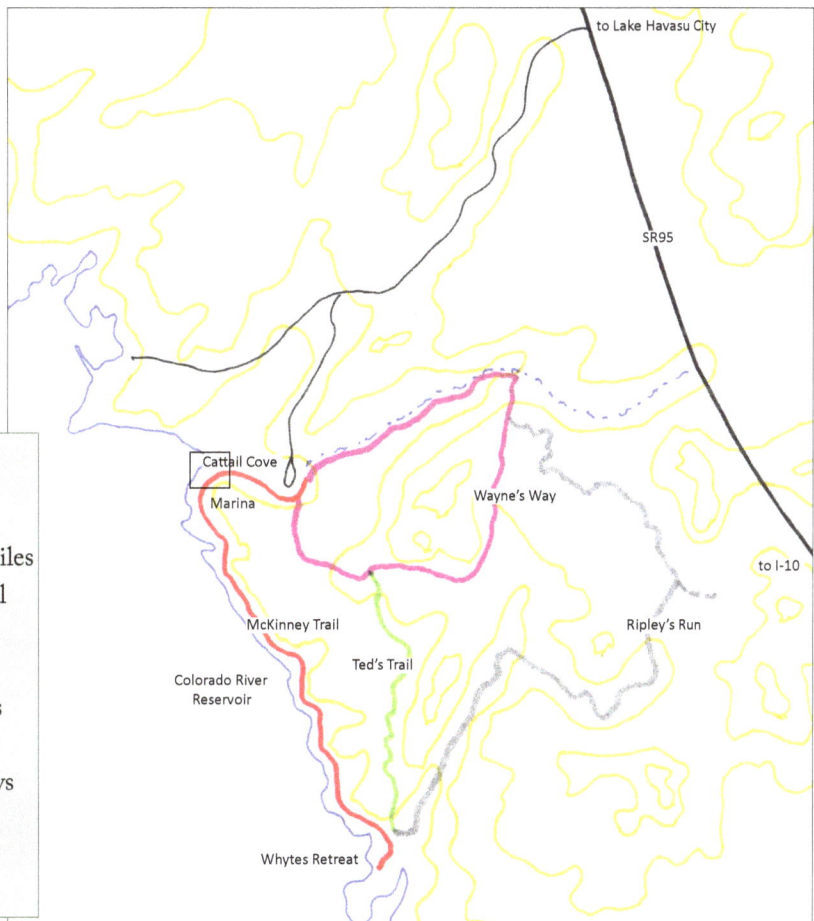

Hiking Distance:
McKinney to
    Whytes Retreat 1.4 miles
Wayne's Way Loop trail
        1 mile
Ted's Trail .5 mile
Ripley's Run   1.5 miles

Map: Arizona Highways
    or the Trail map
    provided by the
    Visitor's Center

to Lake Havasu City

SR95

Cattail Cove

Marina

Wayne's Way

to I-10

McKinney Trail

Ripley's Run

Ted's Trail

Colorado River
Reservoir

Whytes Retreat

47

Buckskin State Park

River Island

Twenty-seven miles south of Lake Havasu City, SR 95 reaches **Buckskin State Park**. The Park has two units. The **River Island** Unit on the north end is named after a small sandbar in the river which provides a back water from the main channel.

The Park office is in the Buckskin Point Unit, south of River Island. Both units offer camping and hookups in the shadow of tall buttes towering over the campgrounds.

At River Island, the Wedge Hill Loop follows the shore line for about a half mile to cliffs along the river. Hikers are discouraged from jumping off the cliffs into the dark waters that obscure rocks hidden beneath the surface. In the early evening this is a cool scenic stroll with lovely views along the river. The trail winds inland before returning to the parking area.

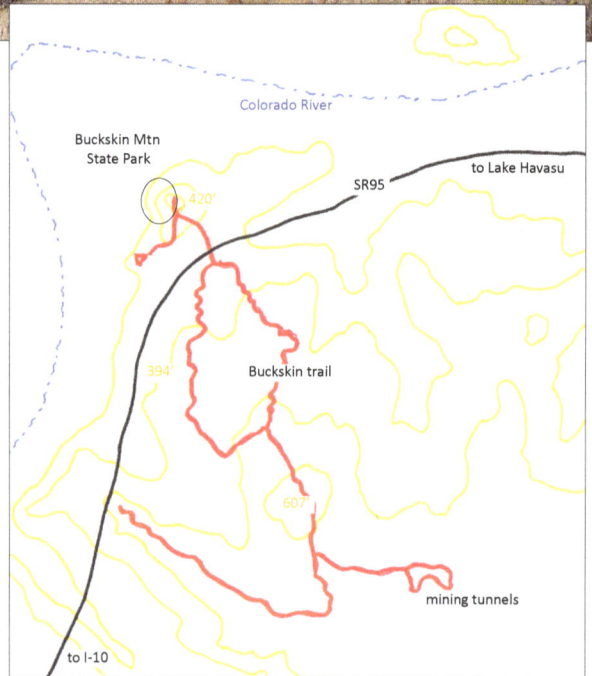

Colorado River

Buckskin Mtn
State Park

to Lake Havasu

SR95

420'

394'

Buckskin trail

607'

mining tunnels

to I-10

Buckskin Point

The trail head is located across from the central office at the Buckskin Point Unit. From the trail head, it is a rigorous climb up a hill overlooking the campground with excellent views of the river and the Buckskin Mountains east of the Park. Descending from the hilltop, a pedestrian overpass takes hikers safely across US 95 to the Buckskin trail. This is part of a loop trail with the left branch a steep climb. At the first junction, the right branch returns to the bridge over SR95.

Those choosing to continue straight reach a second junction. Continue straight to the highway or take the left branch toward the site of several pit mines. Those turning toward the mine sites, find several shallow tunnels before reaching the first mine shaft, the trail winds around the site to a second pit before turning north toward River Island.

The open mine shafts have been fenced in. One shaft is identified as the Skinner mine, depth 28 feet, water level at 17 feet. Therein is a story of how dreams came to a soggy end. Most likely the source of the water is a perched aquifer above the level of the river. Mining is a tough business.

The entire network of trails is exposed with no shade - not the best hiking location during the warmer months.

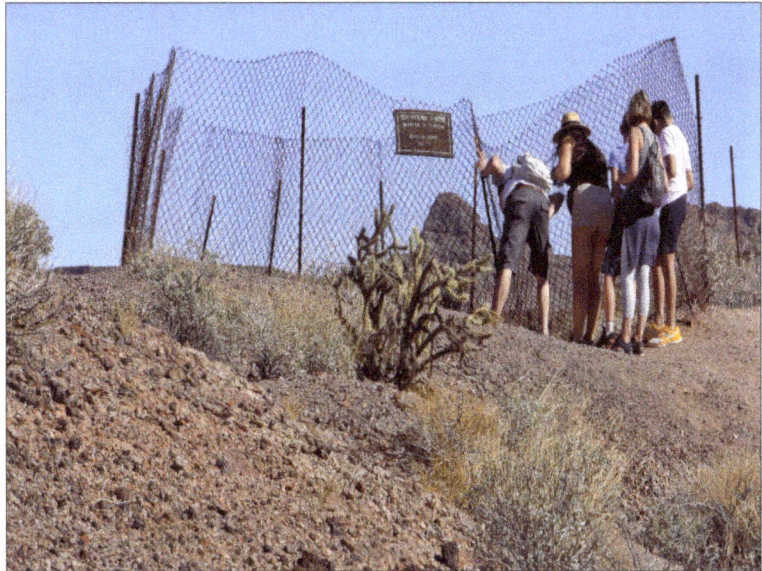

Peering into a mining shaft

Hiking Distance: 1+ miles
Rating: Moderately easy
Elevation: 1000'
Best Season: Winter, spring & fall.
Special Features: Tip-top view from Buckskin trail, old mining district
Precautions: Heat, poisonous reptiles & insects. Take lots of water.
Infomation: Buckskin State Park
(520) 667-3231

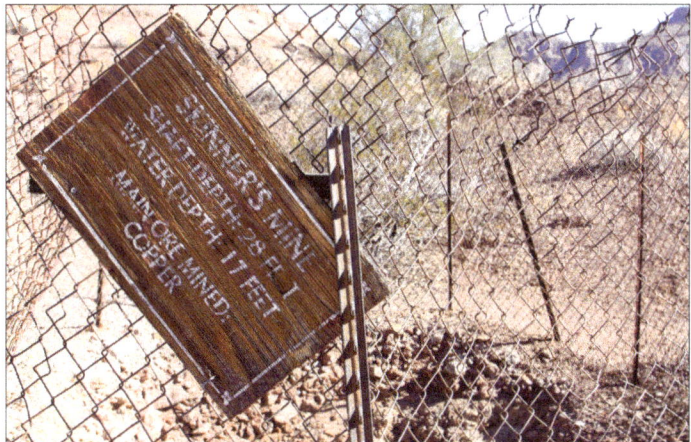

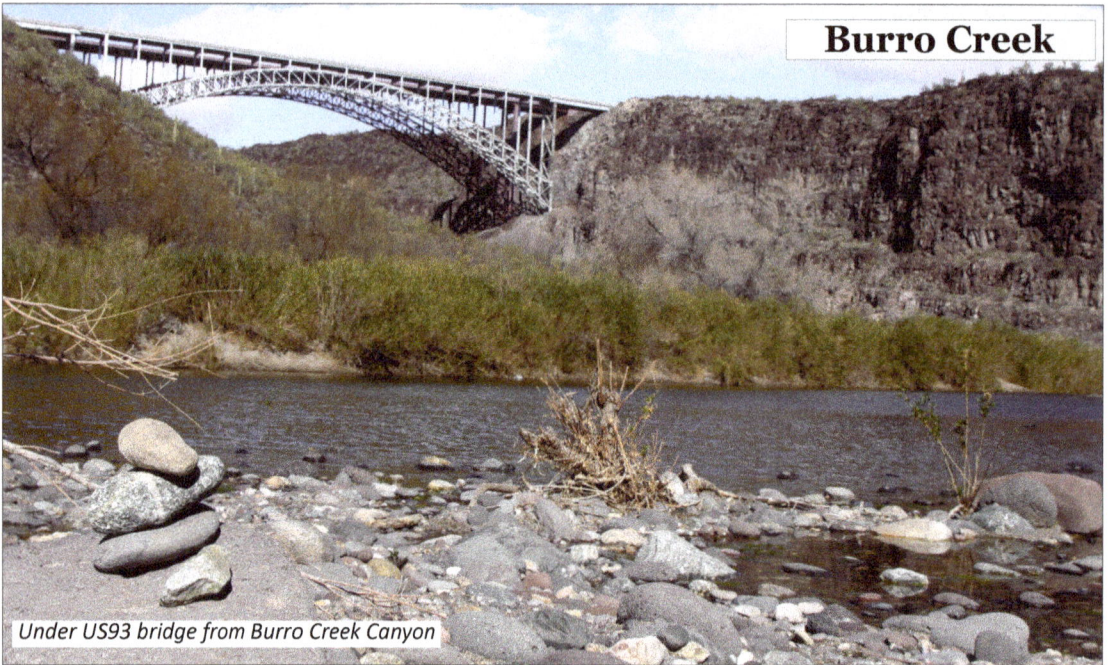

Burro Creek

Under US93 bridge from Burro Creek Canyon

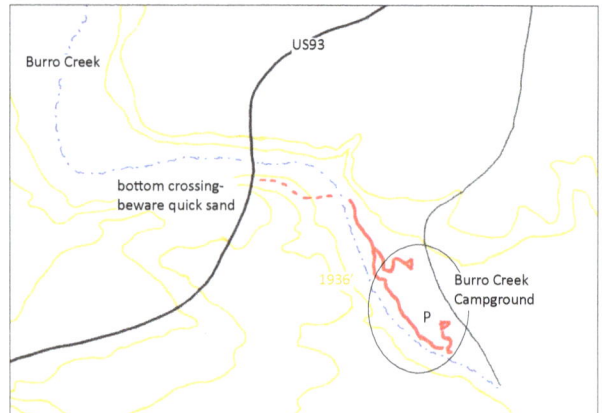

US Highway 93 has long been a popular route for Phoenix residents driving north to Las Vegas. About twenty miles south of the I-40/US93 junction, the highway crosses **Burro Creek** Canyon, a deep gulch carpeted with desert shrub.

Visitors turning west toward the small campground in the canyon, find a pleasant desert retreat with campsites and restrooms. At several points along the campground, trails lead down into a watercourse. During the winter months, a shallow stream fills the canyon floor.

The trail follows the watercourse upstream, passing under the bridge into the narrows. During our last two visits, we were unable to reach the bridge without wading across the stream. Before venturing a crossing, be aware that quick sand may have developed. Proceed one step at a time, helping anyone who may find their progress impeded. This is a pleasant walk along a desert canyon with no particular destination in mind - a good place to stretch our legs and clear our minds.

Driving Distance: 72 miles from Kingman
Hiking Distance: .75 miles, more if wash is dry.
Rating: Moderate
Elevation: 1936'
Best Season: Winter, maybe spring, or fall.
Special Features:
Precautions: Slick rock, poisonous vipers.
Maps: Arizona Highways

Palm Canyon

The Kofa Mountains rise along the eastern exposure of the Colorado River, seeming to form a barrier between the river and the urban areas further east. The mountains are named after the King of Arizona Mine with old mine sites found through out the range.

The mountains are the home of big horn desert sheep and mountain lions as well as the coyotes, desert tortoise and kit fox. In a narrow canyon on the west side of the range, a short hiking trail follows a deep wash to stately palms nestled in pockets high along a ridge.

The Washingtonia palms have sprouted from wind-borne seeds during a wet season. The heavy fronds reminded early settlers of a desert oasis and they hoped the palms would supply fruit. In more recent times, landscapers have made the species popular across Phoenix and Tucson.

Palm Canyon is a good place to stretch one's legs when driving between Yuma and I-10. We would not recommend attempting to climb up the rough terrain to the palms as the slopes are unstable.

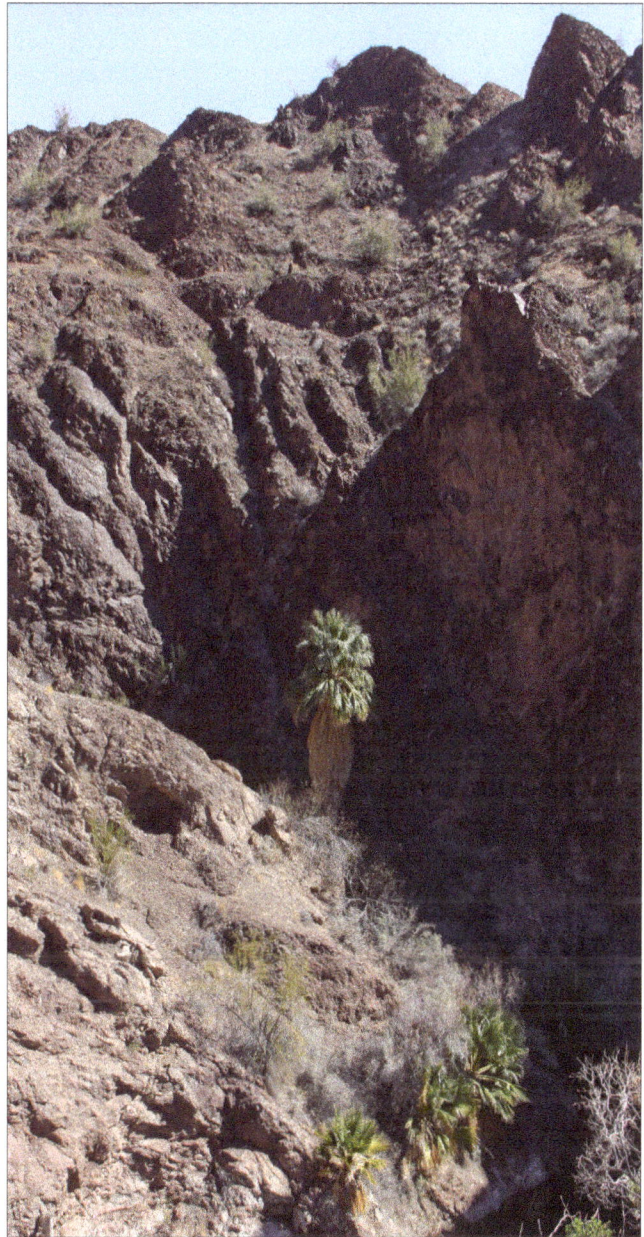

A Washingtonia palm is an isolated desert canyon.

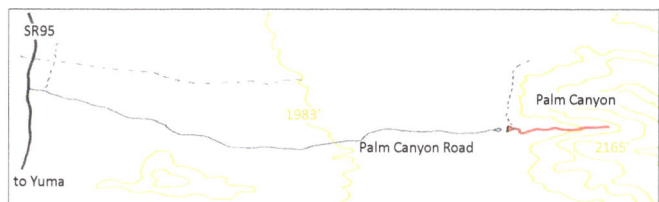

Driving Distance: 66 miles from Yuma
Hiking Distance: .75 mile one way
Rating: Moderate
Elevation: 2100 - 2530'
Best Season: Winter, spring or fall.
Special Features: ancient palm trees
Precautions: Slick rock, poisonous vipers.
Maps: Arizona Highways

Yuma Crossing and the East Wetlands Interpretive Trail

Hiking Distance: .5 to 1 mile
Rating: easy   Elevation: 185'-247'
Best Season: Winter, spring & fall
Special Features: Historic Territorial Prison
Precautions: Yuma is a crossroads for I-8 and
            traffic flowing north from Mexico. Due
            to the presence of migrants and the
            homeless, be extremely cautious!
Infomation: Yuma Territorial Prison
            (928) 783-4771

Telegraph Pass

Yuma residents with strong hearts and young knees regularly hike **Telegraph Pass**, posting the number of times they have climbed on a message board at the summit. While the road to the summit is not particularly scenic, the top offers a good view of the surrounding area.

Drive east on I-8 from Yuma for 16 miles and take the Fortuna Hills exit. Turn north, then east onto the frontage road and drive to a small parking area. Follow the maintenance road to the summit of Telegraph Pass. At the summit, modern communication towers have replaced the telegraph. Distance is just under half a mile.

Photo: Yuma Crossing

The Spanish first came to a crossing on the Colorado River they named after the Yuman Indians who lived along the river. White settlers followed their route in the late 1800's and a small town began to rise along the bank of the river. A military base was built to protect the trade routes that crossed the desert.

At one time, the river could stretch as wide as a half mile, with a braided channel and marshland. A ferry was established to transport traffic across the river. Early settlers found the Colorado River thick with silt, too thick to drink. They would hardly recognize the river today. Upstream, huge dams hold back the waters, allowing the silt to settle and protect Yuma from flooding. The water released into the river bed is cool, clear green.

When politicians began to consider the need for a secure prison in Arizona Territory in the mid 1870's, the original site chosen was Phoenix. Then two unscrupulous legislators came along and quietly removed the name Phoenix and inserted Yuma into the legislation. The bill was passed before anyone discovered the change.

The prison offers several tours a day and the guides give a detailed and colorful history of the prison. An interpretive trail now runs along the river, from the Gateway Historical Park east beyond the Territorial Prison. Near the river, the old freight depot presents displays of Yuma's history.

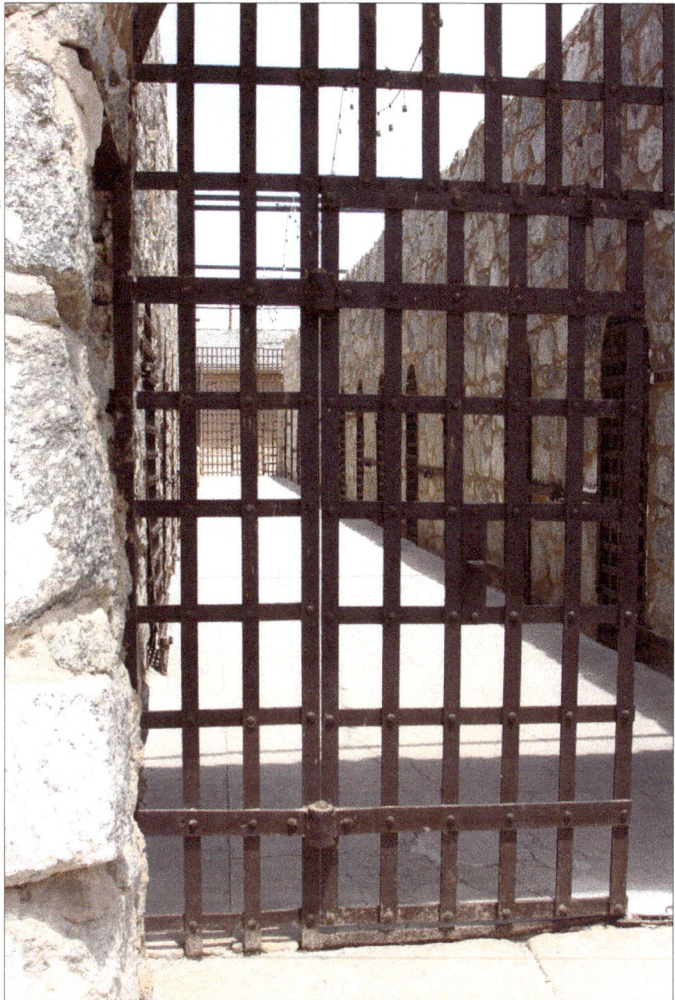

A gate and cells in Yuma Territorial Prison

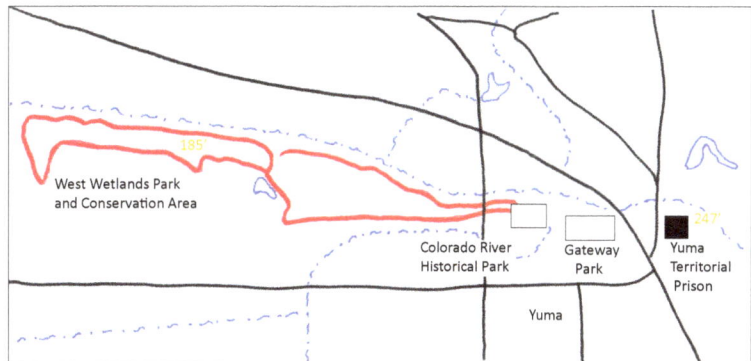

West Wetlands Park and Conservation Area

Colorado River Historical Park

Gateway Park

Yuma Territorial Prison

Yuma

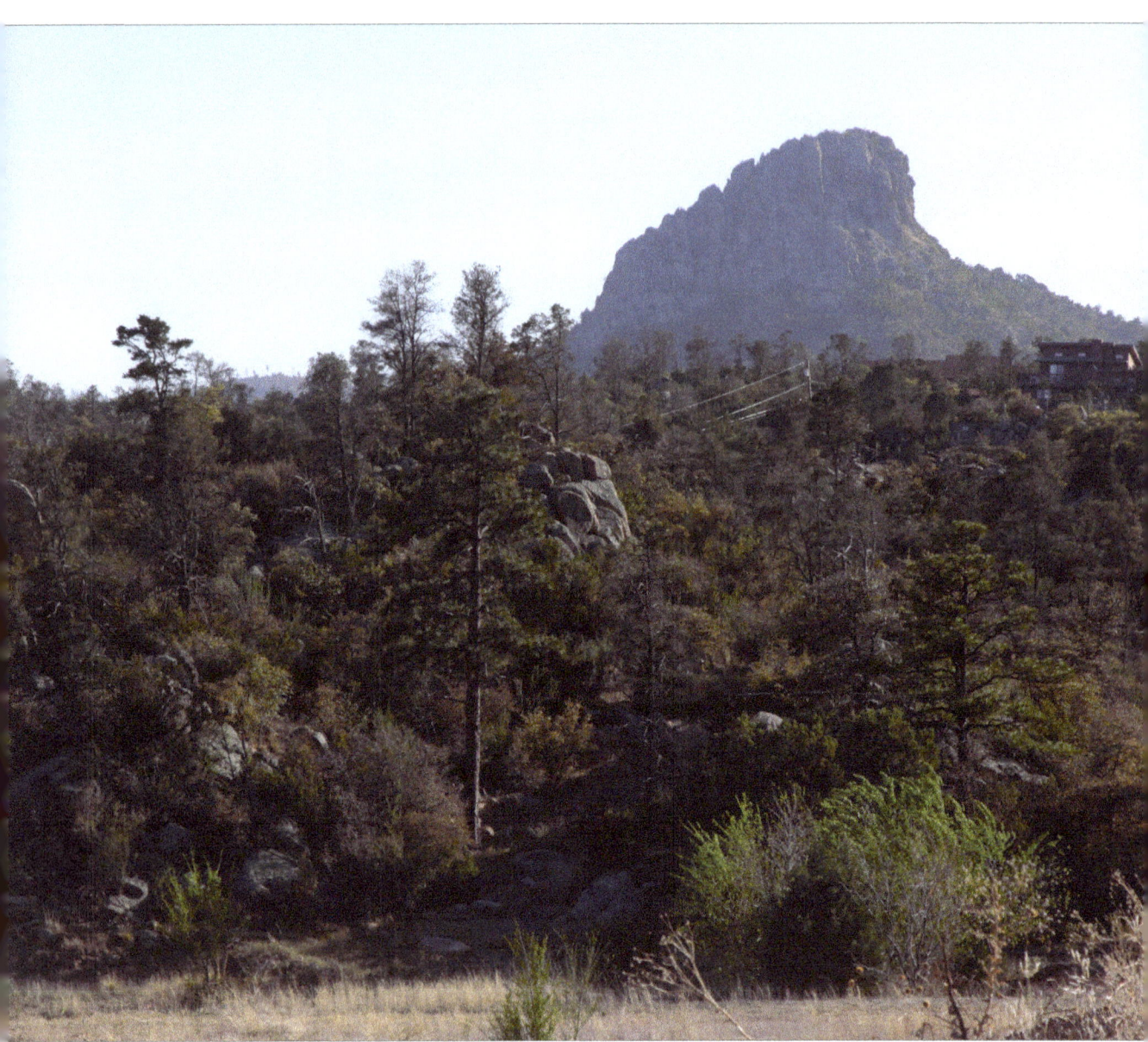

The Thumb

Prescott was once the territorial capitol of Arizona. In the 1800s, the Bradshaw Mountains drew prospectors, merchants and fortune hunters to this town.

the Senator Highway, 16 miles south of Prescott. A high-clearance vehicle is recommended. This was once a stagecoach stop, now used as office space for the Forest Service. There are several old mines and

Prescott & the Bradshaw Mountains

Today, the Bradshaws, along with the Hassayampa River, are favorite territories for those looking to explore and get away from the busy urban centers of Arizona.

The Senator Highway is a popular route for four-wheelers to the summit of the Bradshaw Mountains and the little community of Crown King. Many of the trails along the ridges and valleys of the Bradshaws are steep but reward hikers with expansive views.

We've chosen to feature trails in the lowlands that are easier for novice hikers. One location that may be interesting to those who wish to see a bit of history is Palace Station along

the site of a stamp mill along Senator Highway just before reaching Palace Station.

Numerous side roads tug for attention and a bit of exploration but drivers should be aware that they may be accessing a private drive or possibly a 4WD jeep trail.

The lower elevations around Prescott are located in the woodland zone, with forests of juniper and oak. The hills around Prescott and along the Senator Highway are populated with pondersoa pine, indicating a transition to a higher elevation. Those drawn to water should remember the streams and the lakes in this region are tainted by the chemicals from early mining efforts.

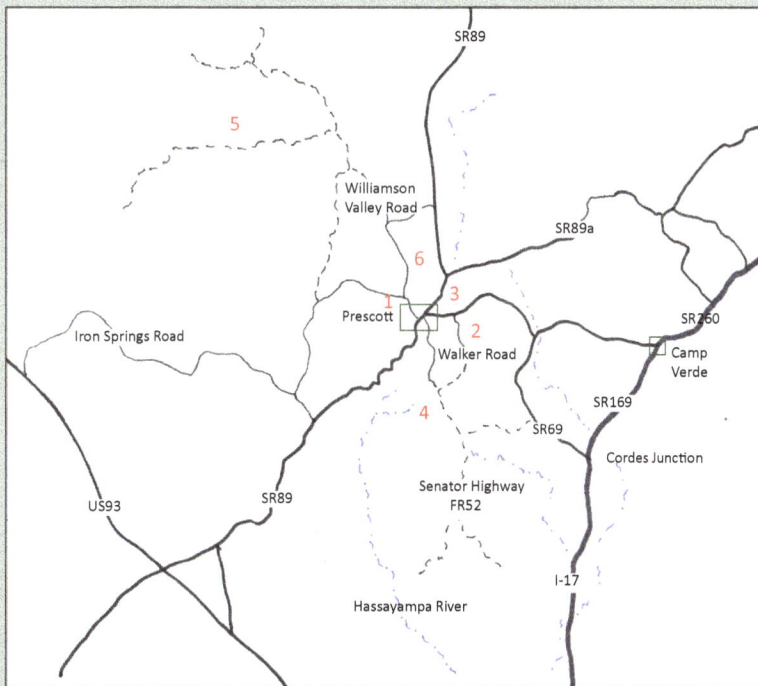

1 Thumb Butte
2 Lynx lake
3 Granite Dells & Watson Lake
4 Wolf Creek Trail
5 Hyde Mountain Lookout
6 Granite Mountain

Thumb Butte Recreational Area

Prescott has spread around the base of **Thumb Butte,** turning the rocky knob into more of an urban park. The trail to the summit is short with a steep grade and great views of the area around Prescott.

To reach the trailhead, drive west through Prescott on Gurley Street. As Gurley makes a sweeping left turn, watch for Thumb Butte Road on your right. The road passes through a residential section before entering the park. At the Thumb Butte Recreation Area, a number of trails spiral out into the surrounding forest.

The Thumb Butte trailhead is on the left or south side of the road across from a parking area. Hikers can climb the loop trail in either direction. The right or west side climbs along a small wash lined with oak, pinon pine and juniper to a saddle with a view of the Prescott area. From the saddle the trail rises steeply toward the basalt outcrop regarded as the 'thumb' extended above clenched fingers. Daring hikers scramble around the rock face to reach the summit. We don't recommend the climb for inexperienced climbers, especially young children, due to the possibility of serious injury.

Hikers complete the loop, descending along the left or east side through a series of switchbacks down to the trail head.

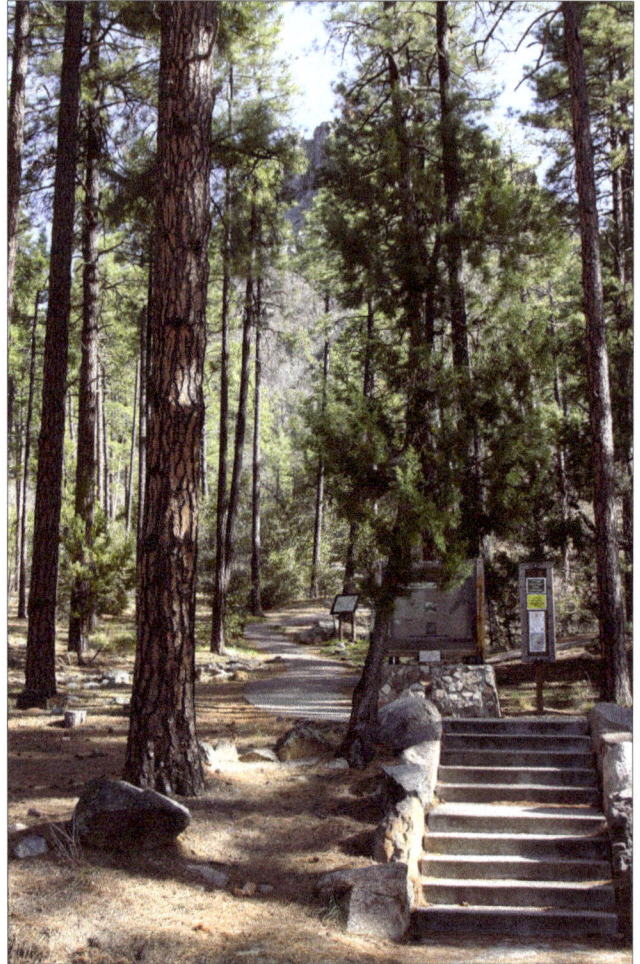

Photo: Thumb Butte trail

Driving Distance: 4 miles from downtown Prescott.
Hiking Distance: 1.75 mile loop
Rating: Moderate   Elevation: 5600' - 6400'
Best Season: Spring, summer & fall.
Special Features: Urban trail to landmark. Great views.
Precautions: Loose rock under foot. Only experienced climbers with proper equipment should attempt ascent up the Thumb.
Maps: City of Prescott Trail map
        928- 777-1590

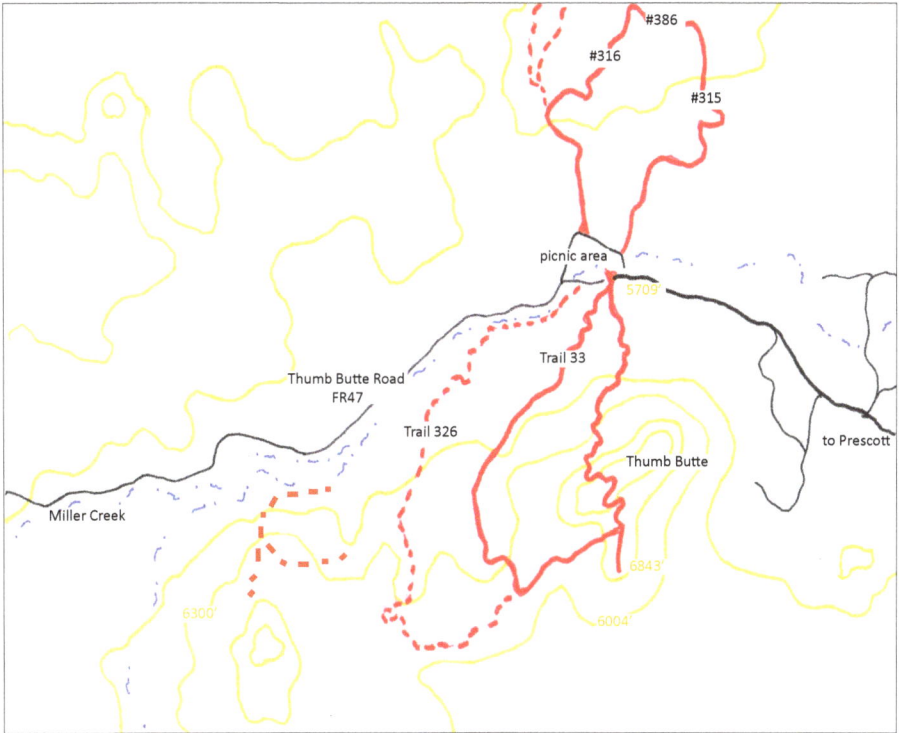

Map labels: #386, #316, #315, picnic area, 5709, Trail 33, Thumb Butte Road FR47, Trail 326, Thumb Butte, to Prescott, Miller Creek, 6843, 6004, 6300

The City of Prescott has developed a network of trails between the Thumb Butte Recreation Area and Iron Springs Road. We recommend picking up a map of the trails around Prescott at the Forest Service office or the Visitors Center if you are interested in exploring other routes.

The Other Loop at Thumb Butte

The **Willow Creek** trail is located at picnic table #8 in the day use area across from Thumb Butte. Follow trail #316 to the junction with trail #386 and turn right. When the trail intersect #315, turn right again to return to the campground.

For a side trip, note the well worn footpath on the right .75 mile from the campground. Shaded by tall pines, the trail drops into the Willow Creek drainage. Make a note of your entrance to the wash for the return trip. Turning downstream, hikers follow the stream bed to a narrow passage through a natural volcanic dike. The water has worn a network of shallow rivelets through the black granite to drop over a low cliff and into a wide canyon. The trail passes close to several homes. Emmanual Pines Camp is nearby and campers regularly visit this special spot. This is a lovely rest stop on a warm afternoon before moving back to the loop.

Hiking Distance: 2 miles round trip
Rating: Easy
Elevation: 5900' - 5700'
Best Season: Summer & fall
Special Features: Fascinating granite formation with seasonal stream.
Precautions: Be respectful of local residents.
Maps: City of Prescott Trail map

Lynx Lake

Swimming is forbidden in the lakes around Prescott as the water has become a chemical stew with mercury and arsenic at levels hazardous to our health. While arsenic may be naturally present in the soil, mercury is definitely a blast from Prescott's mining history. Mercury was used to separate gold from the rock ore in the amalgamation process.

Originally, a dam was constructed in the late 1800's to contain waters for use in gold dredging operations. The original dam was damaged by severe flooding and in 1958 Game & Fish built the current dam to create a trout fishing lake. It has become extremely popular, offering boating and fishing along with hiking, a day-use area and campgrounds. An easy trail winds along the shoreline for 2.5 miles. Along the route a number of footpaths lead up small washes or to campgrounds, inviting hikers to further exploration.

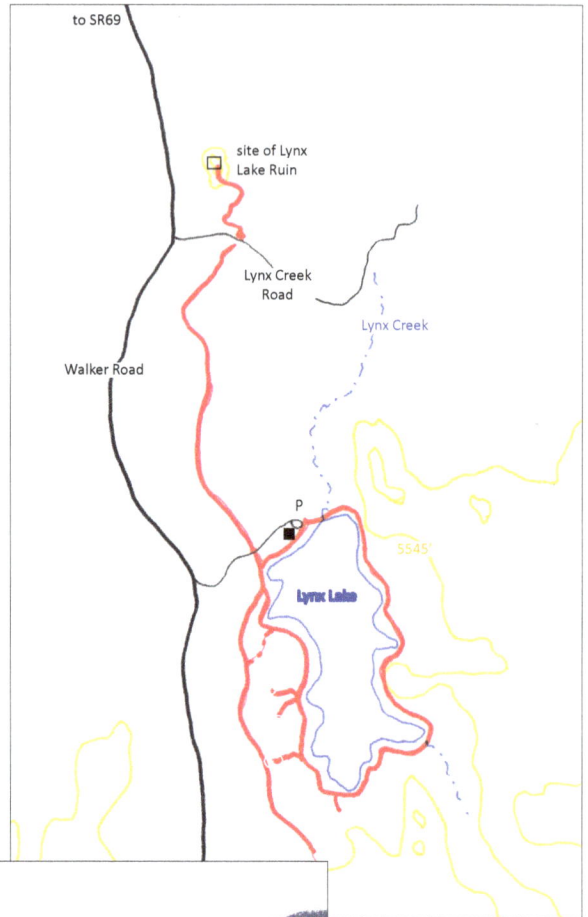

to SR69

site of Lynx Lake Ruin

Lynx Creek Road

Lynx Creek

Walker Road

P

5545'

Lynx Lake

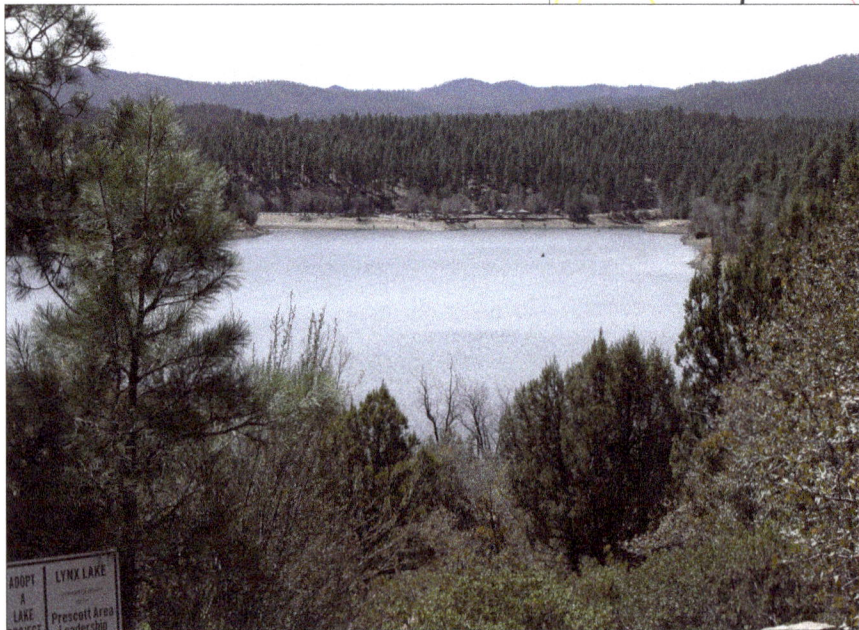

Lynx Lake

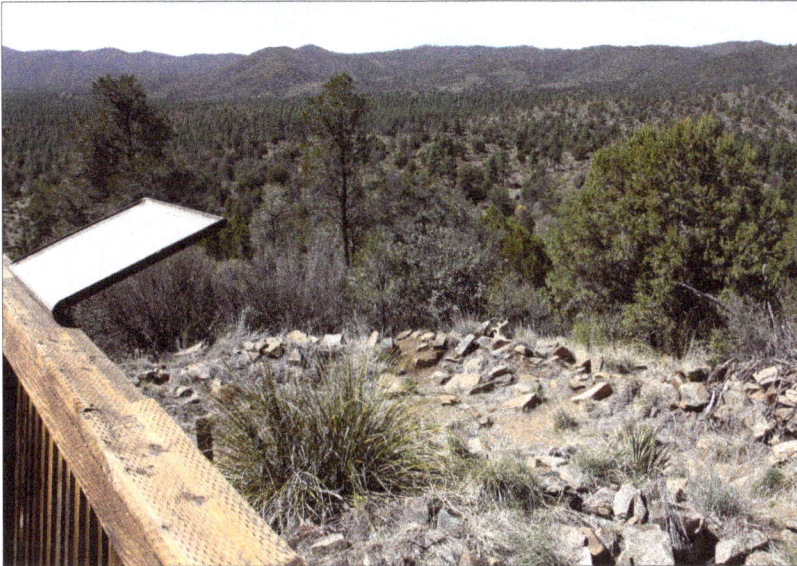

Lynx Lake Ruins

Ancient people once built their homes on a ridge overlooking the canyon above Lynx Lake. They must have found this locale to have a fairly reasonable climate with mild winters and warm summers. A seasonal stream gave the residents water. Hunting was supplemented with fruit from local vegetation. The prickly pear cactus offered seasonal fruit. They harvested berries from the skunkbush and seeds from the pinon pine. The pads of the agave plant were baked in a rock-lined pit.

To visit the site of the **Lynx Lake Ruin**, drive east from Prescott on SR 69, just over four miles, turning right or south on Walker Road. Follow Walker Road about 1.4 miles to the signed turnoff to Lynx Creek Ruins. Turn east to the parking area. The trail to the ruins leads north through scrub oak and alligator juniper. After crossing several small washes, the trail ascends a small hill to an observation deck with views of Lynx Lake, Prescott and the Bradshaws.

Lynx Lake Ruin

Lynx Lake

Driving Distance: Approx. 6 miles from downtown Prescott.
Hiking Distance: 1.75 mile loop
Rating: Moderate
Elevation: 5545'
Best Season: Spring, summer & fall.
Special Features: Water!
Precautions:
Maps: Prescott NFS map or
City of Prescott Trail map

Lynx Lake Ruins

Driving Distance: Approx. 6 miles from downtown Prescott
Hiking distance: .75 mile one way
Rating: Easy
Best Season: Spring, summer & fall.
Special Features: Indian ruins, Lynx Lake nearby.
Precautions: Be careful of loose gravel underfoot on descent.
Elevation: 5545'
Maps: Prescott NFS map
Infomation: Prescott Ranger Station (928) 443-8000

58

Granite Dells and Watson Lake

The City of Prescott, with a little help from those who wander, has developed a whole network of trails around Watson Lake. Granite Dells, on the north end, is a great place to explore with trails dipping down to Watson Lake. It is helpful to pick up the City of Prescott trail map or print the map off the internet to stay on the correct route. For those who don't, each junction is signed with the trail name and a small map that will give hikers a sense of their position relating to the lake.

We suggest starting out along

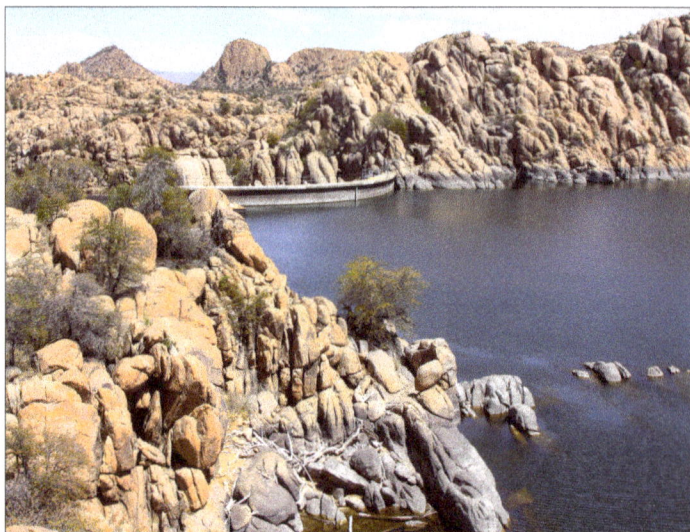

Watson Lake dam

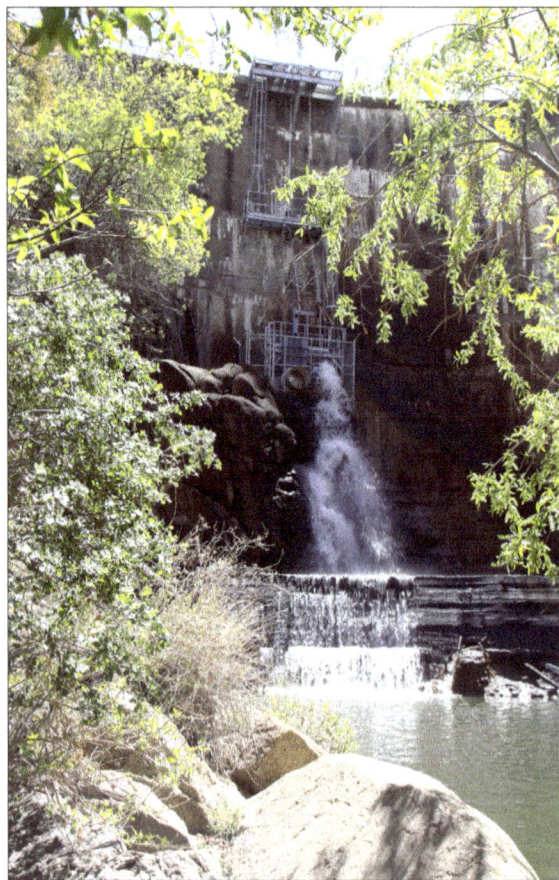

the **Northshore Trail** at the Watson Lake Recreation Area trail head near the boat launch site. The trail follows a series of ledges above the lake then turns inland, passing over a granite peak. Following white dots painted on the rocks along the trail, hikers descend to a small streambed and turn right to cross the stream. Much of the year water is being released from the dam and a side trail takes hikers to the pond formed at the foot of the dam.

Turning back, don't cross the bridge but move ahead to a steep ascent along the **Over the Hill trail** into the Dells, climbing through one summit after another. As you stop to catch your breath, look around and imagine the subterrean force that brought these rocks to the surface. Granite is formed deep underground in the movement of super-heated rock called magna.

From the summit, as hikers begin to descend, a couple of short side trails lead to Hidden Cove along the shoreline. The trail intersects a dirt road to the left - this is the **Peavine trail**. Follow either the Peavine or the **Lakeshore trail** southwest to a junction with a footpath crossing Granite Creek.

59

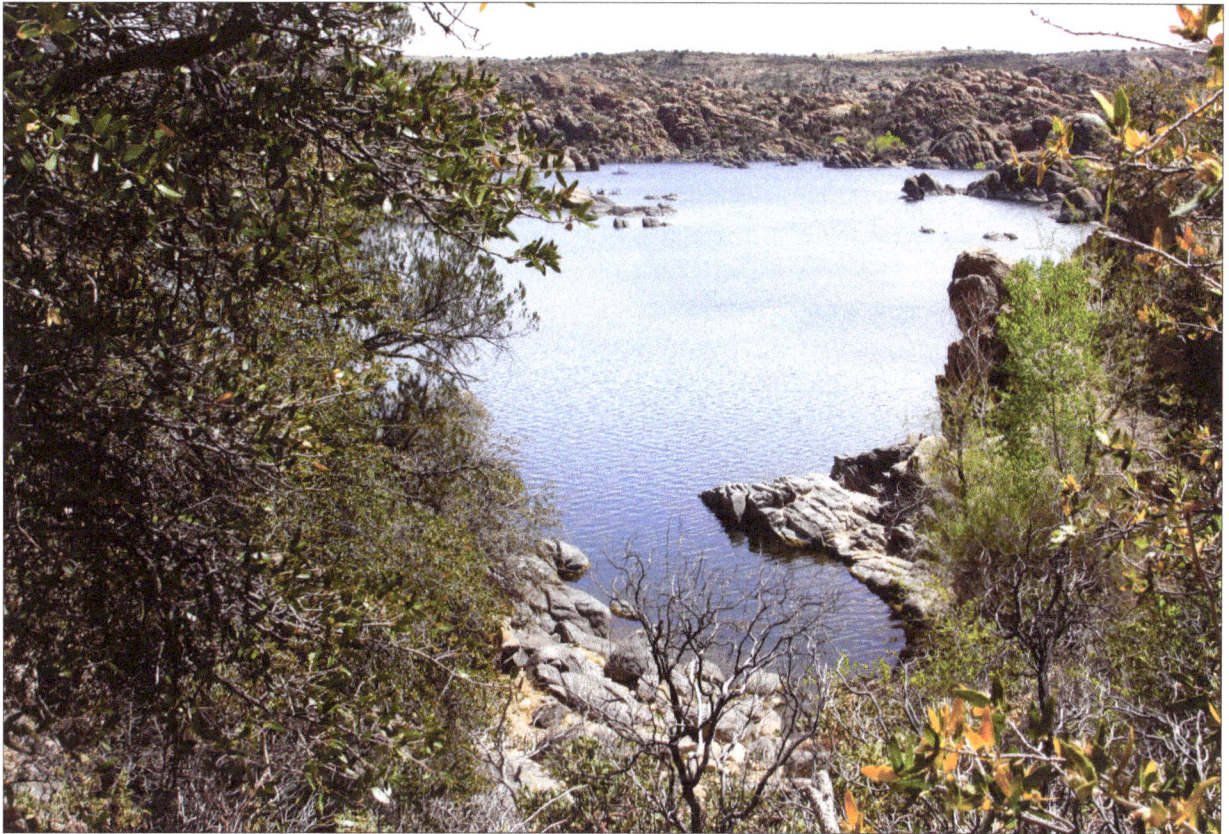

Watson Lake, Northshore trail

The loop is completed with the **Discovery Trail,** returning to the point of departure. Part of the Discovery trail is through a disc-golf course.

Hiking Distance: 4.8 mile loop
Rating: Shoreline easy, Dells moderately
    challenging
Elevation: 5,235' - 5,075'
Best Season: Spring and fall.
Special Features: Granite formations,
    seasonal stream.
Precautions: Watch your step, use your
    hands when climbing if steep.
Maps: City of Prescott trail map.
    928- 777-1590

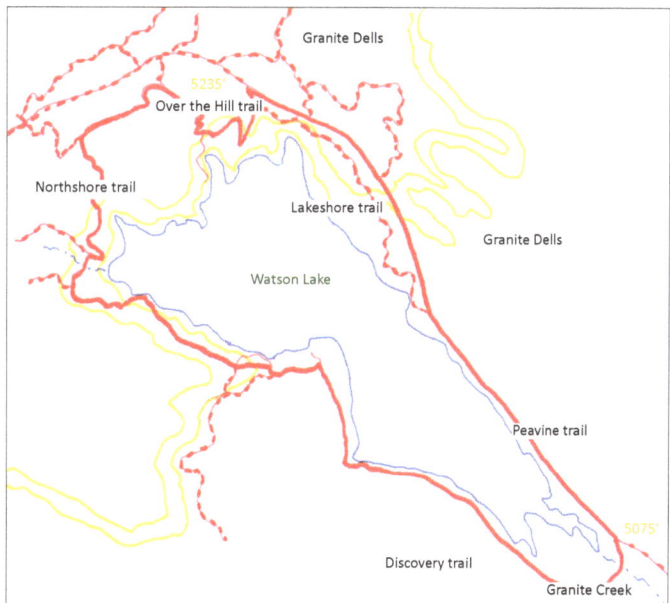

Wolf Creek Trail

Long before hiking boots and mountain bikes lured visitors into the foothills of the Bradshaws, the lure of gold induced early settlers to riffle the rocks and soil found in the washes of the Bradshaws. Miners shoveled gravel onto riffle boards from the Hassayampa River, searching for the gleam of gold. Today, Prescott residents enjoy a creekside stroll and the cool water of the river during the warmer months.

To access the area, turn south from Gurley Street on to the Senator Highway, FR 52. Drive past the turnoff to Pine Summit Campground and Lower Wolf Creek, at 7.3 miles from Gurley Street. The next turnoff is the Mount Trimble Road, or FR79. Turn right and follow FR 79 for 1.3 miles to the crossing of **Wolf Creek**. Vehicles can easily drive across the stream when the water level is low. Park at the junction with **FR 79B**, above the creek. Do not attempt to cross if the water level is high!

FR79B follows Wolf Creek toward FR 74 and the Lower Wolf Creek Campground - I suggest walking FR74. Along the route, several pools call to visitors to enjoy the cool water for an hour - a good way to explore this historic area.

For those interested in historical sites, a short climb up FR 79 brings visitors to a bullet-pocked sign for Kendall Camp. Turn right along a dirt track, walking downhill, to an old orchard tucked behind a rail fence. Notice the shallow pits which were dug with the soil sifted over riffle boards as a miner searched for gold flakes. If you should find old 4x4 beams with glass jars attached, do not disturb. These are legal documents and official notices of mining claims.

Driving Distance: 10 miles from Gurley St.
Hiking Distance:
    Kendall Camp 1.2 mile one way.
    Wolf Creek trail .75 mile
Rating: Kendall Camp - moderate climb.
    River Walk - easy.
Best Season: Summer & fall.
Special Features: Historic mining site, beautiful creek.
Precautions: Flash floods along Wolf Creek can make it dangerous. Do not attempt to cross when the water is high!
Maps: Prescott NFS Map
Infomation: Prescott National Forest
    (928) 443-8000

Opposite page: Wolf Creek along FR74B

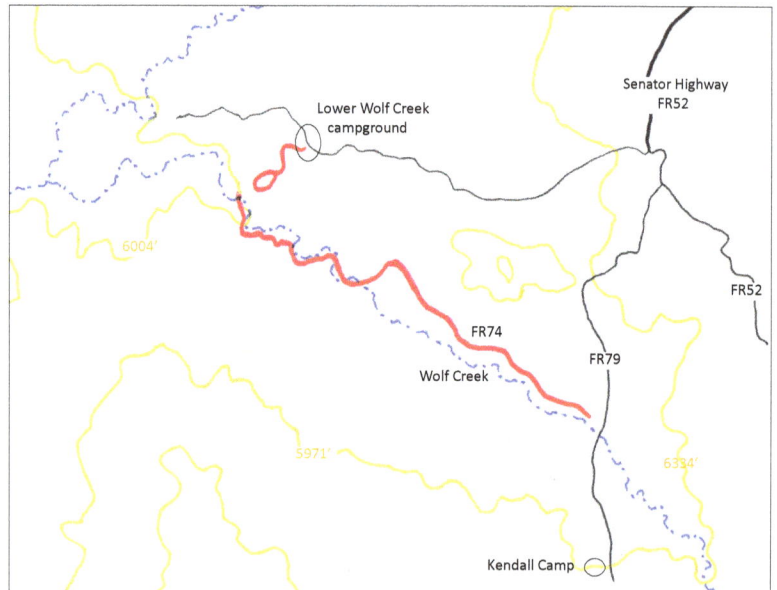

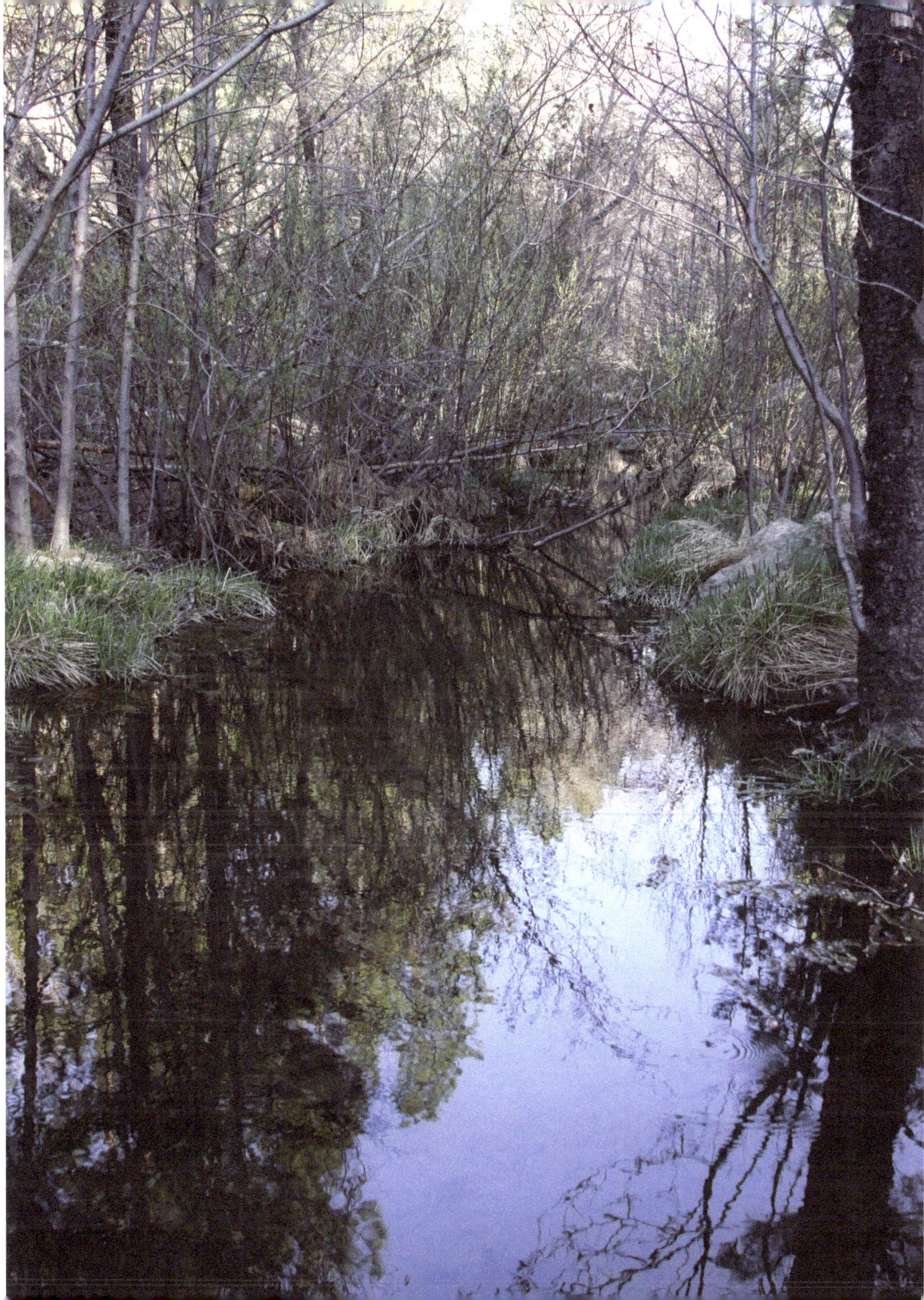

Branching Out: Hyde Mountain Lookout

The **Hyde Mountain** trail climbs to an old fire lookout cabin built by the Civilian Conservation Corp. The long drive out to the trail head limits the number of people using this area compared to the more popular trails around Prescott. Drive north on Montezuma St. from downtown Prescott as it turns to Iron Springs Road. Turn north onto the Williamson Valley Road and drive 22 miles to the turnoff to Camp Wood, FR21. Turn west, drive 16 miles to FR 95. Turning right, drive .3 mile through an open area that used to be the site of Camp Wood. Turn left onto FR 95C, a narrow rough track lined by dense manzanita brush. On our last visit, we found that much of FR95C had been washed out and it was best to park and follow the road on foot. Cross the sandy creekbed and follow the track uphill to the trailhead. The footpath leads to a metal gate. Beyond the gate, the trail forks twice, 1st fork, stay left. At the second fork, stay right. The trail ascends through a forest of juniper and scrub oak toward a saddle between two peaks.

Upon reaching the saddle, the trail turns left to climb a fold between two peaks through a series of switchbacks. After reaching a second saddle, the trail crosses on to the backside of Hyde Mountain for the final ascent to the summit. Just below the summit, the trail forks with the left branch descending to Brown Springs.

A one-room wood cabin stands at the summit. With no access road, building materials and supplies were painstakingly hauled in by pack-mule. The cabin is still used by a conservation group. The isolation, the trail itself and the view all make this a great hike in a remote area.

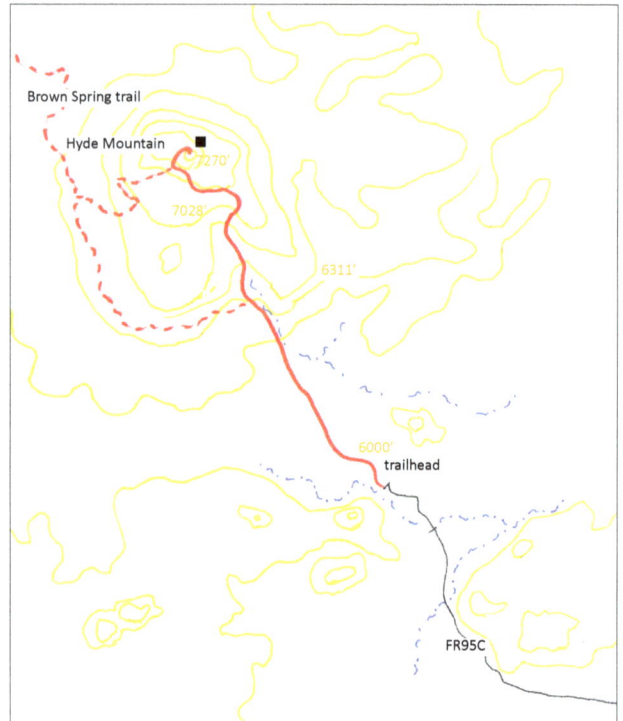

Driving Distance: Approx. 40 miles NW from Prescott

Hiking Distance: 3 miles, including access along road.

Rating: Moderate

Elevation: 5700' - 7272'

Best Season: Spring & fall

Special Features: Old fire lookout on Register of Historic Places.

Maps: NFS Prescott District map

Infomation: Prescott National Forest
(928) 443-8000

Granite Mountain

Granite Mountain rises over the skyline of Prescott with an expanse of gray-leaden rock. One trail leads visitors to the summit while a second takes visitors into the Granite Mountain Wilderness.

From Gurley Street in downtown Prescott, turn right/north onto Montezuma Street. At the intersection of Montezuma and Iron Springs, follow Iron Springs Road to the turn-off into the Granite Basin Recreation Area. The road passes a small lake before the turn-off to the Metate trailhead. The Granite Mountain trail is #261. The trail starts across the road from the trail head, turning away from the lake. At the base of the mountain hikers ascend steep switch-backs, gaining a great view over the Recreation area and the town of Prescott before reaching a saddle. Nearing the top the trail passes through awesome rock boulders, alligator juniper and ponderosa pine. Take the time to explore, checking views to the north-east. Hikers frequently step out onto ledges overlooking the basin below - be careful! Only those with rock climbing experience should attempt scaling the boulder at the summit.

After climbing Granite Mountain, hikers may wish to spend some time along the edge of the little lake, cooling off and dipping a fishing line. Check with the Forest Service for further information.

Driving Distance: approx. 7 miles
Hiking Distance: 3.25+ miles
Rating: Moderate
Elevation: 5500' - 7000'
Best Season: Spring, summer, fall.
Special Features: Pretty lake and
       great views of Granite Basin.
Maps: NFS Prescott District map
Infomation: Prescott Ranger Station
       (928) 443-8000

Caution:
Both hikes are exposed. Carry lots of water during hot weather. Watch for lightning during monsoons and descend quickly from the peak.

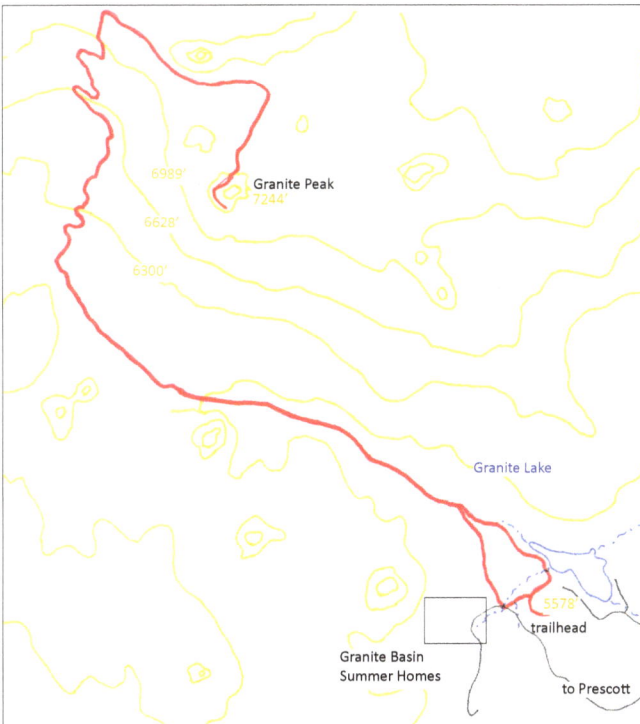

6989'
Granite Peak
7244'
6628'
6300'
Granite Lake
5578'
trailhead
Granite Basin
Summer Homes
to Prescott

Saving Our Forest for Future Generations.

Arizona residents are happy to remind visitors that we don't seem to have tornadoes or earthquakes that amount to much. In turn visitors remind us that we have very hot summers - at least in the southern part of the state.

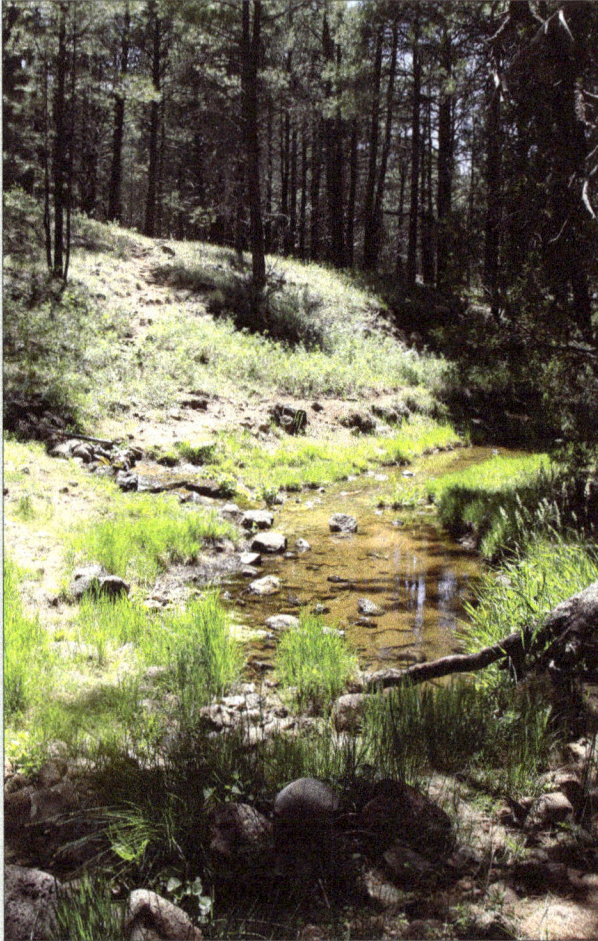

In recent years devastating wildfires have become a much greater concern for those living in the transition zone. To counter this threat, the Forest Service conducts controlled burns. To accomplish this, Forest Service personnel survey a tract of forest, marking trees to be thinned. Crews move in with chain saws and large equipment. Once the trees have been cleared, the brush and litter is swept into large piles and allowed to dry. Later, during cool weather, crews set these piles ablaze, maintaining watch to ensure that the fire remains on the ground and does not reach into the tree tops where it can begin to run wild.

It can be a bit alarming to see a pillar of dense gray smoke rising above the trees. Look at little closer. If the base of the fire, seems to be spread across a broad area, most likely this is a controlled burn. If the smoke rises in a narrow dark column, chances are the fire lookouts have already called dispatch and alerted crews that a campfire or lightning strike is starting to run.

For our part we can honor the fire restrictions. If the Forest Service declares a red flag day or the fire restrictions are in place, don't start a fire. Not even for a barbeque! Most of the large fires in the western United States in recent years, including Arizona, have been human caused.

Flagstaff and small neighboring communities are located on the Coconino Plateau. This plateau was pushed upward by subterranean forces, creating the rift known as Mogollon Rim. The Rim is also a demarcation between the woodlands distinguished by pinon and juniper and the ponderosa pine found around 7,000 feet in elevation. This region sees snow and freezing temperatures each year. At one time skiing and snowshoeing

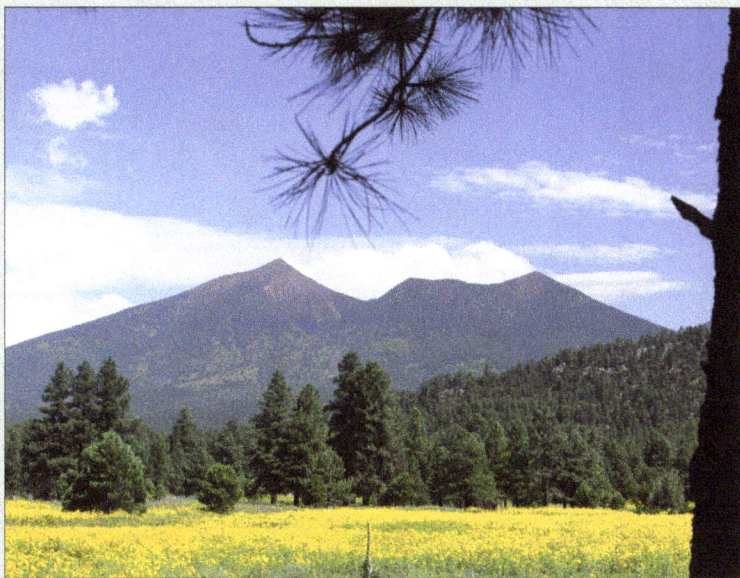

Flagstaff & the San Francisco Peaks

were the predominant outdoor activities durng the winter. Now, it is possible to hike almost 10 months of the year.

The forest around Flagstaff is the home of large herds of elk and deer and other mountain wildlife. This ponderosa forest is a dry zone with small man-made ponds providing water to wildlife. Perennial streams are rare. As the population of Arizona grows, the high country has become a popular place to visit during the warmer months in southern regions. The mountain stretching across Arizona have seen huge, devastating fires in recent years. Please exercise every precaution when hiking and or camping.

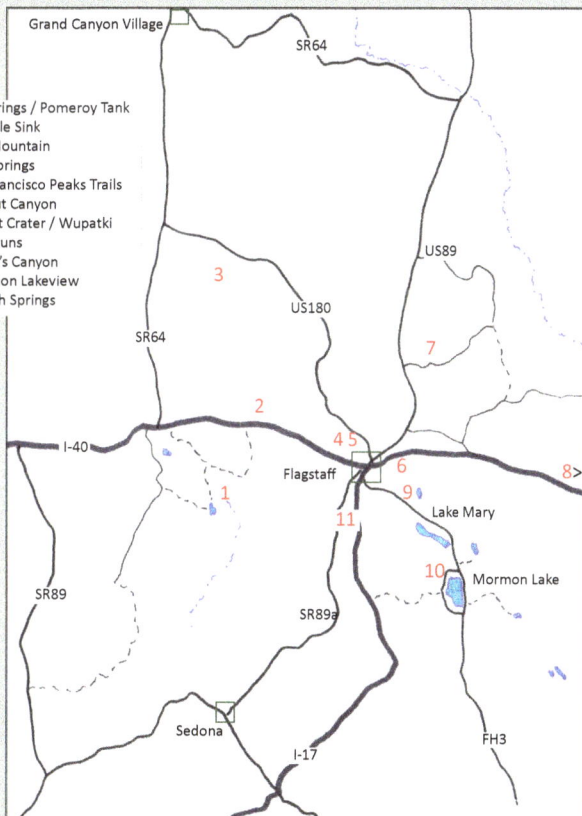

1 LO Springs / Pomeroy Tank
2 Keyhole Sink
3 Red Mountain
4 Veit Springs
5 San Francisco Peaks Trails
6 Walnut Canyon
7 Sunset Crater / Wupatki
8 Two Guns
9 Sandy's Canyon
10 Mormon Lakeview
11 Griffith Springs

Sycamore Canyon Rim

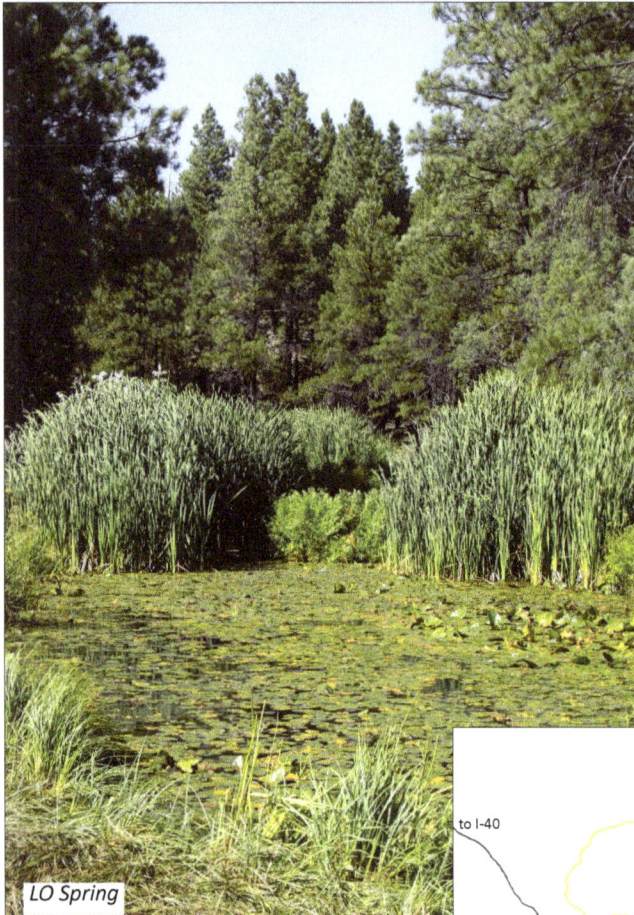

LO Spring

LO Springs is a historic site dating back to the history of logging in Arizona.

To reach the Dow Springs trailhead, exit I-40 at mp178 and turn south onto the Garland Prairie Road/FR141. Drive 9.5 miles to FR131 and turn left. In .4 of a mile, the trailhead is on the right.

The trail parallells an old railroad bed before turning to drop over the edge of Volunteer Canyon to Dow Springs. This spring usually has water flowing March through May.

Below the rim, the trail follows the drainage to the left toward LO Springs. The first pond usually has water year round with lilly pads in the warmer months. Beyond the pool, the trail descends to a second pool before returning along the trail to the parking area.

Driving Distance: 28-35 miles depending on freeway exit taken.
Hiking Distance: 1.5 miles
Rating: Easy
Elevation: 6726' - 6700'
Best Season: Spring & fall
Special Features: Site of old mining camp, natural springs.
Maps: NFS Kaibab / Challender District
Infomation: Kaibab Chalender District Ofc. (928) 635-8200

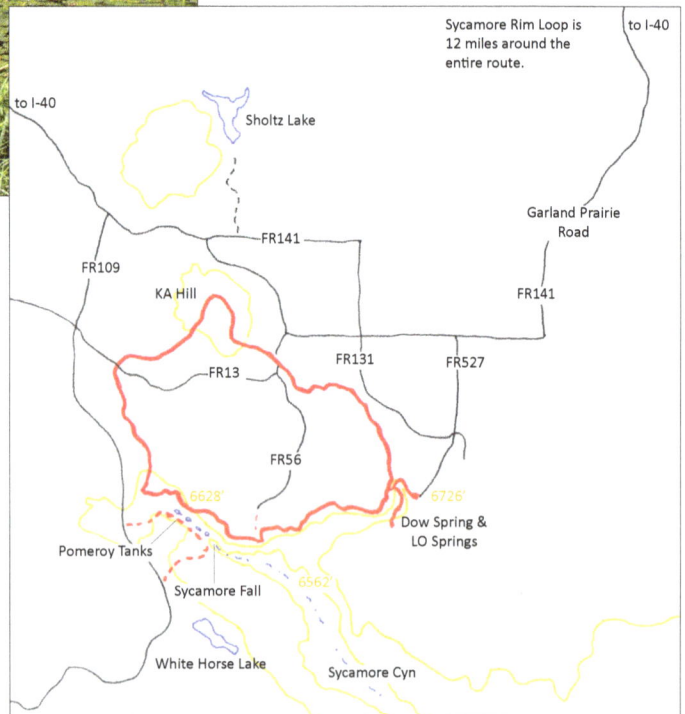

Sycamore Rim Loop is 12 miles around the entire route.

to I-40

to I-40

Sholtz Lake

FR141

Garland Prairie Road

FR109

FR141

KA Hill

FR13

FR131

FR527

FR56

6628'

6726'

Dow Spring & LO Springs

Pomeroy Tanks

Sycamore Fall

6562'

White Horse Lake

Sycamore Cyn

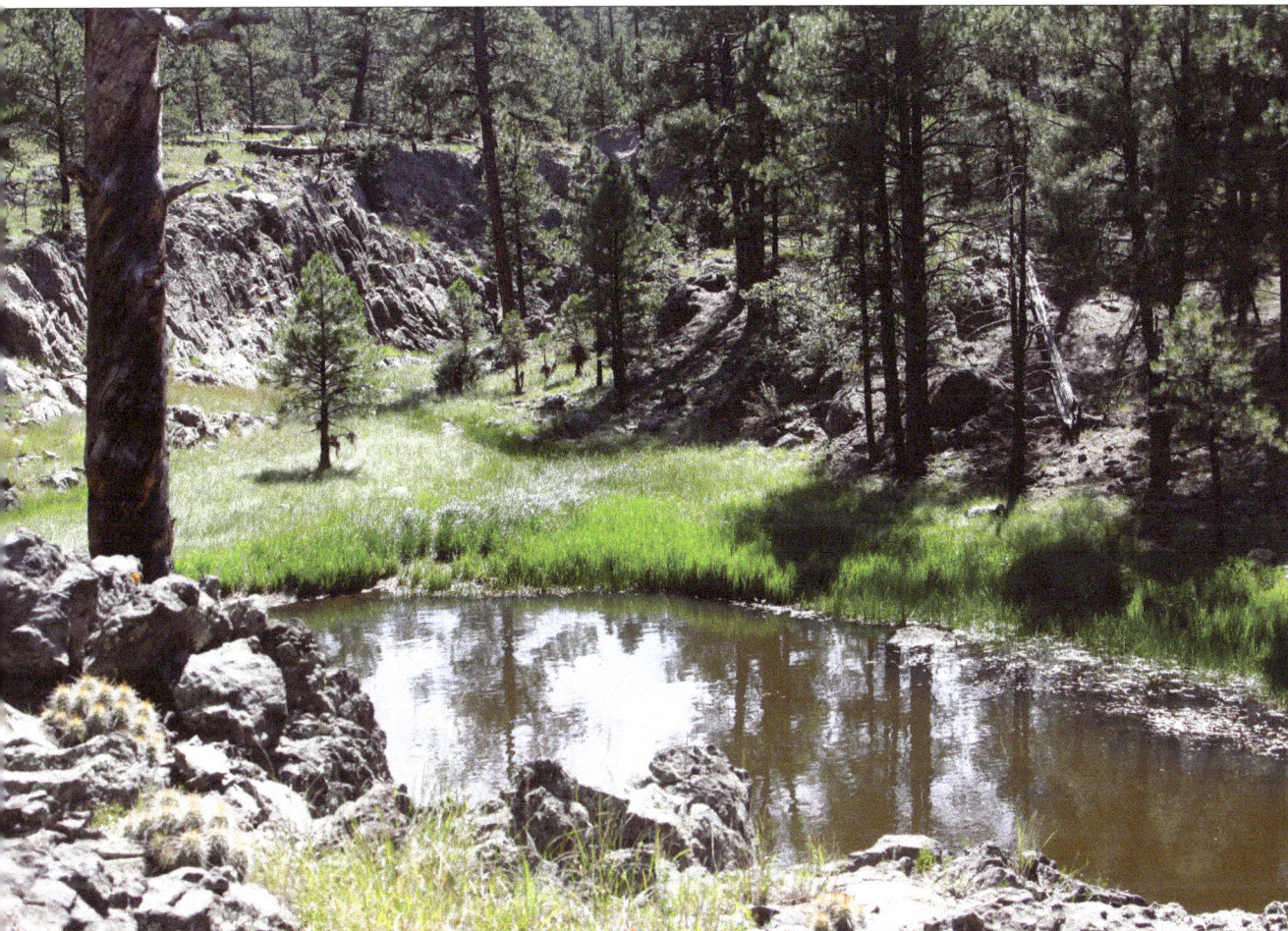

One of the Pomoroy Tanks

Pomeroy Tanks is a series of ponds set along a fault line in a shallow canyon just north of White Horse Lake. Turn south off I-40 at exit 171. Follow FR141 to the junction with FR109, turn right. Two miles further, there should be a trailhead sign on the left side of the road, park and begin walking east cross-country toward a small drainage. The ponds are spread over a half mile with the lowest of the ponds a short ways above Sycamore Falls. The waterfall only flows during the spring and the corduroy rock cliffs are a popular climbing area. It is helpful to mark this location on your map app on your cell phone before leaving home. This will help you know when you are getting close to the trailhead.

Driving Distance: 16 miles from Williams, 33 miles from Flagstaff.
Hiking Distance: 1.5 miles
Rating: Easy
Elevation: 6750' - 6725'
Best Season: Spring & fall
Special Features: Natural spring, seasonal waterfall.
Maps: NFS Kaibab / Challender District
Infomation: Kaibab Chalender District Ofc. (928) 635-8200

Keyhole Sink

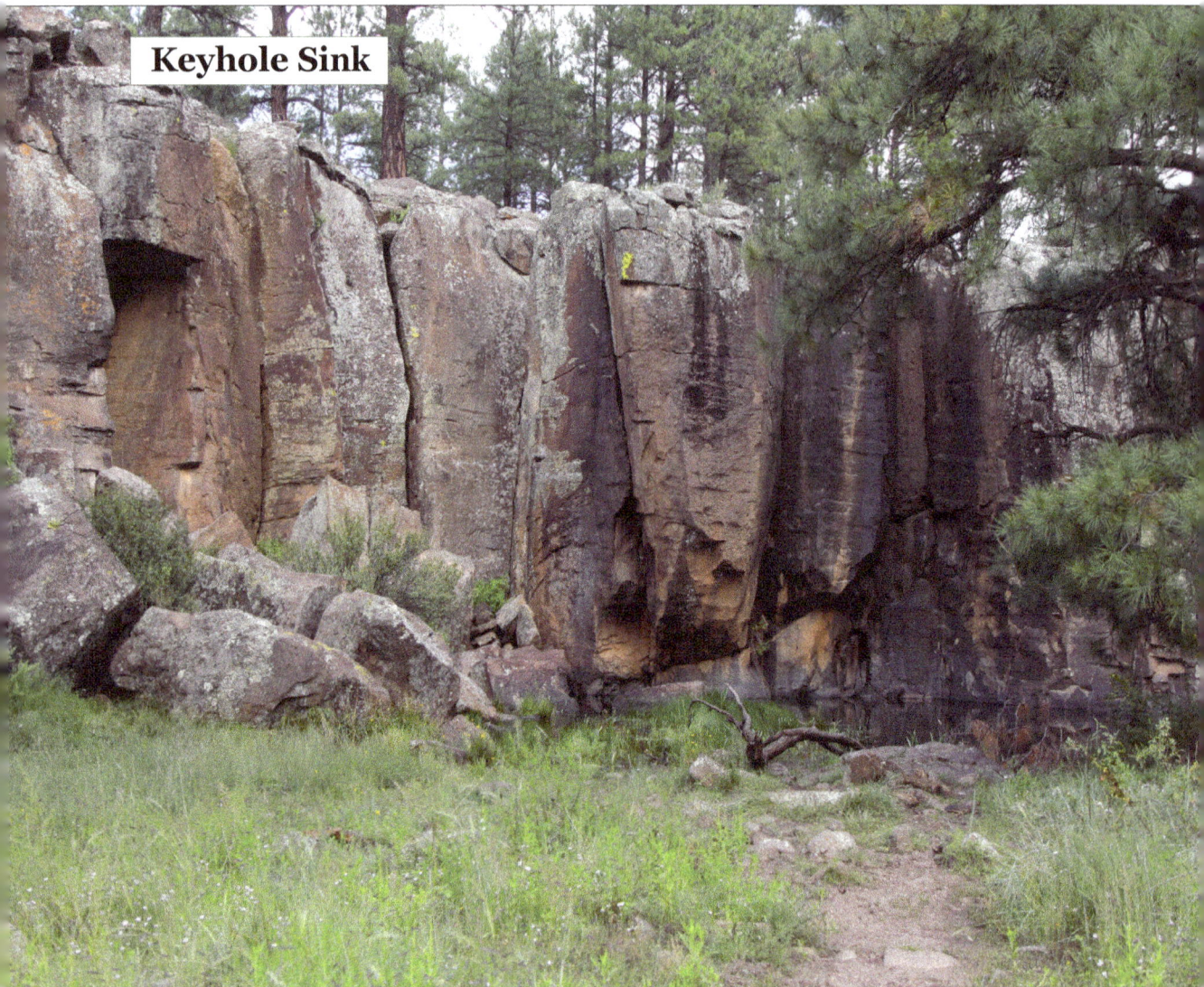

Within Keyhole Sink, a small pond forms at the foot of rhyolite cliffs from both snow melt and summer rains. This hike is best in the spring before the mosquitos hatch.

Set in a grove of quaking aspen, **Keyhole Sink** is a quiet niche with a seasonal pool of water and tall rhyolite cliffs with prehistoric art. It is a place for hikers to retreat from busy schedules to sit quietly and soak up warm sunshine. Visitors may search for two panels of petroglyphs etched on the cliffs by early Americans.

The cliff are part of a ridge that encircles the north and east sides of the sink. In the spring, water pours over the cliff from a small tank unseen by visitors below the cliffs. Please be respectful of the sink as it is an important source of water to the wildlife. Please do not deface the panels of rock art - this has become more of a problem in the last few years.

Many families find this a great place to spend the afternoon with a picnic lunch spread on the lush grass. Other hikers choose to explore the forest beyond the sink. We've found that springtime is usually the best season to visit as there is water in the pond and the mosquitos are still getting established. In late summer, you might carry mosquito repellant.

To visit, drive west from Flagstaff on I-40 to Parks Exit #178 and turn right. At .1 mile the road intersects old Highway 66. Turn left and drive through Parks. At 4.3 miles turn left and park at the Oak Hill Snow Play Area. Across the road, a trail sign designates the path to Keyhole Sink. The trail passes the site of a recent burn which has been thinned and harvested. Closer to the sink, the trail passes through mature ponderosa pines and around the point of the ridge, descending into a streambed. In about a mile, visitors pass through a rail fence that encloses the sink.

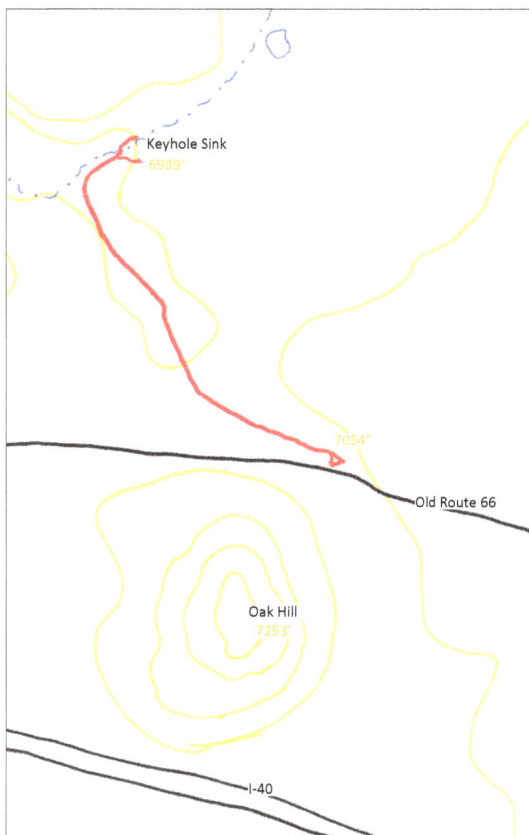

Driving Distance: 22 miles from Flagstaff
Hiking Distance: 1 mile one way
Rating: Easy
Elevation: 7000'
Best Season: Late spring, summer & fall.
Special Features: Petroglyphs, seasonal pool of water, beautiful meadow and aspen grove.
Precautions: Be considerate of others who may inhabit the same space at the same time.
Maps: Kaibab National Forest Map
Infomation: Chalender Ranger Station
(928) 635-8200

Red Mountain

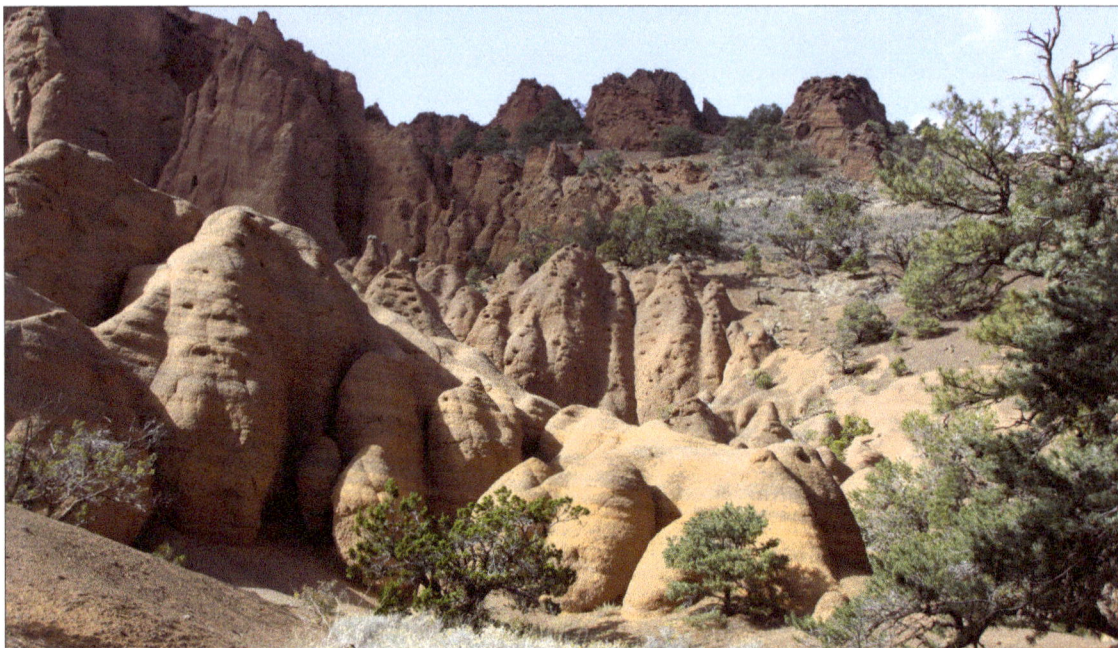

Hoodoos within Red Mountain

Surrounding Flagstaff are dormant cinder cones, most carpeted with wild grass and ponderosa pine. Imagine being able to walk into the center of one of these cones. How different would the mountain core be from the placid exterior? To travelers driving north on US 180, **Red Mountain** looks as if a giant knife has sliced into the mountain's interior, revealing a tumultuous past.

To reach Red Mountain, follow US 180 north from downtown Flagstaff. Approximately 32 miles from Flagstaff at mp 247, turn left onto FR 9032V and follow it .5 mile to a parking area for the Red Mountain Geological Area.

A clearly defined trail leads west through a forest of pinon pine and juniper toward Red Mountain. At .85 mile the trail drops into a wash, winding into the heart of the mountain. It is a good idea to mentally note where the trail enters the wash for the return trip.

As hikers approach Red Mountain, the sides of the wash begin to rise. At one point black rock formations jut from the wash walls, contrasting with the light brown and red interior.

After hiking 1.4 miles, hikers reach a dam across the wash. In the years since construction, silt washed from the hillside filled the dam. Note that a pipe extends from the base, allowing water to escape after infilterating the cindered fill.

A ladder allows hikers to climb to the top of the dam and proceed into the heart of Red Mountain. The entrance through a gap in a black volcanic dike is a startling contrast to the red rock of the interior.

An alternate route is to climb the hillside to the right of the dam, sliding along the black cinders. Topping the rim, hikers descend a slope into the interior. The descent is a match for the most agile hiker. Some hikers simply sit and slide down the hill, risking a hole in the seat of their pants. Most visitors opt for the route over the dam.

Entering Red Mountain, there is an air of mystery surrounding the giant trees and rock hoodoos. Wind whispers through the pines and the rocky ridges reflect the warmth of the sun. Unlike the black cinders at the entrance, the rock in the interior is shades of buff to red as if witness to its fiery inception. The noise of the outside world is muffled as awed hikers explore the hidden niches among the rocky mounds.

Returning to the trail, it is almost as if visitors return from another land, another time.

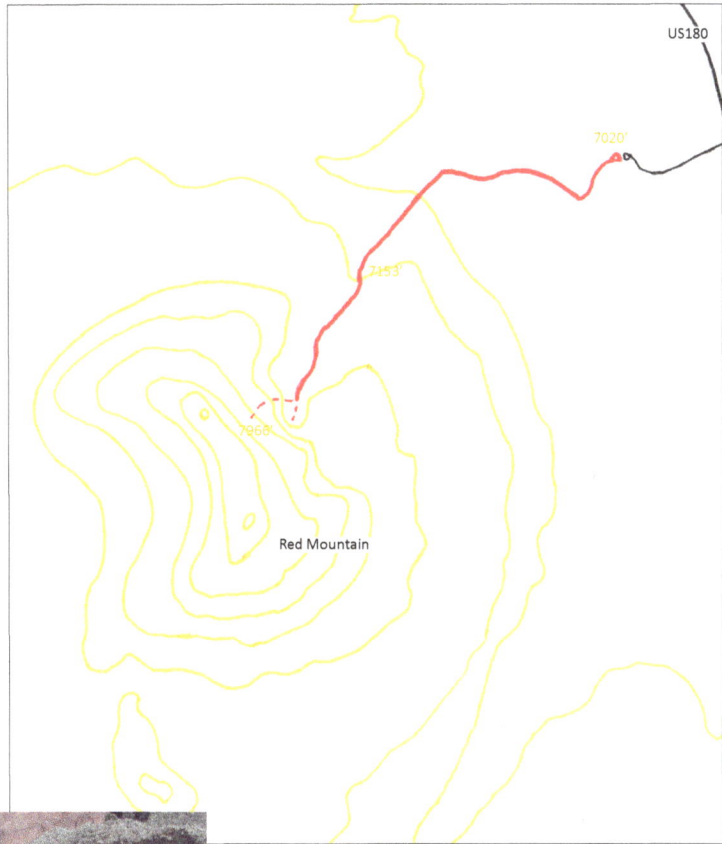

Driving Distance: 32 miles from Flagstaff
Hiking Distance: 1.4 miles one way
Rating: Moderately easy
Elevation: 6950' - 7200'
Best Season: Summer and Fall
Special Features: Hoodoos cut from the heart
   of the mountain by rain, ice and wind.
Precautions: Use caution descending
   cinders and in climbing through rock
   formations. Help is a long way off.
Maps: Coconino NFS map
Infomation: Peaks Ranger Station
   (928) 526-0866

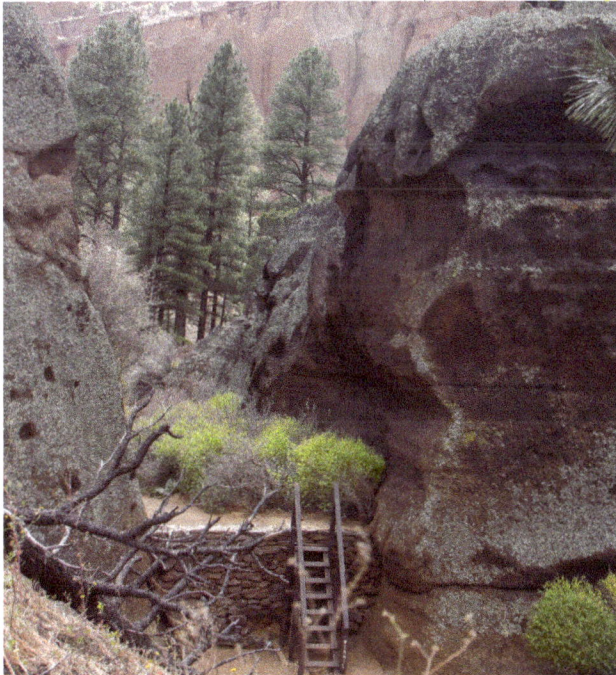

The entrance to Red Mountain

Veit Springs & the Lamar Haines Wildlife Refuge

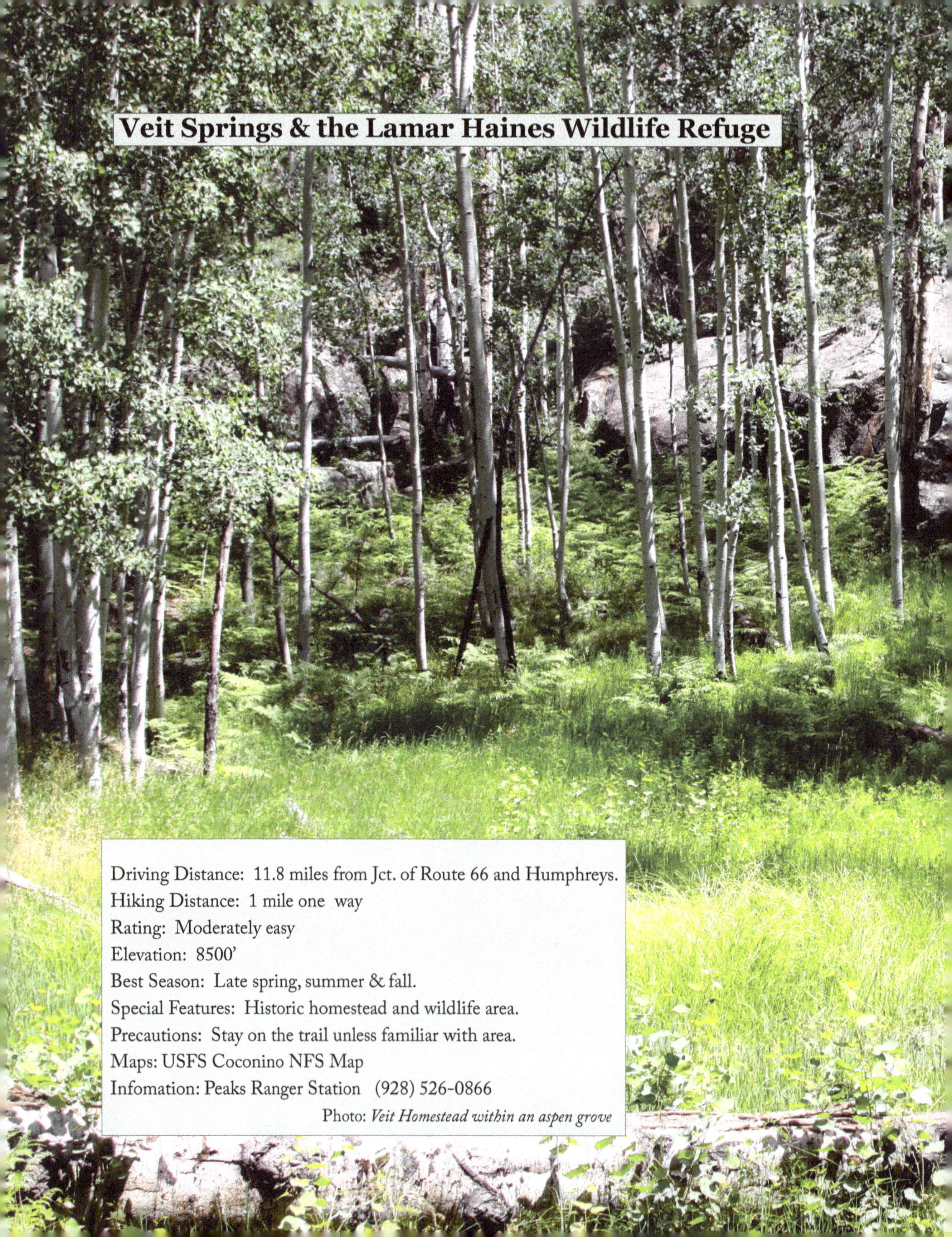

Driving Distance: 11.8 miles from Jct. of Route 66 and Humphreys.

Hiking Distance: 1 mile one way

Rating: Moderately easy

Elevation: 8500'

Best Season: Late spring, summer & fall.

Special Features: Historic homestead and wildlife area.

Precautions: Stay on the trail unless familiar with area.

Maps: USFS Coconino NFS Map

Infomation: Peaks Ranger Station   (928) 526-0866

Photo: *Veit Homestead within an aspen grove*

At one time homesteads dotted the northwest side of the San Francisco Peaks. In 1892, Ludvig Veit built a cabin and spring-house to capture water flowing from a fracture in a rock wall. He was not the first to appreciate this source of water on the San Francisco Peaks. Petroglyphs on the cliff above indicate early native Americans valued this spring too.

Drive north on Humphreys from the junction with Route 66 in downtown Flagstaff, turning left onto Columbus/US 180. Just over seven miles from Route 66, take a right onto the Snowbowl Road which ascends the peak to the Arizona Snowbowl Ski Resort. Turn right into a small parking area 4.5 miles from US 180.

A sign proclaims this is the **Lamar Haines Memorial Wildlife Area**. Just beyond the gate, turn right along a footpath to follow the fence line. The trail drops into a small valley, passing through a meadow and thick groves of aspen and spruce. This area is especially popular when the aspen leaves begin to turn a brilliant yellow in the fall. The trail winds past a small tank and then briefly follows the fence line again. Upon reaching a second gate, the trail turns left toward the **Veit Homestead**.

Approaching the ridge, a path leads up to two small spring houses built of native rock. The cabin has been removed and the USFS has carved two tanks to catch water for wildlife during dry spells. Following the base of the basalt ridge to the left, the water flows from a narrow passage in the cliff. Take a moment to examine the pictographs on the rock cliff above the spring and to enjoy the beauty of this isolated home site.

Some hikers are more comfortable in returning the way they came. Others cross the meadow below the ridge to follow the electric lines to a trail that rejoins the passage below the entrance.

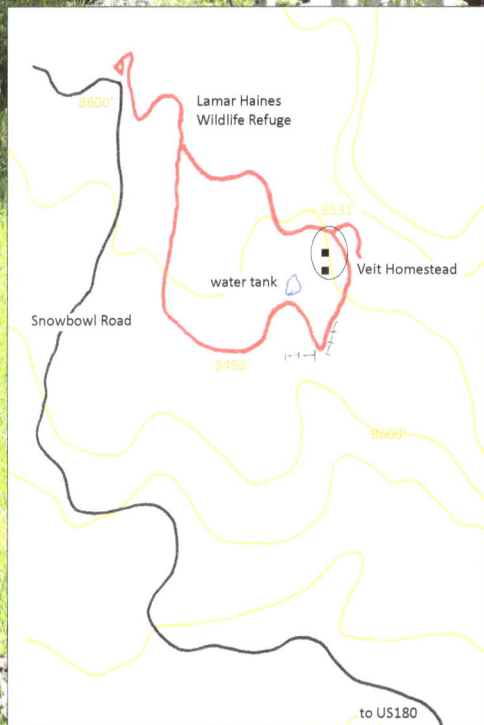

Lamar Haines Wildlife Refuge

water tank

Veit Homestead

Snowbowl Road

8600'

9531'

8498'

8600'

to US180

San Francisco Peaks and the Kachina Peak Wilderness

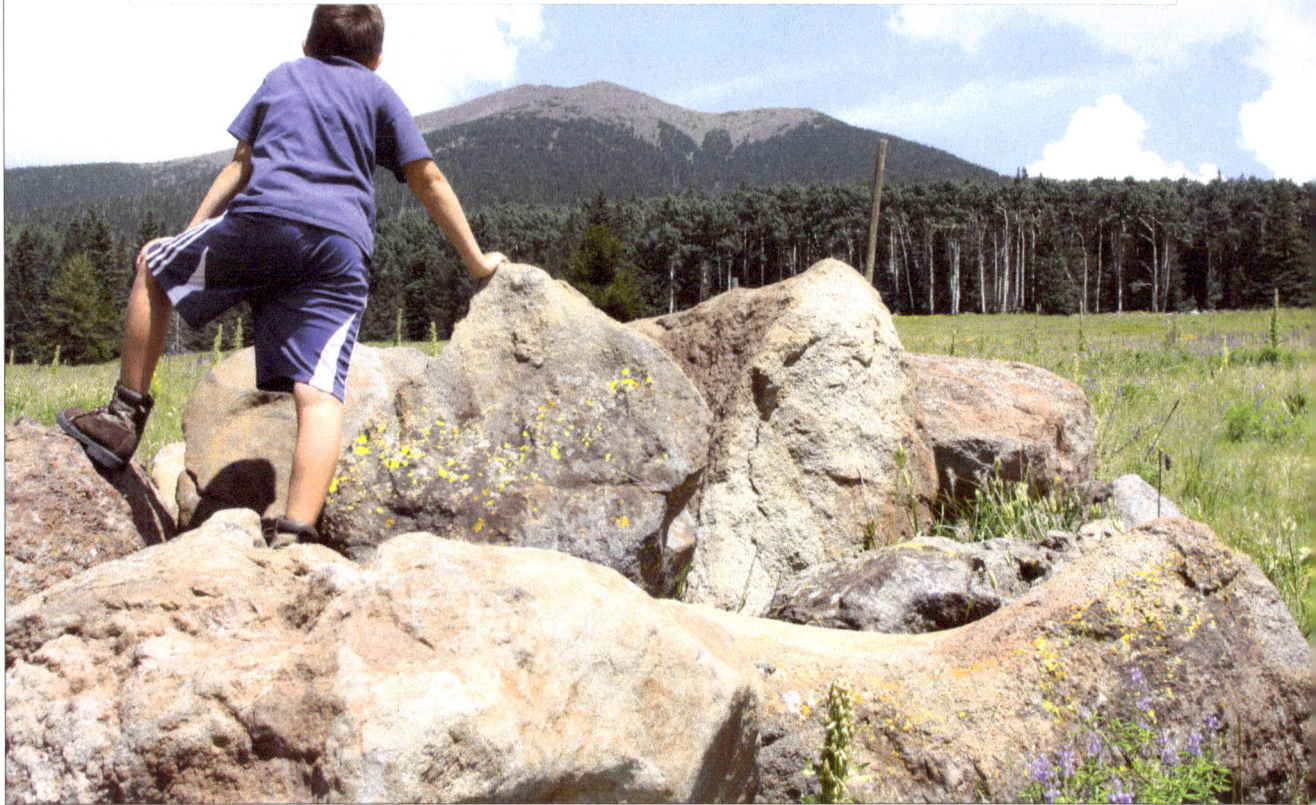

The San Francisco Peaks dominate the Coconino Plateau. Several popular trails take hikers across the peak. **Humphreys Peak** trail starts at the Arizona Snowbowl and allows hikers to reach the summit. **The Inner Basin** trail allows hikers to explore the ancient crater created when the volcano lost tons of rock during a series of eruptions.

The **Shultz Pass/Weatherford** trail ascends the eastern side of the mountain, passing three of the four peaks before intersecting the Humphreys peak trail a half mile below the summit.

I have a love-hate relationship with the **Abineau-Bear Jaw loop** on the northwest side of the peaks. The steep ascent along Aubineau is a breath stealer but the trail leads to the site of an old avalanche with huge ponderosa tossed horizontally like toothpicks. The site helps us understand the tremendous power that a snowslide can exert as it picks up speed moving down the steep slope.

The **Kachina trail** drops from the Arizona Snowbowl, passing below Fremont Peak to the Weatherford trailhead on FR522.

Two shorter trails are popular with day hikers futher down the slopes from the summit. The **Veit Homestead** trail is a loop off the Snowbowl Road.

Bismark Lake is a short hike to a small reservoir off the poular Hart Prairie Road that funnels visitors along the base of the Peaks.

During the fall months, many visitors find dirt tracks leading into the aspen groves at the 8,000 foot level, losing themselves in a shower of golden leaves.

Humphreys Peak

Driving Distance: 14.5 miles from
        Flagstaff
Hiking Distance: 5.4 miles one way
Rating: Difficult, at elevation
Elevation: 9238' - 12,633'

Inner Basin

Driving Distance: 21 miles from
        Flagstaff
Hiking Distance: 5.4 miles one way
Rating: Difficult, at elevation
Elevation: 8,640' - 9,385'
Access off FR552 & SR89

Shultz Pass/ Weatherford

Driving Distance: 15 miles from Flagstaff
Hiking Distance: 10.7 miles one way to
        saddle below summit.
Rating: Difficult, at elevation
Elevation: 11,000' - 12,633'
Access off US180 to Shultz Pass Road

Kachina Trail

Driving, north end: 14.5 miles
Hiking Distance: 5 miles one way
Rating: Moderate, at elevation
Elevation: 9,250 ' - 8,795'
Access at Arizona SnowBowl, east parking lot

Aubineau-Bear Jaw Loop

Driving Distance: 20 miles from Flagstaff
Hiking Distance: 5.4 miles one way
Rating: Difficult
Elevation: 9238' - 12,633'
Access: FR151 & FR418

Bismarck Lake

Driving Distance: About 15 miles
        Flagstaff
Hiking Distance: 5.4 miles one way
Rating: Difficult
Elevation: 8,600' - 8,790'
Access off FR151

See Veit Homestead on previous page

Photo: Hart Prairie, looking up at the summit of the San Francisco Peaks

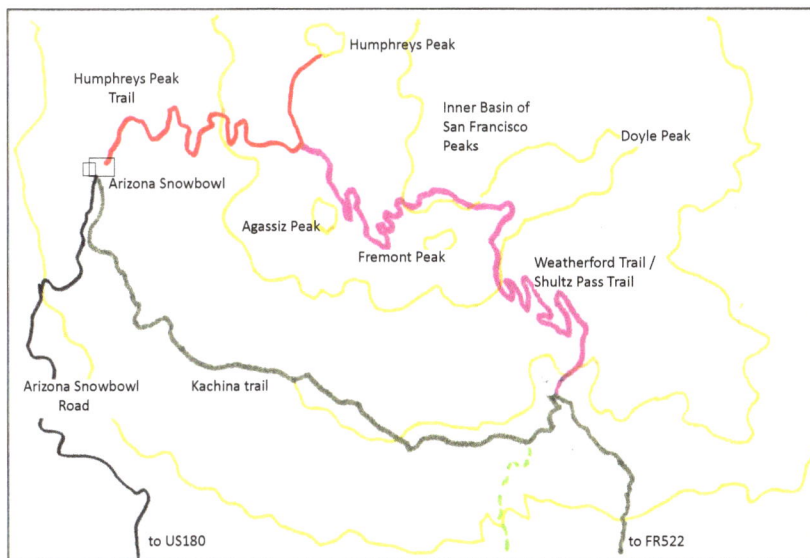

*The **Lava River Cave** has long been popular. The cave was created when the exterior of a lava flow cooled even as the interior kept moving. Unfortunately, the site is being overwhelmed with visitors. On a recent visit, visitors were carrying dogs, their paws unsuited to the sharp rocks inside. There are reports of people urinating within the cave. I can no longer recommend this site until the Forest Service institutes better management practices.*

Walnut Canyon

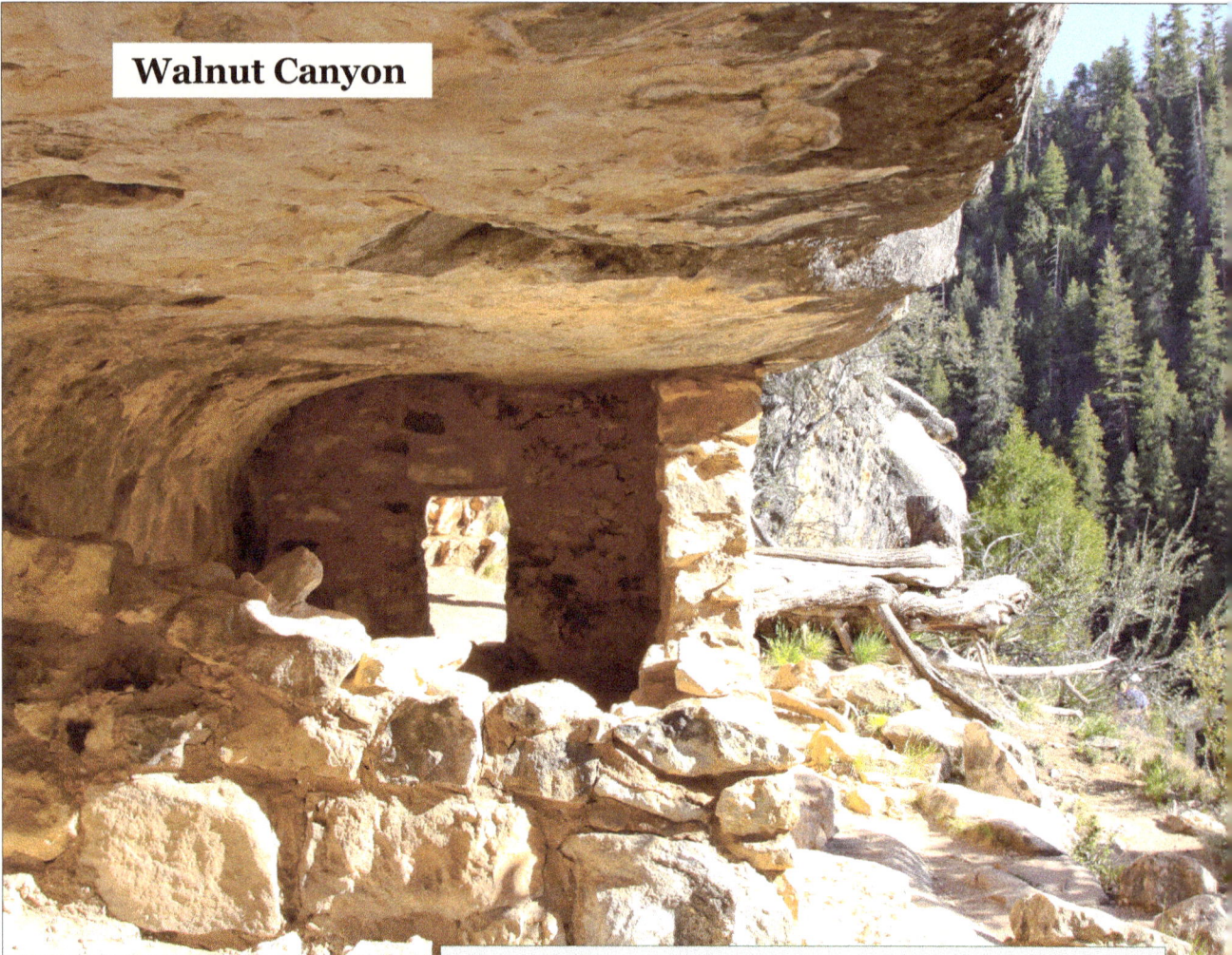

Imagine living in a cave dwelling on an island of rock high above a canyon floor. For kids it is the stuff adventures are made of; for parents a nightmare as their young children learn to walk. This is the home of the ancient Sinagua in Walnut Canyon National Monument.

Photos: Ruin within Walnut Canyon

Driving Distance: 15 miles from downtown Flagstaff

Hiking Distance: Rim trail, .4 mile / Island trail, .8 mile

Rating: Rim trail - easy / Island trail - moderate

Elevation: 6700' - 6400'

Best Season: Summer & fall.

Special Features: Well preserved native American ruins along unique peninsula jutting into a pristine canyon.

Precautions: Spring weather may leave ice on trail. Due to steep climb, those with a heart condition or oxygen deprivation should probably not take this trail.

Maps: Arizona Highways map.

Infomation: Walnut Canyon National Monument   928-526-3367

The Walnut Canyon National Monument is located off I-40 at exit 204. Drivers turn south and drive three miles to the Visitors Center, perched on the canyon rim. The rim trail follows the canyon's rim with signs describing the plants and animals of the area and their use by Native Americans.

The island trail descends from the Visitors Center, dropping 185 feet into the canyon along 230 steps. Scientists believe that centuries earlier this area was covered by water with layers of lime and shells deposited on the bottom of an ancient sea. Once the sea receded, water seeped through joints in the rock cap, dissolving the limestone and forming ledges the native Americans would use for their homes. The trail follows these wide ledges around the peninsula high above the canyon floor. Here, the Sinagua had access to water, wild plants and game animals. Early residents were around five feet tall - shorter than most people today but they still had to stoop to enter the dwellings.

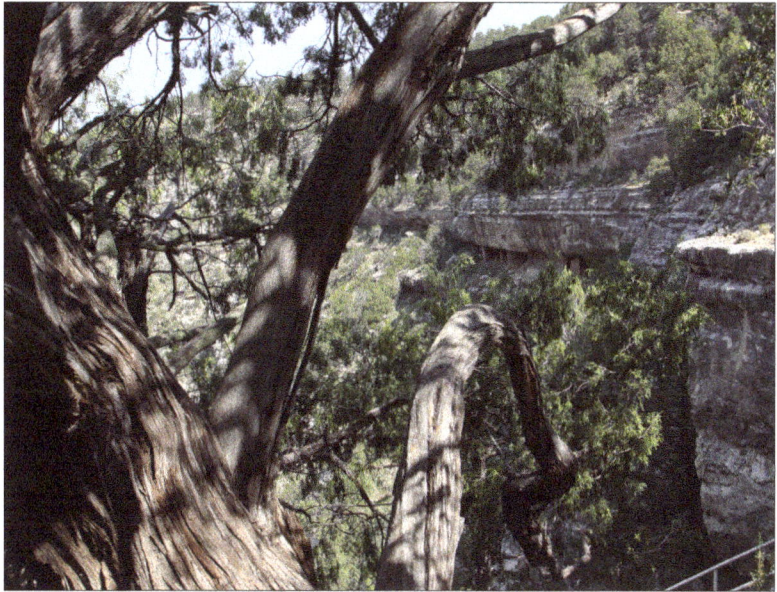

Most of the dwelling entrances are closed due to vandalism and the threat of hantavirus but a few remain open due to the disintegration of the original walls. Across the canyon, other ruins, give us a perspective for how high we stand above the canyon floor.

Small signs tell us what plants provided nourishment and materials for the residents. One of the most popular, the agave, provided both edible fruit and fiber for clothing and baskets.

From the far point of the peninsula, the trail swings back to the Visitors Center. There's a temptation to race up the steps. We suggest taking it easy. As with the story of the tortoise and the hare, slow steady progress wins the day.

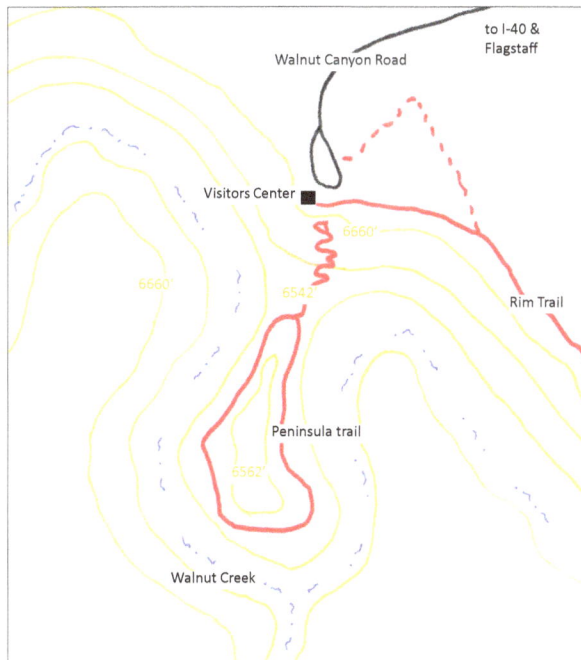

A thousand years ago a river of fiery rock crept across the landscape of what would become **Sunset Crater National Monument**. Over the centuries wind and rain have made little impression on the waves of black rock, leaving us a vivid picture of a lava flow. Dating the flow from the charred remains of pit houses, scientists know Sunset Crater erupted in late 1064 or early 1065 AD.

To visit Sunset Crater, drive north on US 89 from Flagstaff. Turn right at mp 430.3 toward Sunset Crater National Monument and drive 2 miles to the entrance fee booth. At the Visitors Center, educational displays and park rangers give visitors a good understanding of how volcanoes form and shape the landscape.

A short trail 3.5 miles beyond the Visitor's Center leads hikers through the lava flow. A guide booklet helps visitors identify plants and unique features. Good hiking boots support feet and ankles across the rocky surface.

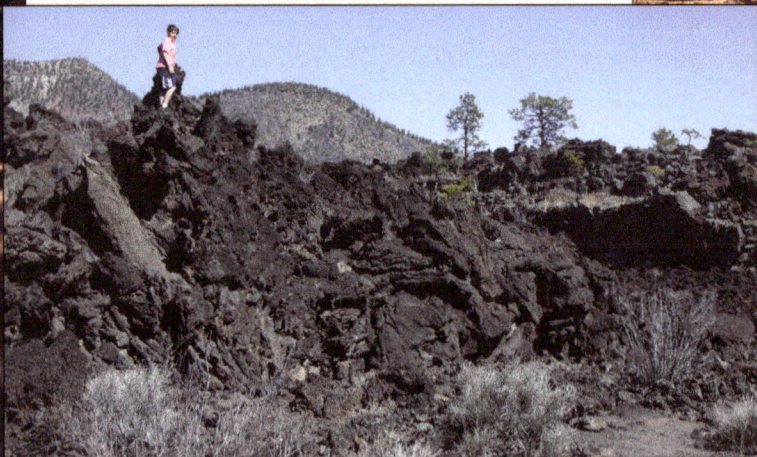

Sunset Crater National Monument

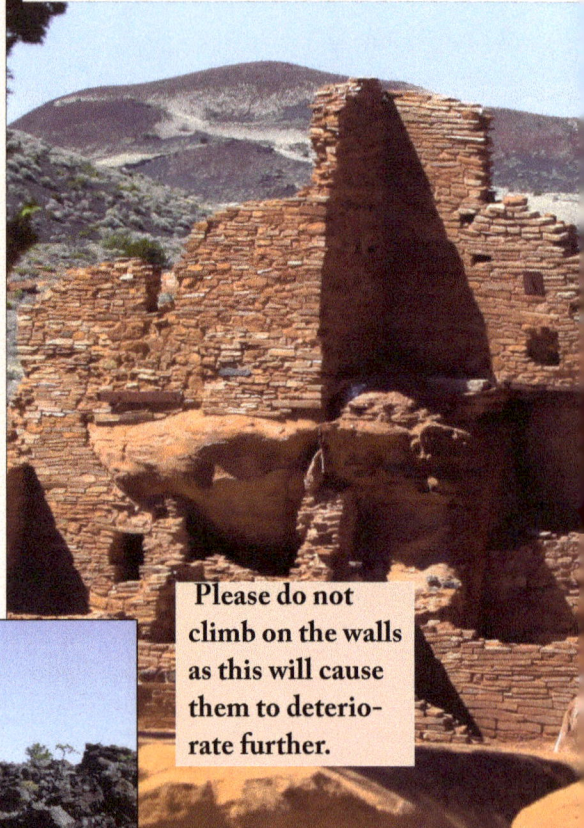

Please do not climb on the walls as this will cause them to deteriorate further.

At one time it was possible to climb Sunset Crater and walk among the pines growing inside the crater. In the 1970's the Forest Service closed the crater to the public due to severe erosion to the cone. Be aware that if driving off the paved main road, it is easy to become stuck in the cinders on side roads.

Driving: 22 miles from Flagstaff
Hiking Distance: 1 mile
Rating: Easy   Elevation: 7000'
Best Season: Spring, summer, fall.
Special Features: Stunning view of massive lava flow frozen in motion.
Precautions: Rough volcanic rock can be nasty in a fall so take it easy and watch your footing.
Maps: Arizona Highways map
Infomation: (928) 526-0502

Wupatki National Monument

The well-preserved pueblo at **Wupatki National Monument** gives us a look at how early native Americans lived on the Colorado Plateau. Pueblo residents could easily see visitors approaching and the pueblo was close to a natural spring. The pueblo has withstood the ravages of our cool climate through the centuries.

The trail from the Visitor's Center descends past the large pueblo to an ancient ball court and blow hole. Arenas like this are found throughout the southwest; the ball game pitted opponents from neighboring villages in a contest where the losers lost clothing and possessions. The object of the game was to hit the ball through a ring mounted sideways on a wall overlooking the court. Participants used all parts of their bodies, except possibly their hands. Spectators cheered the players on, making wagers of their own on the sidelines. Near the ball court is a blow hole. During the cooler hours it takes in air, releasing it during the warmer daylight hours.

To visit the Monument, follow US 89 north from Flagstaff. At mp 430.3, turn right onto FR 545. This road makes a loop through Sunset Crater and Wupatki National Monuments before returning to US 89. Both entrances charge a National Park fee.

Driving: Approx. 37 miles from Flagstaff
Rating: Easy   Elevation: 4900'
Hiking Distance: .4 mile loop
Best Season: Spring, summer or fall.
Special Features: Pueblo ruins & ball court; blowhole.
Maps: USFS Coconino NFS Map
Infomation: Wupatki Nat'l Monument
(928) 679-2365

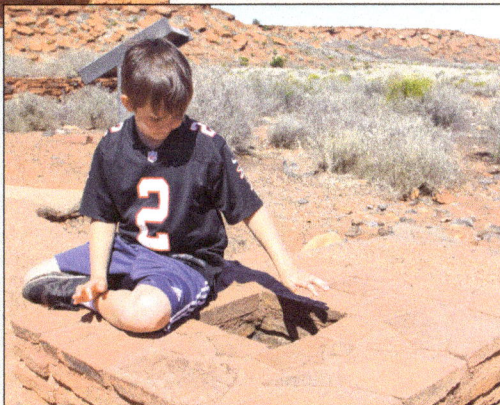

Two Guns Ruin

Canyon Diablo was once a major obstacle for western expansion. A small community was built on the rim of the canyon three times, before its demise as a travelers rest stop.

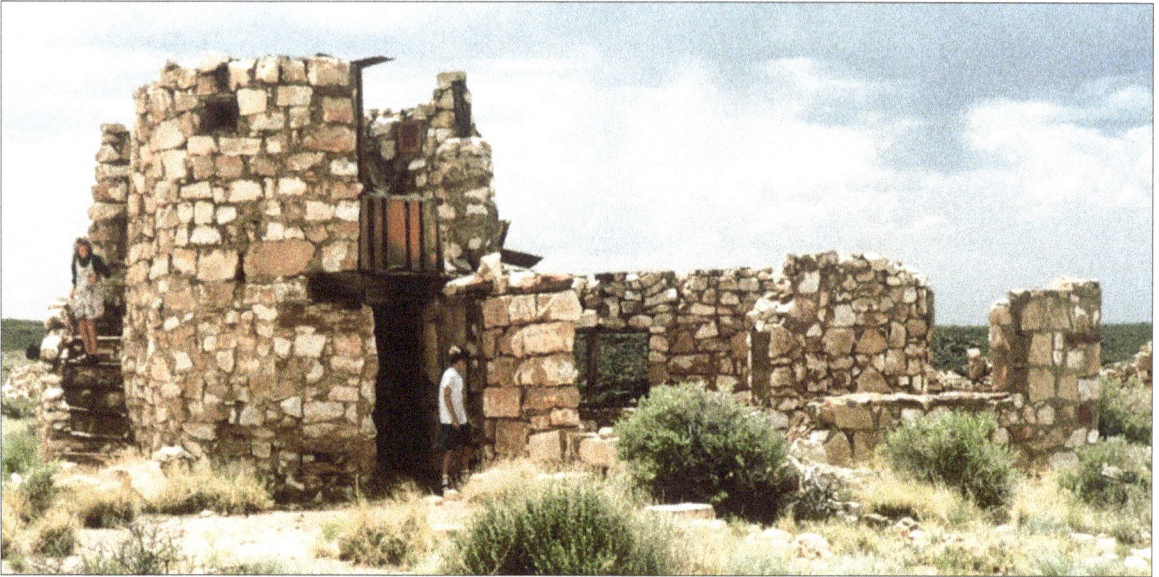

Located half way between Flagstaff and Winslow at exit 230 on Interstate 40, the ruins overlook Canyon Diablo. An old bridge spans the canyon as a link on the Old Trails Highway which was later renamed Route 66. Fire destroyed the first settlement on the southside of the canyon and it was re-built on the north side. The bridge between the two sites is now listed on the National Historic Registry.

The proprietors of the settlement on the north side offered travelers a taste of the west with a small zoo. Visitors can still see the faint lettering over the main entrance proclaiming the presence of mountain lions. Walking under the arch, visitors wander past small cages where the animals lived. By our standards today these cages seem inhumane but sightseers must have been enthralled to stand so close to the cougars of western fiction.

The ruins include a two-seat outhouse and a small observation tower - climb this only at your own risk. A narrow pathway leads down into the canyon and the rocky entrance to the legendary cave of Two Guns. The legend of this cave goes back to the 1700's when Navajo camps were repeatedly attacked by hostile Apaches. Recovering from the surprise attacks, Navajo warriors raced ahead to cut off the Apaches. However, after each attack the Apaches simply vanished. In their search, the Navajos were surprised to hear voices as they rode along the rim of Canyon Diablo. They discovered a large crack in the rim revealing a narrow passageway to a cave that was large enough to conceal the raiders and their horses.

The Navajos, after learning that the captives had been killed, exacted their revenge by sealing the entrances with brush and setting it on fire. The

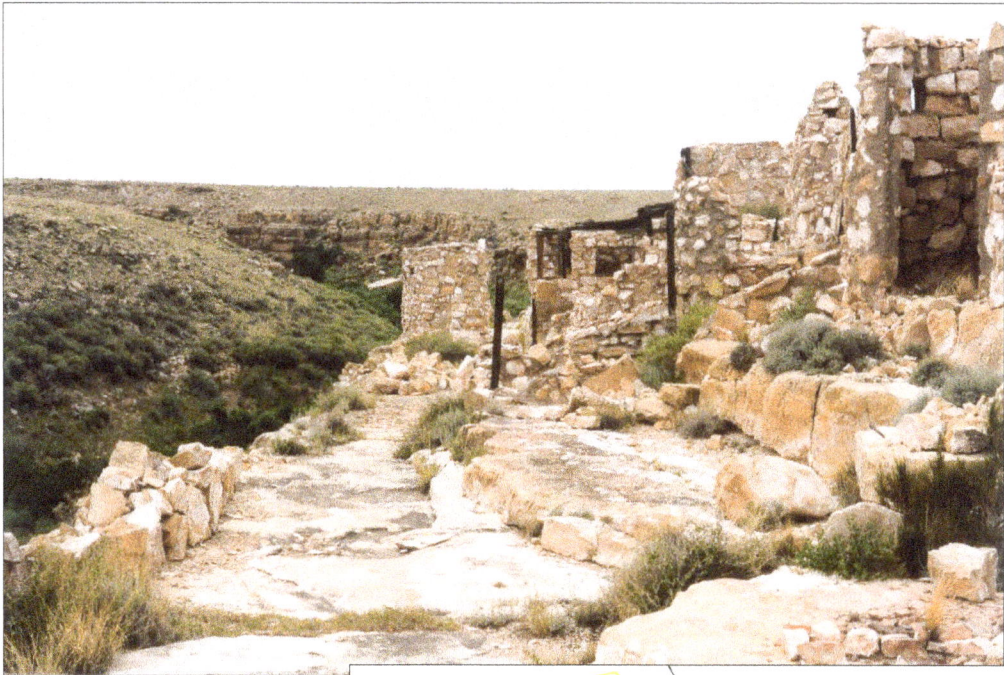

Photos: Two Guns Ruins

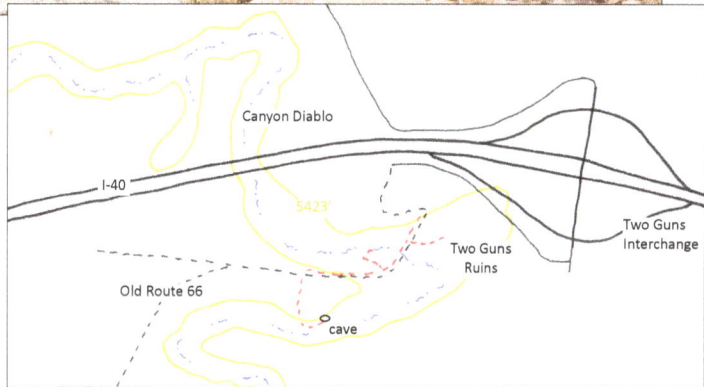

Apaches and their horses perished. When white settlers reached the area, they learned the story from the Navajos and came to believe that those who entered the cave were struck by a curse. The unfortunate deaths of two previous owners of Two Guns helped add validity to the story of the curse. Some believe that ill gotten gain from a robbery may be hidden in the cave as well.

Along with visiting the ruins, visitors may descend into Canyon Diablo to explore the narrow paths along the canyon bottom.

Hiking Distance: .25+ mile exploration

Driving Distance: 30 miles east of Flagstaff, 22 miles west of Winslow. Additional .5 mile into ruins from station.

Rating: Easy   Elevation: 5423'

Best Season: Spring, summer & fall. Winter visits are possible but visitors may encounter snow storms.

Special Features: Colorful western history, ruins to explore with hidden cave.

Precautions: The cave and ruins are frequented by rattlesnakes. If you see a snake, give it lots of room.

Maps: Arizona Highways map

Sandy's Canyon to Fisher Point

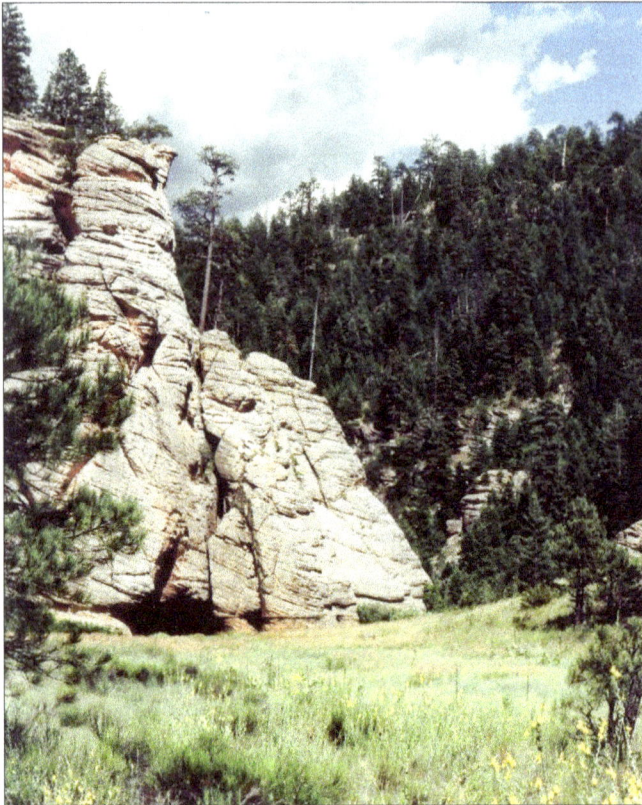

Hiking Distance: 3 miles one way
Driving Distance: 3.5 miles from
    Jct. US 89a and Lake Mary Road
Rating: Easy
Elevation: 6,726' - 6,690'
Best Season: Spring, summer & fall.
Special Features: Sandstone cliffs with
    small alcove. Beautiful canyon.

Cave hidden beneath the sandstone cliffs at Fisher Point.

Fisher Point is a popular destination, but for me the trail through Sandy's Canyon is the highlight of this hike. The canyon can be accessed from a trailhead 3.5 miles from US89A on the south edge of Flagstaff or by parking at a small campground just north of lower Lake Mary off Lake Mary Road. The trail is located between these two trailheads with the trail dropping into Sandy's Canyon about half way between the trailheads.

Watch your step descending into the canyon as the trail is not well maintained. Upon reaching the canyon bottom, the trail follows the streambed for Walnut Creek. The upper end of the canyon is the spillway for lower Lake Mary but in recent years with the drought, the streambed is usually dry.

For the first mile, the trail passes through groves of aspen, oak and pine before becoming more exposed to the open sky. Hikers can see the sandstone cliffs of Walnut Canyon well in the distance and at the base of the cliffs a low alcove is the signature of Fisher Point. On the ridge overhead, a second trail allows hikers to peer into the valley below.

From the Fisher Point, those turning right into Walnut Canyon will pass a second cave before reaching a fence. This is the boundary of the National Monument - No Trespassing.

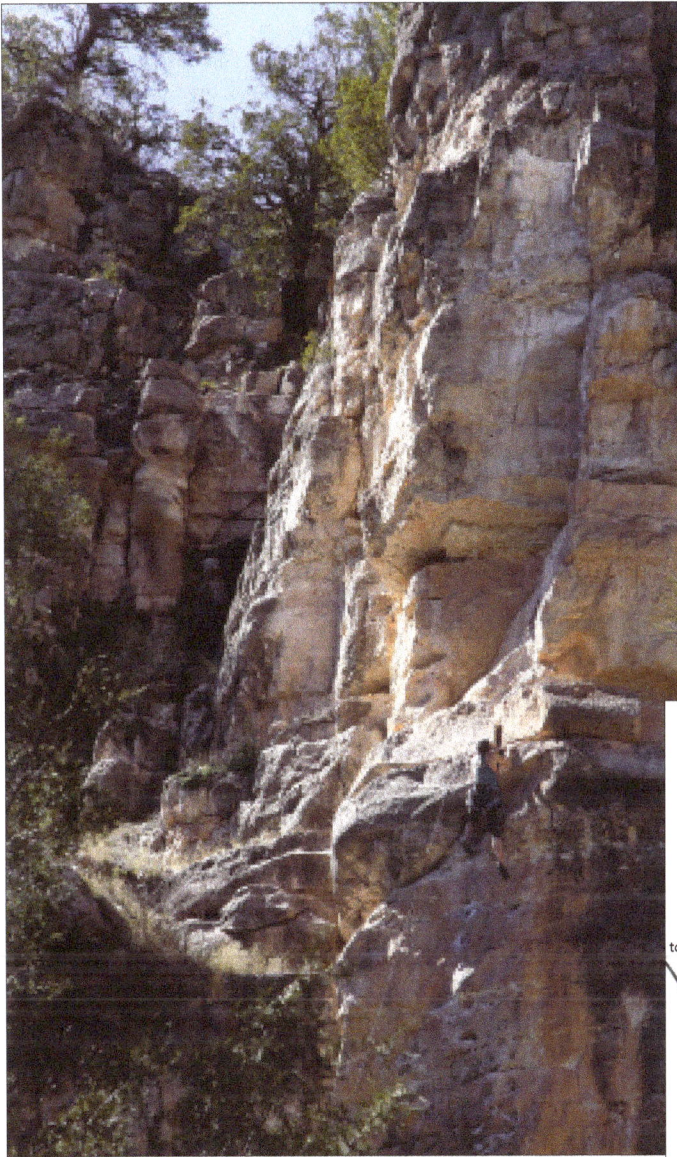

The Pit is accessed from a trailhead just beyond the little campground north of the Lake Mary Market and lower Lake Mary. At a trail junction east of the campground, turn to the right and descend into the canyon. The trail to the left follows the rim toward Sandy's Canyon and a second trailhead. Some hikers choose to explore the canyon floor while others watch the climbers make their way up the sandstone cliffs. Do not attempt to climb the cliffs without proper equipment and training. If you choose to watch, please observe quietly without disturbing the climbers.

A climber choosing his route up the sandstone cliffs of the Pit.

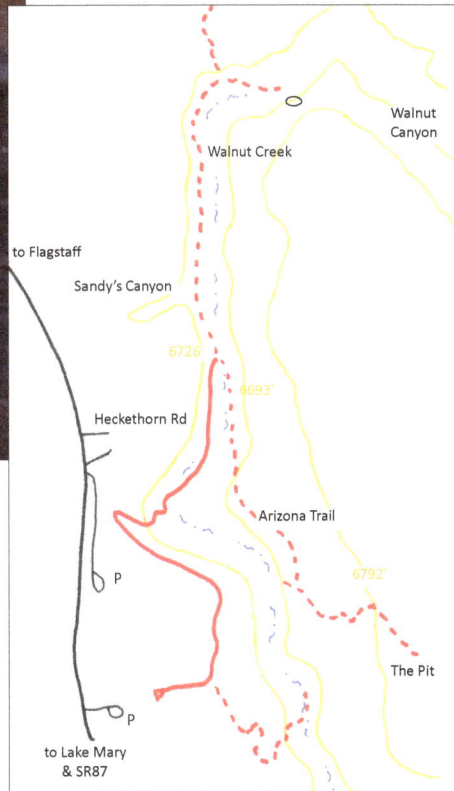

Walnut Canyon

Walnut Creek

to Flagstaff

Sandy's Canyon

6726'

6693'

Heckethorn Rd

Arizona Trail

6792'

P

The Pit

P

to Lake Mary & SR87

Griffith Spring

The Griffith Spring canyon offers a lovely trail just off US89A south of Flagstaff. From the junction of I-17 and I-40, drive about 5 miles south on US89A. Just past the MCS Stables, look for the signed trailhead on the east side of the road.

From the parking lot, hikers follow the trail as it switchbacks into the canyon to a trail junction. Turn to the left and the path leads to Griffith Spring, the output of a small perched aquifer.

Turn right and the trail divides with the upper route following the rim of the canyon. The route into the canyon follows the streambed just over half a mile to a large culvert - kind of a disappointing end but good for bouncing echoes through the pipe.

In the spring, a stream flows through the small pools along the drainage with multiple stream crossings. Along the path is a second spring, evident from the reeds that grow at the base of the ridge. At times, wildlife are drawn into the canyon to quench their thirst - hike quietly to have any opportunity of seeing a deer or other small creatures.

Climbers have begun climbing a rocky cliff about half way down the canyon. Do not attempt this without proper equipment and training.

Water flowing from Griffith Spring

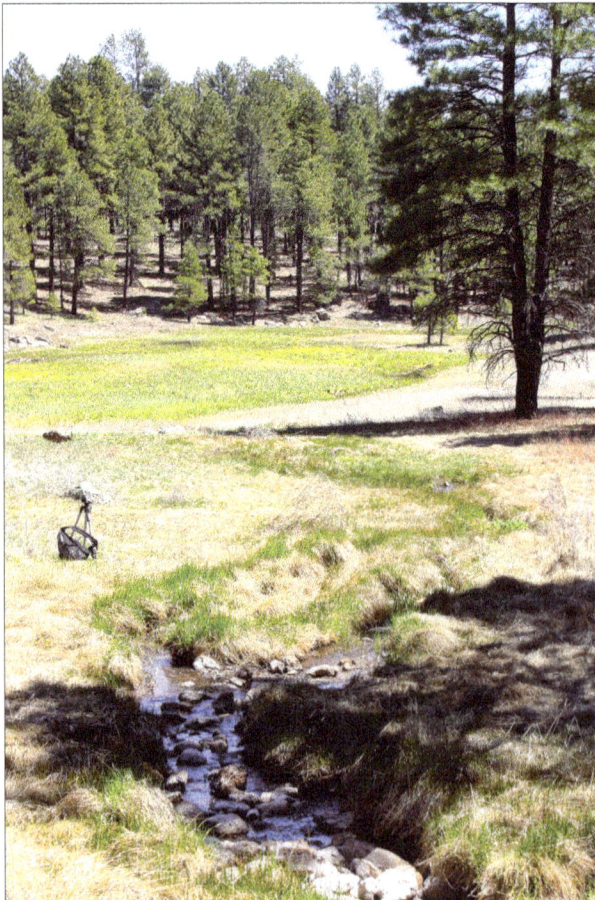

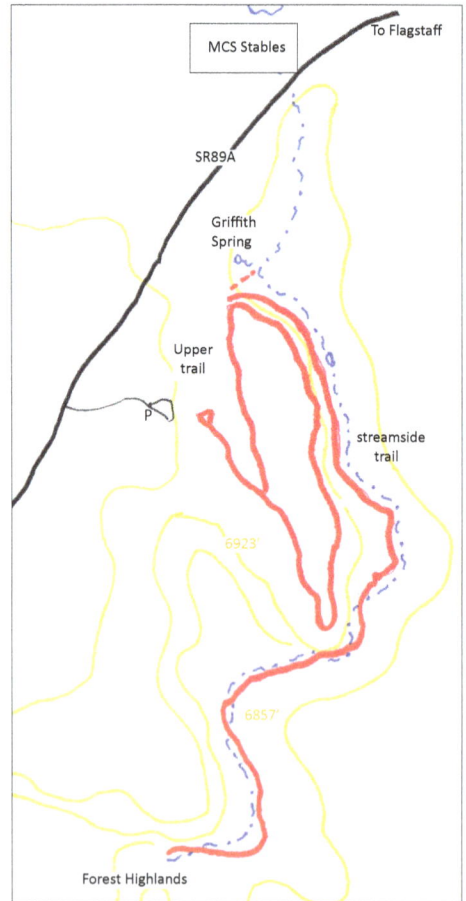

Mormon Lakeview Trail

Three trails enter the forest at the Mormon Lake campgrounds. Double Springs campground has the trailhead for the **Lakeview trail.** This trail is an easier ascent than the one named for the mountion. It is named for the ledges that jut out from the hillside overlooking the lake. The views are crowded with ponderosa but hikers still get a glimpse of the lake below.

The trail seems to end at Windsor Tank though hikers could explore further along dirt roads. I much prefer this trail over the Mountain Mountain trail for the view and the less demanding ascent.

Distance: 1.2 miles one way to Windsor Tank

The **Ledges trail** also begins at Double Springs and follows a route north, crossing the

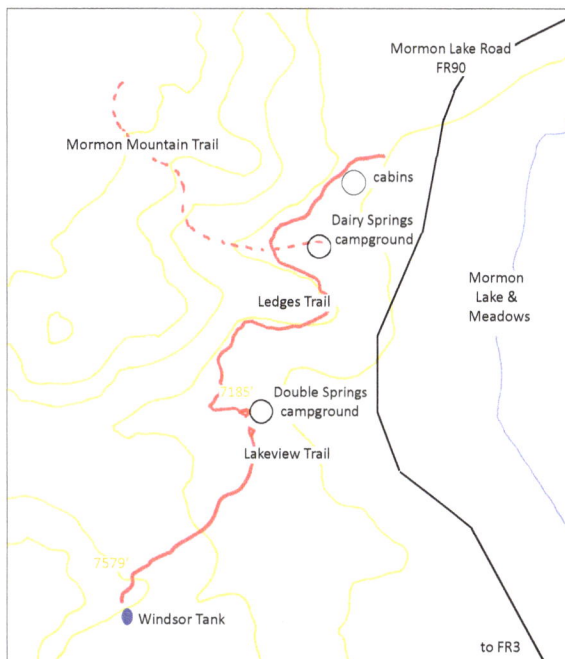

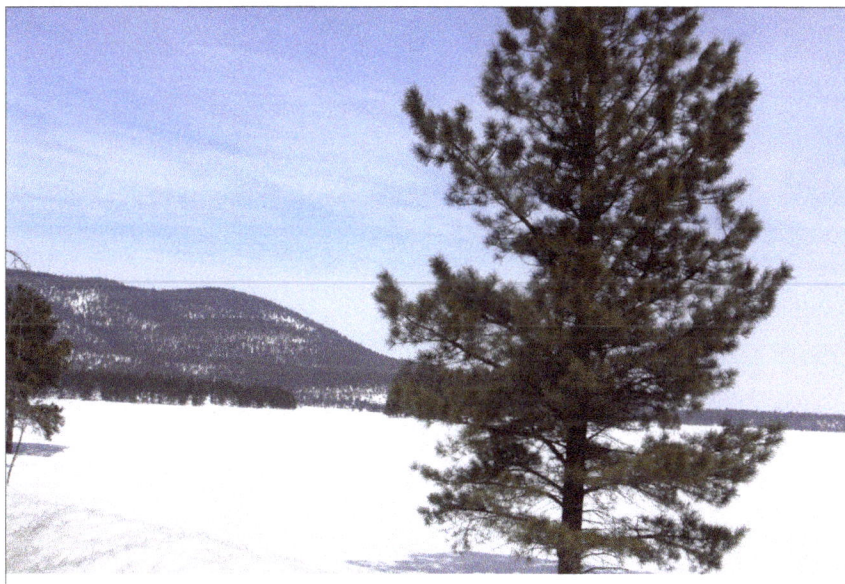

Looking across Mormon Lake to Mormon Mountain. When snow buries hiking trails in the northland, hikers pull out the snowshoes and challenge the snow drifts along familiar routes.

Mormon Mountain trail before emerging on a rock ledge overlooking the lake. This is the least demanding of the three as there is little change in elevation. Distance: 1 mile one way

Mormon Mountain trail, the most demanding of the three, begins at Dairy Springs campground. The trail begins to climb steeply and never quite lets up. There are no viewa cross the basin below. I've yet to find a satisfactory end to this trail, it just peters out into brush and ponderosa pine.

Distance: 2.5 miles one way to last meadow.

Oak Creek Canyon

to Flagstaff

Pine Flat campground

Cave Spring campground

Bootlegger Day-use Site

Banjo Bill Day-use Site

Halfway Day-use Site

*Red Rock Pass
required for parking*

Slide Rock State Park

Encinosa campground

Indian Gardens

Wilson Mountain

Grasshopper Point
Day Use Area

Bridge

to Sedona

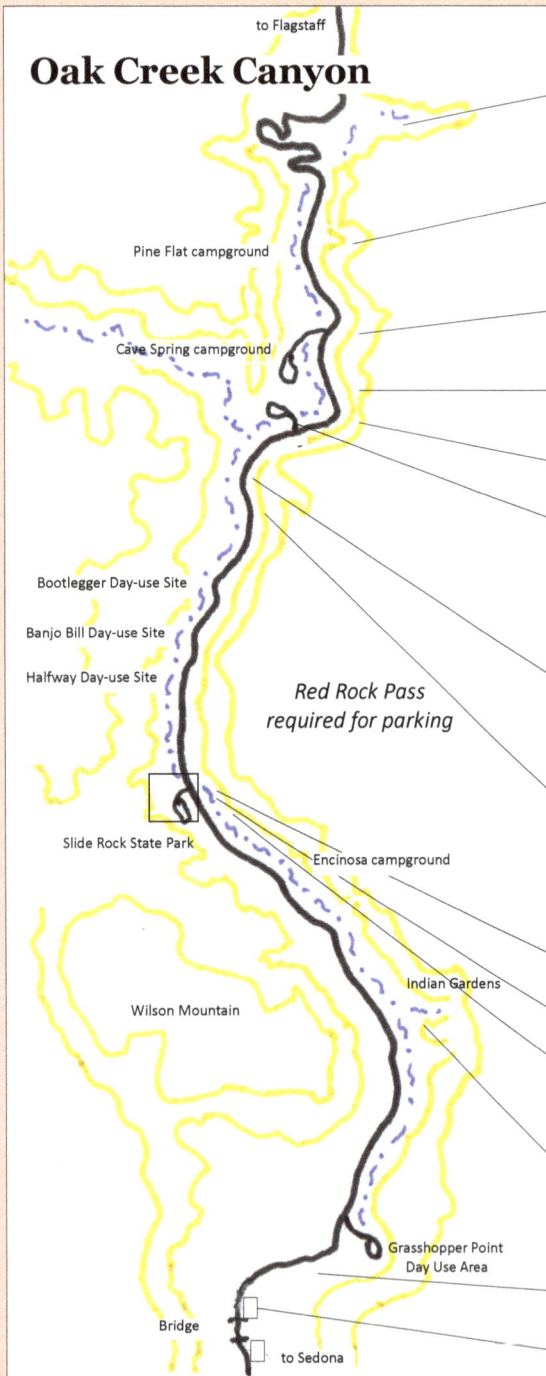

Other Trails in Oak Creek (north to south)

Pumphouse Wash   mp 387.7 at Pumphouse Bridge; 1+ mile through creek bed when water isn't running, moderate.

Cookstove Trail   mp 386.9 at Pine Flat CG; .75 mile up east wall; moderately strenuous.

Harding Spring Trail   mp 385.6 at Cave Spring CG .8 mile up east wall; strenuous.

Telephone Trail   mp 385.1 - 1.25 miles up east wall; strenuous.

Thomas Point   mp 384.7 - 1 mile up east wall; moderately strenuous.

West Fork   mp 384.7 in the parking area; 3 - 12 miles, trail follows creek south from parking area to side canyon of Oak Creek. North end of canyon accessed above rim.

A.B. Young/East Pocket Trail   mp 383 at Bootlegger CG   1.6 miles up west wall; moderately strenuous; access East Pocket Fire Lookout Tower

Purtyman Trail   mp 382.6 at Junipine Resort/Fire Station 1 mile up east wall; very strenuous.

Slide Rock State Park mp 381.1 at Slide Rock Park .5 mile along popular stream; recreation area.

Brown House Canyon mp 381.1 at Slide Rock Park .3 mile up canyon away from park; moderate.

Thompson's Ladder, Indian Gardens up Munds Canyon. Public access is closed.

Allen's Bend   mp 376.5 at Grasshop per Point .5 mile along Oak Creek; easy.

Wilson Canyon   mp 375.9 at Midgley Bridge; 1.5 mile along canyon; moderate

Central Arizona - Verde Valley

The **Verde Valley** is becoming increasingly popular for recreation with both Phoenix residents and Northland residents, each group escaping the extremes in temperature. If you check out the USFS trail map for the Sedona area, a network of trails spreads out from the major traffic arteries.

When tourist stop in at the USFS office or the Sedona Visitors Centers, they are often directed to the Bell Rock and Cathedral Rock trails. Along with these two popular areas, several other trails in the Valley draw more than the average number of visitors due to some unique feature. Take Devils Bridge as an example. The parking lot is overwhelmed with the number of visitors on any given weekend. Vehicles line the road up to a half mile outside the parking lot. I'll grant you that Devil's Bridge is spectacular but the crowds are not. There are so many trails in the Verde Valley and many of them may offer views of the red and white cliffs as well as other special niches. Listen to the suggestions of others and decide what interests you most.

The trails we've listed are popular. We've even included Devil's Bridge though you would be well advised to be at the trailhead at the break of dawn!

Despite the crowds that flock to its campgrounds and recreation areas, Oak Creek Canyon remains a scenic pocket set apart from the remainder of Arizona as a place to marvel at creation and the creator. Red cliffs rise through green pines above a silvery stream caught in a rocky creek bed choked with blackberry bushes.

A number of trails climb above the traffic of Oak Creek Canyon. Most of them are brutally steep as the the trail builders seemed intent on reaching the rim by the shortest route.

In the pages that follow, we look at two trails that are particularly noteworthy, West Fork and Sterling Pass. West Fork has become overcrowded and restrictions are placed on the number of people who can visit each day. Vehicles line the roadway north of the parking area during the day.

Those out for a bit of adventure might try Pumphouse Wash, one of the loneliest spots off Oak Creek. Hikers may run into rock climbers but rarely other hikers.

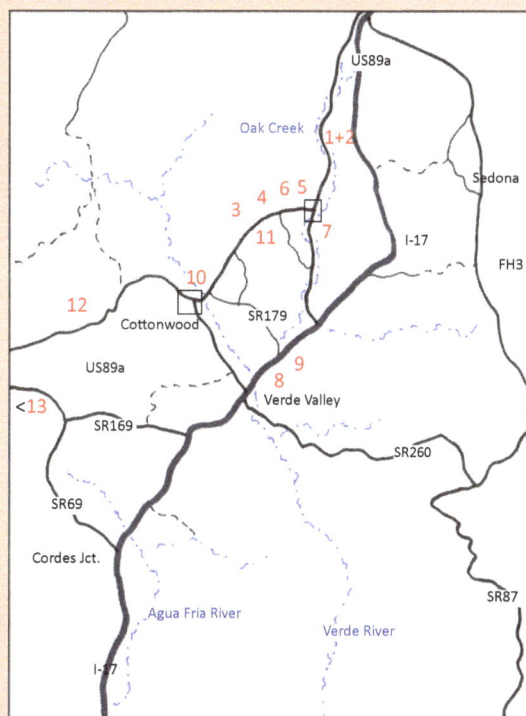

1 West Fork
2 Sterling Pass
3 Native American Ruins
4 Boynton & Fay Canyons
5 Soldiers Pass
6 Devils Bridge
7 Submarine Rock
8 Montezuma Well
9 Beaver Creek &
    West Clear Creek
10 Dead Horse State park
11 Red Rock State Park
12 Parson
13 Woodchute

West Fork of Oak Creek

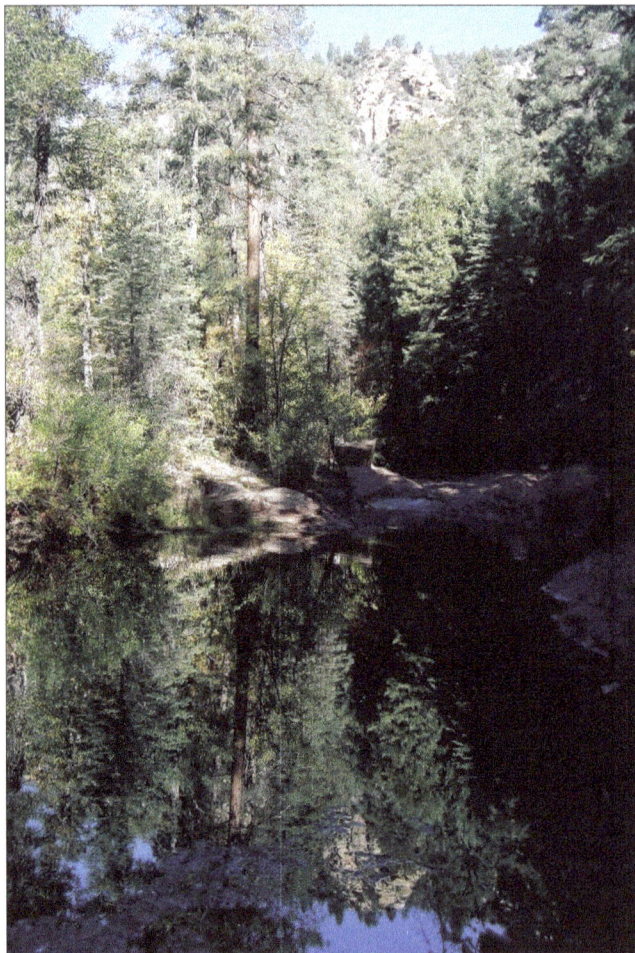

West Fork Canyon is famous throughout the state for casual hiking along a lovely creek. Visitors come to this canyon for the beautiful white and red cliffs that dwarf hikers as well as the cool, clear water. Of all the trails branching out of Oak Creek Canyon, this is one of the busiest and most loved. Unfortunately, easy access and scenic notoriety has left the canyon overrun with visitors. Overflow frequently leaves vehicles lining US89A above the parking area.

The trail crosses Oak Creek along a foot bridge and turns south toward the entrance of the canyon. Hikers approaching West Fork, pass the ruins of Mayhew's Lodge, one of the earliest lodges for visitors to Oak Creek Canyon. The landmark burned down in the early 1970s. A few walls remain along with an old chimney and the orchards that supplied fruit to guests and the Thomas family.

From the ruins, the trail turns west into West Fork canyon between immense cliffs lining a narrow stream bed. Over the next four miles the trail repeatedly crosses the stream bed. It is easily fordable when the water is low. When the water is high, come prepared to get your feet wet.

A mile or so up the canyon the trail passes the narrows where the water flows through a narrow slot into a deep green pool. Good place to swim on a hot day. The trail enters the streambed around four miles from the parking lot. Hikers wishing to proceed further walk in the stream. Hikers may make the 12-mile hike down from Woody Mountain Road on the Rim but it is a rugged hike over fallen trees and through deep pools of water with a maze of side canyons.

Driving Distance: 10.5 miles from Sedona at mp384.7 on US89a.
Hiking Distance: 3+ miles one way.
Rating: Easy
Elevation: 5200'
Best Season: Spring, fall & winter.
Precautions: Rocks can be slippery when wet! Always test your footing.
Maps: Coconino NFS map
Information: Red Rock Ranger Station 928-282-7722

Sterling Pass

Like most of the trails climbing out of Oak Creek Canyon, this ascent was hewn out of rock by the early settlers. The trail to **Sterling Pass** starts a half mile south of Slide Rock State Park at mp 380.5 and is marked by a knee-level metal sign on the roadside. Only a couple of cars can squeeze into parking roadside.

At first, the trail follows a wash westward, gently climbing through an open forest of pine and decidous trees. Drawing near the face of the ridge, hikers find the trail beginning to ascend steeply, seeming to steal their breath at every rise. The ascent encourages hikers to stop and admire the beautifully sculpted sandstone rock cliffs and green pines while catching their breath.

Just over 1.5 miles, the trail tops out at Sterling Pass. Hikers may choose to pass beneath an arch of bowed oak limbs, descending the other side of the ridge to Vultee Arch and FR 152. Or hikers may call it a day and return along the trail to cool off in the waters of Oak Creek at a nearby campground or day-use area.

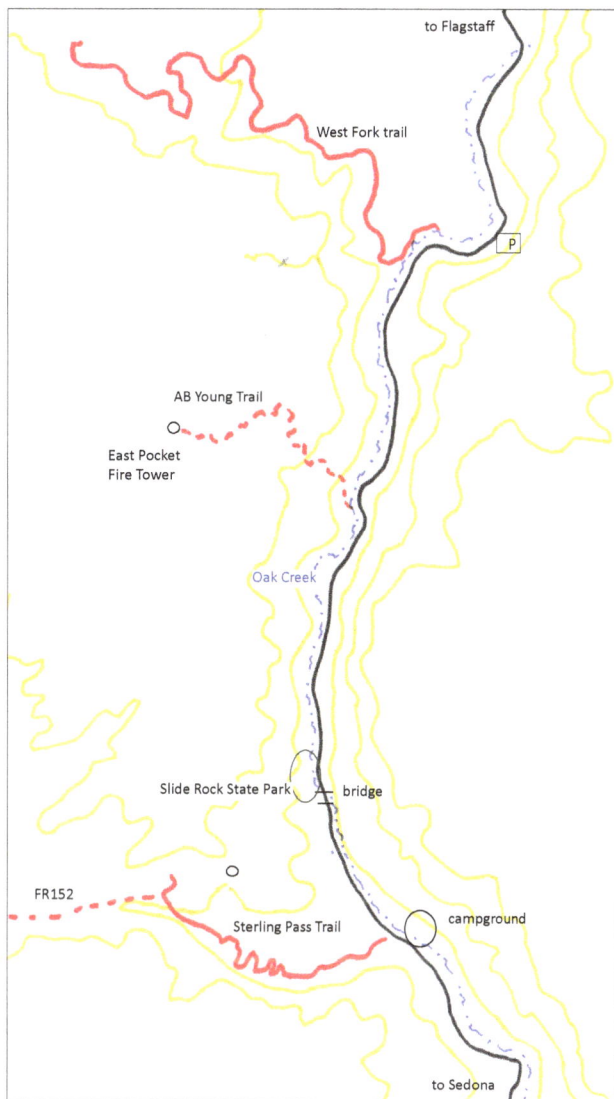

Driving Distance: 6 miles from Jct. SR179/US89A in Sedona

Hiking Distance: 1.65 miles one way to Pass
2.6 miles to Vultee Arch, one way

Rating: Moderate

Elevation: 5,000 - 6,000

Best Season: Spring and fall.

Special Features: Beautiful climb through sand stone rock formations with sandstone arch as destination.

Precautions: Maze of trails on west side of Pass, loose rock underfoot.

Maps: Coconino NFS map

Information: Red Rock Ranger Station
928-282-7722

Verde Valley Native American Ruins

Palatki and Honanki Historic Sites

These ruins hidden at the base of the cliffs along Bear Mountain once sheltered an ancient people. The ruins of early white settlers and a modern ranch house stand nearby, also in the shadow of the red cliffs.

From the junction of US89a and SR 179, drive west to Dry Creek Road/FR152. Turn north and drive 4.5 miles to Boynton Pass Road. Turn southeast (left) onto Boynton Canyon Road/ FR152C. In just over 4 miles, turn right onto FR525 and drive north to **Palatki** and on to **Honanki Ruin**s. Both sites have pueblo ruins. Honanki has small petroglyphs on the cliffs around the ruin.

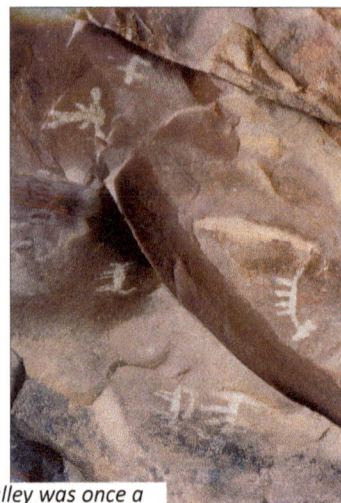

The Verde River valley was once a busy center of commerce and agriculture due to its moderate climate, access to water and fertile fields.

Driving Distance: 17 miles from Jct. US 89A & SR 179.
Hiking Distance: Honanki .5 mile loop; Palatki .5 mile round trip.
Rating: Easy
Elevation: 4800'
Best Season: Spring, fall & winter; summer is hot.
Special Features: Indian ruins in a pretty pocket.
Maps: Coconino NFS map
Information: Sedona Ranger Station
(928) 282-4119

Tuzigoot National Monument

Unlike the pueblo ruins at Honanki and Palaki, **Tuzigoot** may have been a hill-top fortress. Visitors ascend a low hill from the Visitors Center to circle a cluster of rooms around a two-story structure. A stairway allows visitors to climb to the second story for a view across the Verde Valley.

Follow US89a from Sedona or SR60 from I-17 to Cottonwood. Drive along Main Street through Old Town as it turns to Broadway. The road climbs toward Clarkdale but visitors turn right onto Tuzigoot Road and drive to the Visitor's Center.

Hiking Distance: .25 mile one-way

Top photo: Honoanki gyphs, bottom: Palatki Pueblo

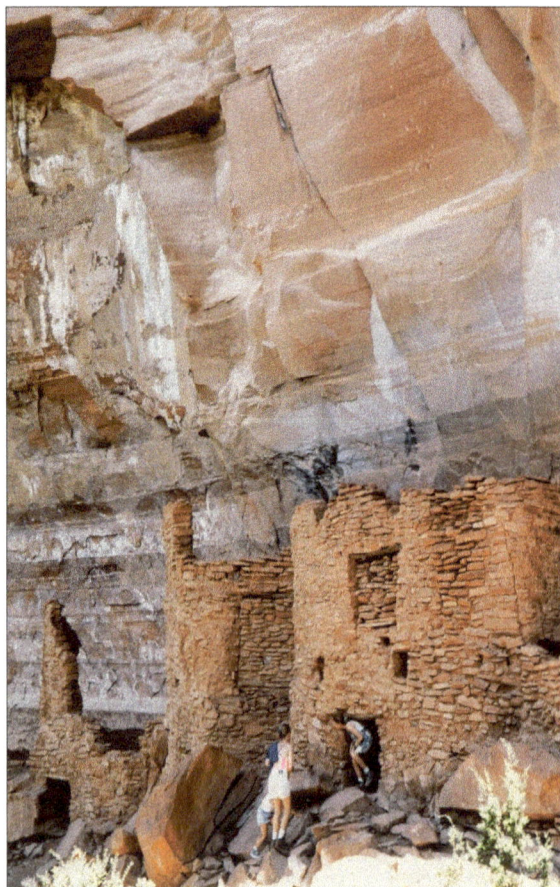

Boynton and
Fay Canyons

Boynton and Fay Canyons are both beautiful with footpaths leading visitors deep into their shady depths. Unfortunately, visitors to Boynton must make a long detour around a resort before entering the canyon. In hot weather, this detour can be a bit prohibitive.

Boynton is a favorite with those who believe this canyon is a vortex site and we've found some unusual sculptures as well as an oversized prayer wheel in the depths of the canyon. The Forest Service discourages meddling with the natural landscape. Side trails lead out of Boynton to some of the finger ridges that overlooks the canyon depths.

Fay Canyon is a shorter hike but still popular. Just beyond Fay Canyon is a parking area for Doe Mountain, a short but rigorous climb up a red rock butte. The trailhead for Doe is also the trailhead for Bear Mountain, a much more challenging climb - make sure you're on the trail you intend to explore.

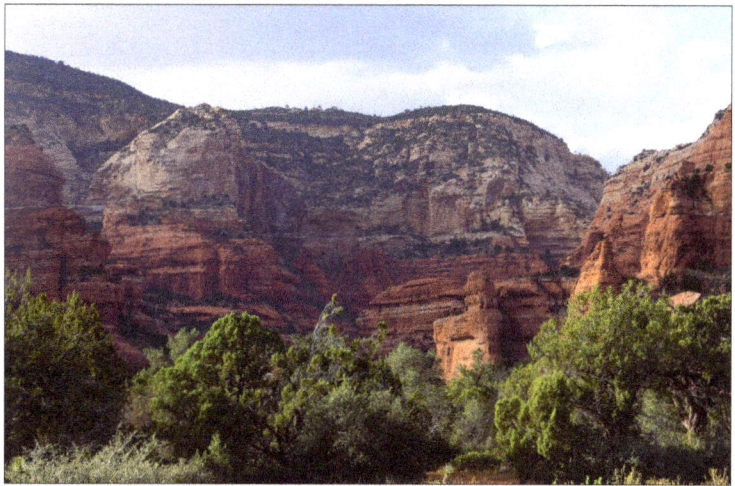

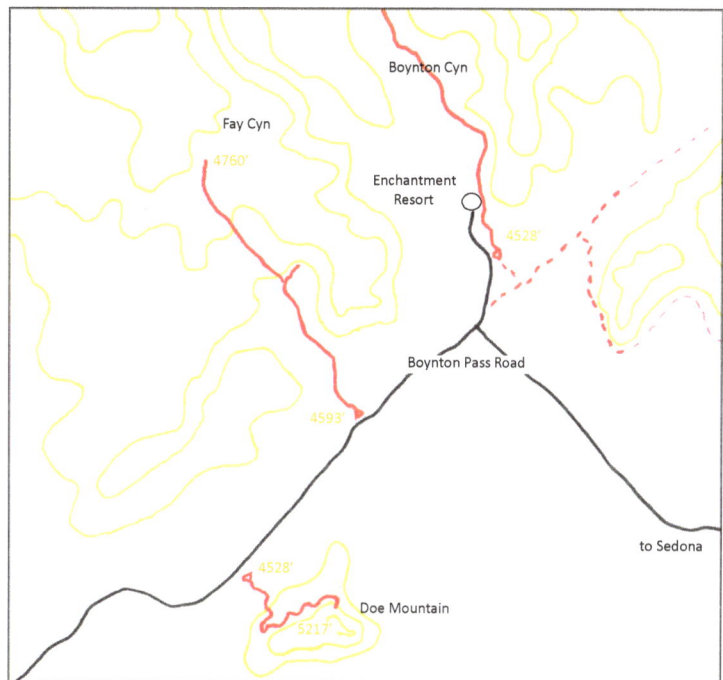

Driving Distance: 4.75 miles from corner of Dry Creek Road and US89a.

Hiking Distance: Fay 2.5 miles out and back; Boynton 3.6 miles out and back; Doe. 1.2 out and back.

Rating: Moderate

Best Season: Spring & Fall Special Features: Beautiful red rock canyons Precautions: Long detour around resort - do not recommend this trail during summer months.

Maps: Coconino National Forest

Information: Red Rock Ranger Station 928-282-7722

Soldiers Pass

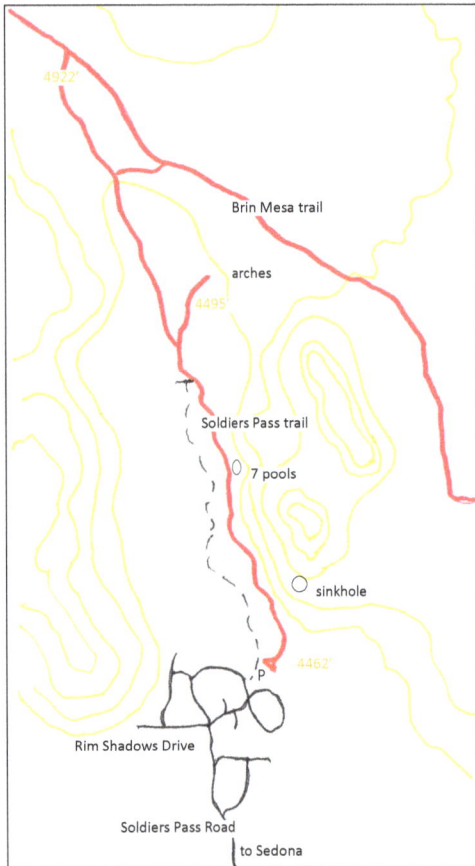

Soldiers Pass has several features that have made the trail one of the most popular in Sedona. To reach the trailhead, turn north onto Soldier Pass Road, 1.25 miles west of the junction of SR 179 & US 89A in Sedona. Drive 1.5 miles to the first intersection with Rim Shadows, a loop road. Turn right and follow Shadow Rock Drive to the intersection with Canyon Shadows. Continue straight through the intersection. Just past the corner house, turn left onto a dirt track leading into the trailhead parking lot. If you miss the turn, Canyon Shadows makes a loop, returning to the same intersection.

Within the first quarter mile, hikers climb to the rim of an active sinkhole. Once an underground cavern, huge blocks of sandstone have collapsed inward, creating the sink hole. We are left wondering about the rock under our feet.

The trail continues to the left of the sinkhole almost a half mile to a series of pools descending a rocky ledge. These depressions were hollowed out of the sandstone and filled with water running off off the mesa above. Early native Americans would have used the pools though they did not consider them sacred as suggested by tour guides. Their depth is progressive from right to left, upstream to down.

Returning to the trail, the path bypasses a jeep trail to follow a wash upward toward the rim of Brins Mesa. A secondary trail branches to the right to climb the red rock toward three arches cut into the side of the mesa. This trail almost disappears across the slick rock, marked only by cairns. Some climb up to an inner shelf to peer through a window or marvel at the sliver of light that falls between the rock walls. Returning across the slick rock the trail climbs to Brin Mesa.

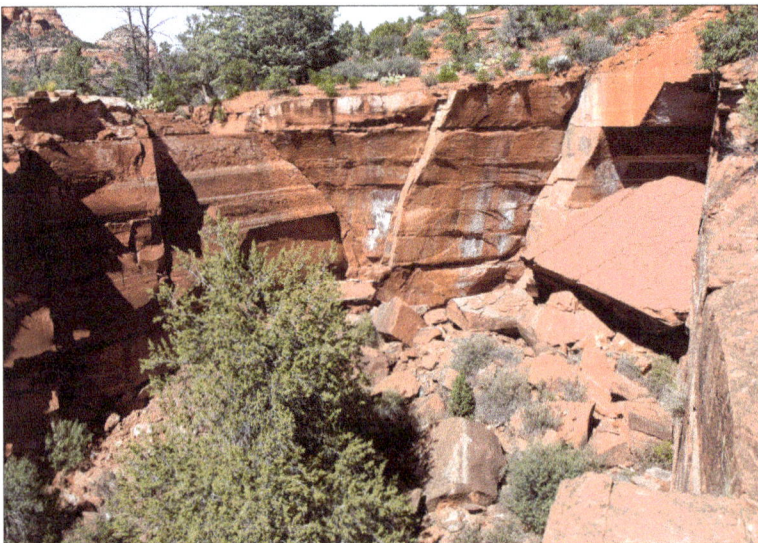

Driving Distance: 3 miles from the
    Jct. of 89A & 179 in Sedona.
Hiking Distance: 1.1 miles one way,
    2.8 miles with loop.
Rating: Moderate   Elevation: 4500'
Best Season: Spring or fall
Special Features: Sinkhole, cienegas &
    three beautiful arches.
Precautions: Don't drink the water! The
    rock within the arch is unstable.
Maps: Coconino NFS map
Information: Red Rock Ranger Station
                928-282-7722
Photo: Seven Pools of Soldiers Pass

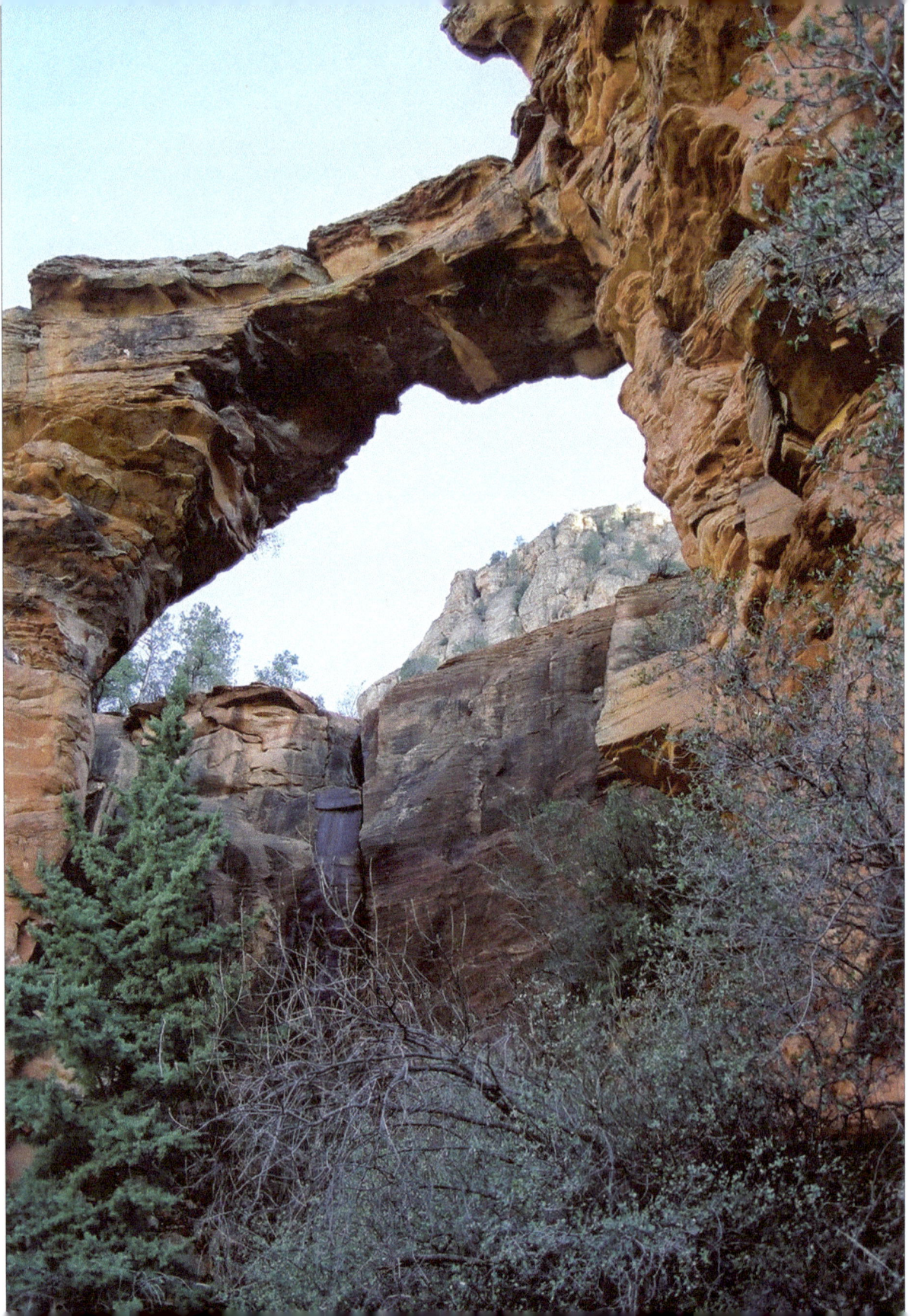

Devil's Bridge

Devil's Bridge, one of the largest arches in the Sedona area, is an awesome sight. Visitors can hike to the top of the arch as well as stand under the sandstone span.

To reach the trailhead drive west 3.2 miles on US 89A from the junction with SR 179 to Dry Creek Road / FR 152. Turning north or right, drive 2 miles to the junction of Boyton Pass Road and FR 152. While hikers could have once driven further, due to the traffic in this area and the poor condition of the road, drivers must park in the large lot at the junction. All-terrain vehicles and tour jeeps easily proceed further. Hikers follow the road 1.4 miles to the turn off for Devil's Bridge and hike an additional mile up to the arch.

Devil's Bridge is located in a canyon off the west side of Capitol Butte. Approaching the arch, the trail splits with the left side dipping down into a wash beneath the arch. The trail to the right climbs a series of steps to a rock ledge with a great view over the plain. A second set of steps takes the hiker up behind the arch with a great view above the arch. Even as hikers admire the view, they must watch their footing on the loose rock as it is a long way down.

For dare-devils, the trail leads around and on top of the arch. Considering how sandstone fractures, this may not be for everyone! There are opportunities for additional hiking up Capitol Butte and along the wash past the arch.

Driving Distance: 6.6 miles

Hiking Distance: 2.4 miles from Mescal
      trailhead one way

Rating: Moderate

Elevation: 4600 - 5000'

Best Season: Spring and fall;
      summer is hot so go early.

Special Features: Impressive sandstone
      bridge.

Precautions: Steep climb - watch your
      footing.

Maps: Coconino NFS map

Information: Red Rock Ranger Station
      928-282-7722

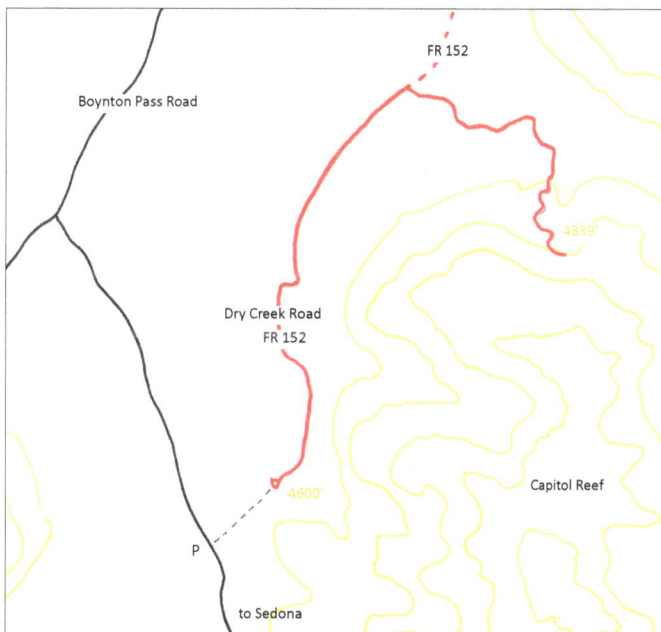

Robber's Roost: I hesitate to mention this unique cave on the side of a sandstone butte south of Sedona due to the vandalism that has begun to occur in the region. Other books will give you directions. The entrance is a bit deceiving due to the thick brush.

The butte is accessed by Red Canyon Road to FR 525 to FR 525c to FR 9530. If you're the sort to appreciate the beauty of our back country without the need to leave your mark, go with a friend who has entered the site previously. The entrance is not for anyone afraid of heights and slick rock.

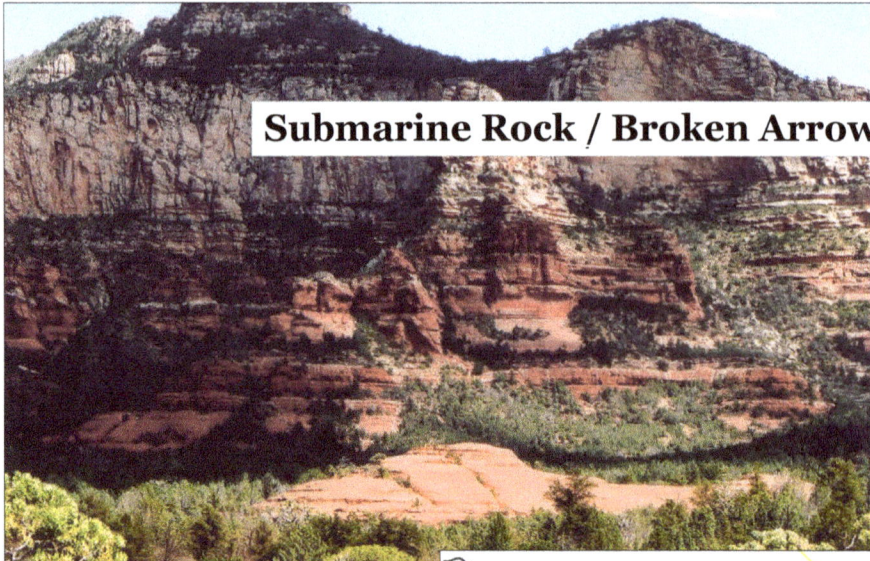

Submarine Rock / Broken Arrow Trail

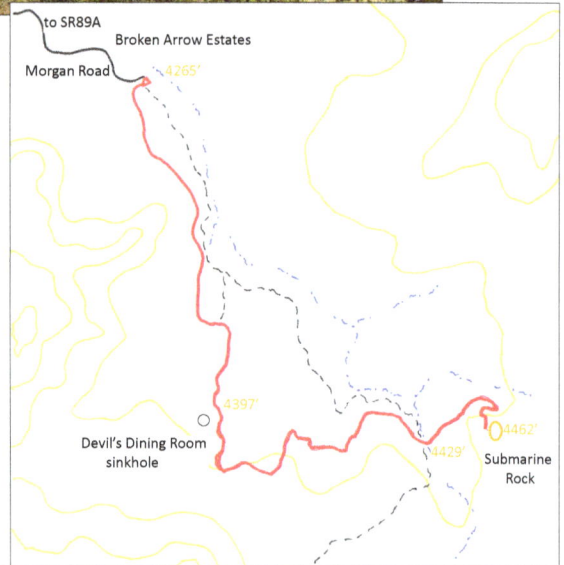

With the proliferation of jeep tours in the back country, this hike may leave you feeling like an exhibit along the trail.

From SR179 and US89A, drive south just over a mile. Turn left onto Morgan Road and drive through Broken Arrow Estates to the trailhead. At first, hikers follow the trail as it parallels a jeep track toward a low ridge. Just under a half mile from the trailhead, the trail passes the Devil's Kitchen sink hole. The pit is fenced to keep visitors from edging forward and falling in.

From the sinkhole, the road climbs a low rise and drops into a shallow valley populated with juniper and pinyon pine. From the overlook, visitors can spot a red rock formation that resembles a submarine rising amid the *sea* of juniper and pinyon forest. The trail divides with the left branch dropping toward **Submarine Rock**.

Returning to the main trail, the route climbs to Chicken Point, a low saddle in the ridge ahead and beyond to SR179.

Photo: Submarine Rock in foreground

Driving Distance: 2 miles from the Jct. of SR89A & SR179

Hiking Distance: .4 mile to the sinkhole, .8 mile to Sub Rock, 1.5 miles to Chicken Point

Rating: Easy   Best Season: Spring or Fall

Special Features: Sink hole and rock formation

Precautions: Keep an eye out for cruisin' jeeps and mountain bikes!

Information: Red Rock Ranger Station
928-282-7722

Montezuma Well

For years I avoided Montezuma Well, regarding the encircled pond as boring. After doing some research on Arizona's springs, I learned that this limocrene spring is very unique.

A short trail takes visitors from the parking area and over a rise to stand above the well. The surface appears undisturbed but 55 feet below the surface is another story. Cameras lowered into the pool revealed undulating waves of sand. Down another 60 feet and scientific instrument extend into inlets where water is forced upward through rock fractures by subterreanean pressure.

The water is released from the well along a subterreanean passage. A short trail descends along the interior wall to this outlet. The main trail descends es around the well to the point where the water emerges from under the limestone, flowing along a channel down to Wet Beaver Creek.

The well is sacred to many of the tribes in the region with a history reaching back to prehistoric ages. When the white settlers first arrived, they found the Verde Valley was heavily populated by native people with ancient ruins scattered along the Verde River. Archeologists theorize that the Verde Valley was an active trading center with traders arriving from tribes to the south, the east and north to exchange trade goods.

The hike is short but worthwhile when we understand the historical and natural significance of this spring.

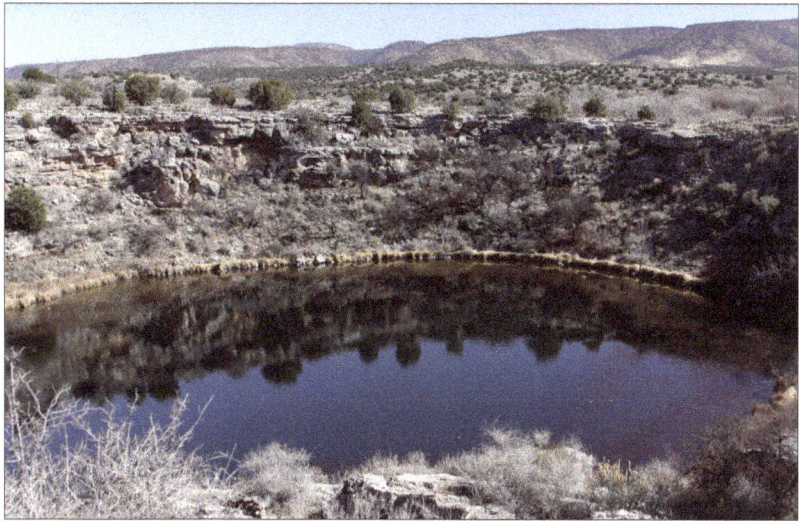

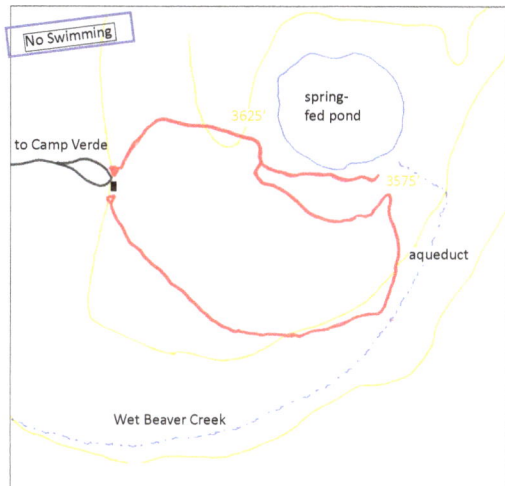

Photo: Montezuma Well

No Swimming

spring-fed pond

to Camp Verde

3625'

3575'

aqueduct

Wet Beaver Creek

Driving Distance: 5 miles from Camp Verde
Hiking Distance: .3 mile to the sinkhole,
.5 mile along channel
Rating: Easy
Best Season: Spring or Fall
Special Features: Sink hole
Precautions: Don't drink the water!
Information: Red Rock Ranger Station
928 (282) 4119
or Montezuma Castle Nat'l Monument
928 567-3322

Bell Trail at Beaver Creek

The **Bell trail** on Beaver Creek is one of the most popular hikes in the state. Visitors flock to popular swimming holes along the stream in the warm months. From I-17, take the exit for SR179. Turn east to follow FR618, driving two miles past the overflow parking to the trailhead for Beaver Creek and turn left into the parking area. A dirt track leads northeast across the plateau, remaining above the creek.

Bell Crossing is 3.5 miles from the trailhead. About one hundred yards beyond Bell Crossing is a large pool known as the Crack. Visitors should carry lots of water as this trail is exposed and very hot during summer months when the cool water of the stream is most welcome. Many hikers come early and spend the day, hiking back only after the temperatures cool off a bit. Please pack your trash out - no maid service.

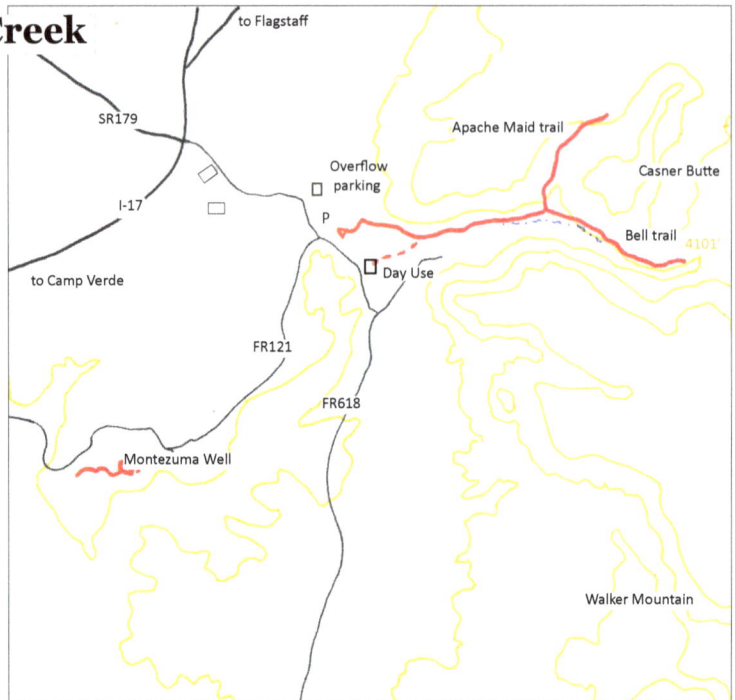

Driving Distance: 14.7 miles from Jct.
        SR 179 and I-17.
Hiking Distance: 1-3 miles
Rating: Easy   Elevation: 3600'
Best Season: All, summer is hot.
Special Features: Beautiful stream and riparian
        area, red cliffs.
Precautions: Poisonous insects, reptiles
        and high summer temperatures.
Maps: Coconino NFS map
Information: Verde Valley Ranger Station
        928-567-4121

The White Mesa trail and the Apache Maid trail both fork off the Bell Trail; both are steep and rocky. The Weir trail diverts to a flow measurement station.

The Blodgett Basin trail is another alternative to the West Clear Creek Trail with great views and far fewer hikers than the area along the creek. The trail descends along a three mile route from FR 214 to the parking area for West Clear Creek. To reach the trailhead, from FR618 turn east onto FR 214 and drive almost 4 miles to the trailhead. Access is clearly marked on the Coconino NFS map. We recommend a two car shuttle between the two trailheads.

The head waters for Clear Creek lie in the hills above Camp Verde. The creek flows southwest to a junction with the Verde River. Along that route, off SR260, are several trailheads leading back to places known as the Hanging Gardens. Check AllTrails online for further information.

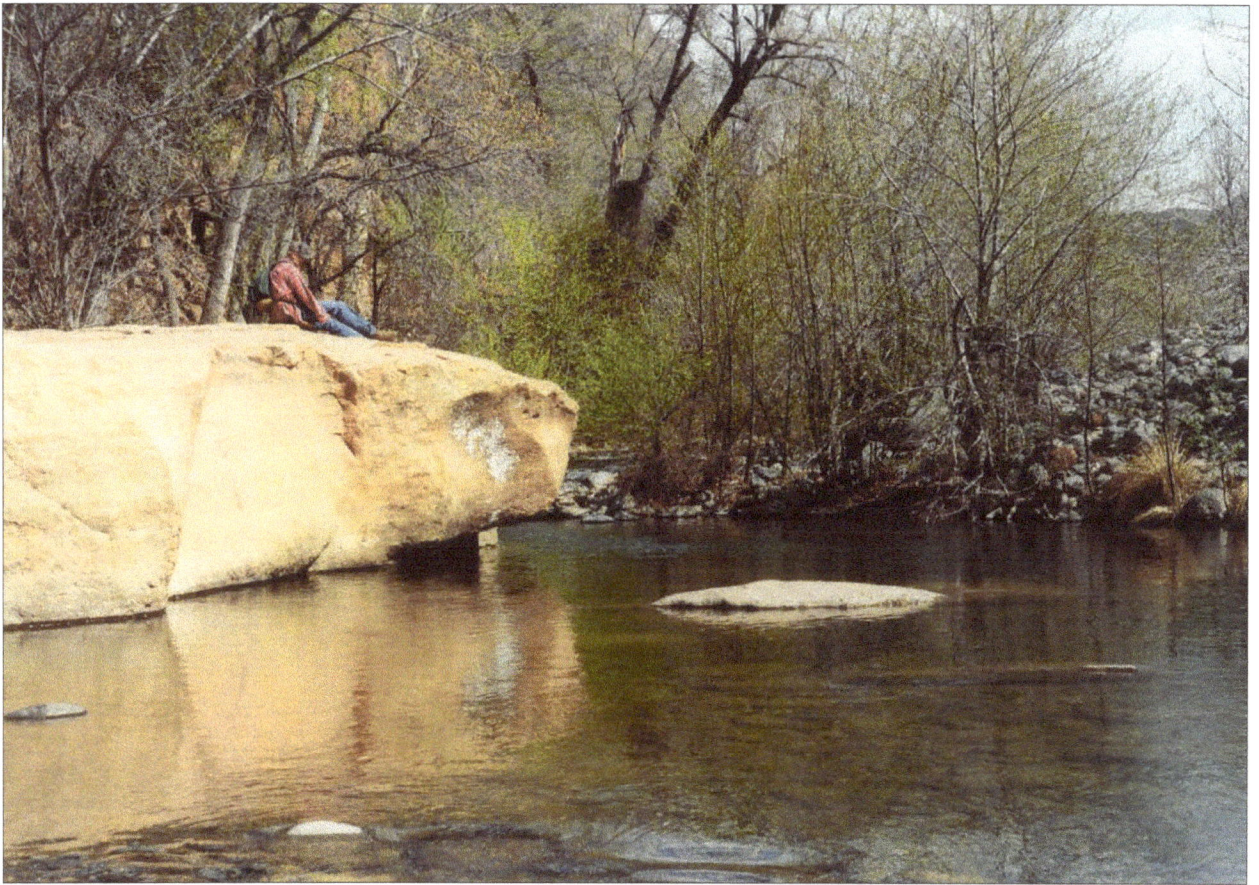

West Clear Creek

The rocky cliffs and cool, green water along West Clear Creek makes it a favorite location for hikers and fisherman. For decades, this entrance to West Clear Creek, began through private property. When the State purchased this land, the public gained access to this popular location.

From the junction of I-17 and SR 179 at Exit 298, turn east along FR 618. FR 618 passes the popular Bell trail before reaching the bridge over Beaver Creek. Just past the bridge, the pavement ends and the road forks, stay right. Drive 11.5 miles from I-17 and turn left on FR 215. This can be a rough road with a wet crossing as it drops into the West Clear Creek drainage.

Pool in West Clear Creek, above crossing.

The road passes a small campground on the right to end at a gate. Find a parking spot and walk through the gate under massive cottonwoods. A dirt track crosses the dry plain and follows the bluff above the creek. High on the left stands a rock cabin with prickly pear cactus sprouting from the roof.

In one mile the road dips down to the creek where footpaths follow both banks. Upstream there are several pools where swimmers can enjoy swimming. The West Clear Creek trail is on the opposite bank and moves away from the creek for the first mile. We chose to find a good spot to spend the day playing in the cool water.

State Parks of Verde Valley

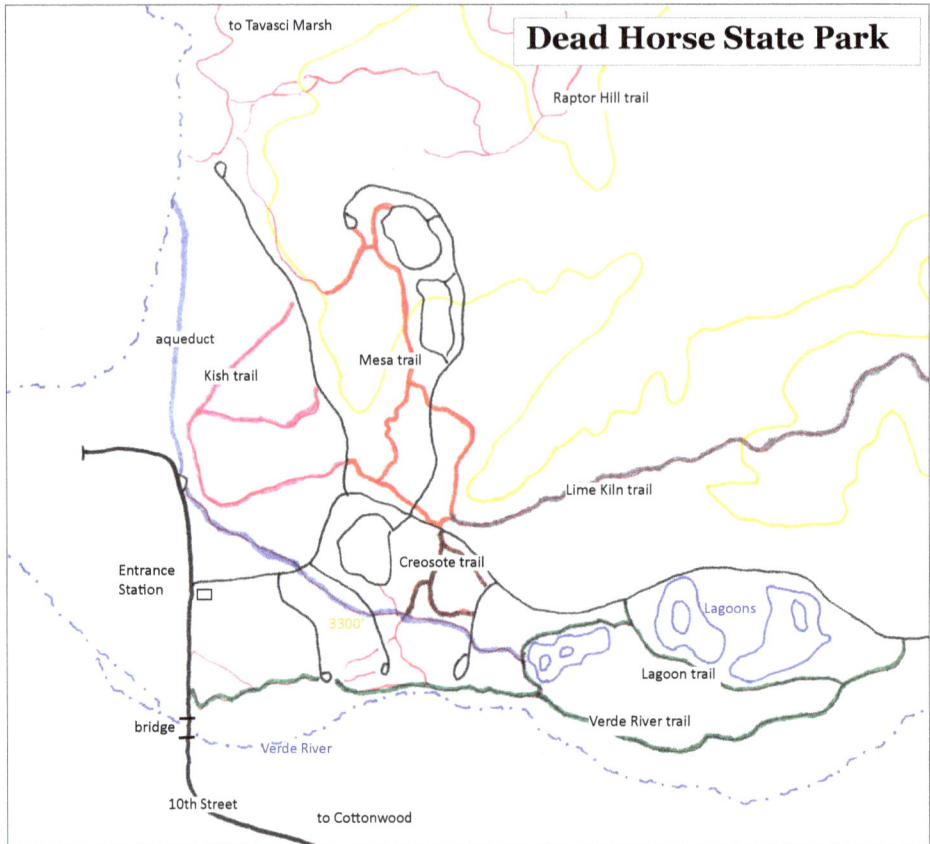

Despite its name, **Dead Horse State Park** is one of the most popular recreation areas in the Verde Valley. Follow US 89A or SR 260 onto Main Street and drive through Cottonwood. Turn right on 5th Street to cross the bridge over the Verde River. Dead Horse State Park and the Visitors Center are on the right. Day visitors pay a user fee. The Park's large campground fills up quickly on weekends during the spring and fall. A map of the Park shows the day use area along the river, the lagoons and Tavisci Marsh with the trails connecting each feature. The trails aren't strenuous.

The State of Arizona, the City of Cottonwood and private parties have developed areas along the Verde River for recreation. Some hikers like to combine a day hike with kayaking for a couple of hours on the Verde River.

Hiking Distance: .5+ mile
Rating: Easy   Elevation: 3300'
Best Season: Year round, summer is hot!
Special Features: Lagoon & River access, hiking
       trail along flume.
Precautions: Heat, Poisonous insects & reptiles,
       current in river.
Information: Dead Horse State Park
              (928) 634-5283

Red Rock State Park

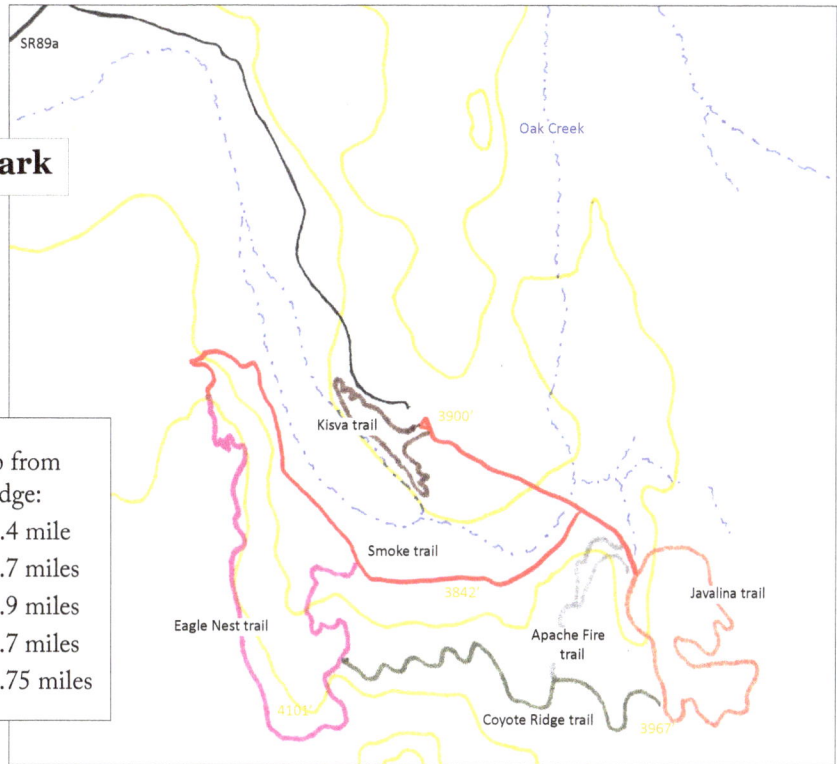

Oak Creek

Kisva trail

3900'

Smoke trail

3842'

Eagle Nest trail

Javalina trail

Apache Fire trail

4101'

Coyote Ridge trail

3967

Trail mileage round trip from Visitors center via bridge:	
Smoke Trail	.4 mile
Kisva Trail	1.7 miles
Eagles' Nest Trail	1.9 miles
Apache Fire Trail	1.7 miles
Javalina Trail	1.75 miles

The Visitors Center at **Red Rock State Park** combined with a network of hiking trails and scenic Oak Creek host a beautiful scenic state park. Throughout the Park, visitors may have the opportunity to see some of the wildlife that favor this area.

Follow US 89A, either east from Cottonwood or west from Sedona to mp 368.6. Turn south along Red Rock Loop Road driving 3 miles, to the entrance station. From the parking lot visitors descend to the Visitors Center built into a bluff overlooking the Oak Creek flood plain. A wide trail leads from the Visitors Center to a foot bridge crossing Oak Creek and the network of trails through the park.

The **Eagles' Nest Trail** climbs a ridge overlooking the Park while the **Apache Fire trail** loops over the ridge around the House of Apache Fire. Access is restricted to this former vacation home.

The **Javalina** and **Yavapai Ridge trails** both lead into back country while the **Kisva trail** parallels Oak Creek. **Coyote Ridge** is a connector between the **Apache Fire** trail and **Eagles' Nest**. The **Smoke Trail** parallels the north side of the creek. As tempting as the water looks on a hot day, swimming and wading are prohibited.

The Center offer hikes by the light of the full moon during the warmer months. Check with the Visitors Center for more details.

Driving Distance: 8.5 miles from 'Y' in Sedona.
Rating: Moderately easy   Elevation: 3900'
Best Season: Winter, spring and fall. Summer is hot!
Special Features: Creek, possibly wildlife and historical features.
Precautions: Poison reptiles & insects, poison ivy.
Information: Red Rock State Park
(928) 282-6907

Parson Trail

The Parson Trail on the southern end of Sycamore Canyon is a popular place for hiking and swimming on a warm day. The creek is lined with sycamores and cottonwoods.

From I-17, drive north 12 miles along SR 260 to the junction with US 89. Continue on through Cottonwood as SR 260 becomes Main/Broadway Street to the turnoff to Tuzigoot National Monument. Turn east and drive .4 mile. Turn left or north on FR 131 just past the bridge over the Verde River. Follow FR 131 as it first parallels the river and then breaks away cross-country toward the parking area on the rim of Sycamore Canyon. Two forks in the road are well-signed as is the trailhead on a high bluff overlooking the river.

The trail drops steeply into the canyon, following an old jeep road. When the trail forks near the bottom, stay right to follow the river. The left branch crosses the riverbed.

It is inviting to spend the day playing in the first large swimming hole but hikers can follow the stream 4 miles to Parson Spring. The large shade trees and vegetation make this a green oasis in the high desert. Beyond the spring the trail gets a bit rough and hard to follow. Those drawn by the allure of water will find a good spot to stop and spend the day before returning to the parking lot.

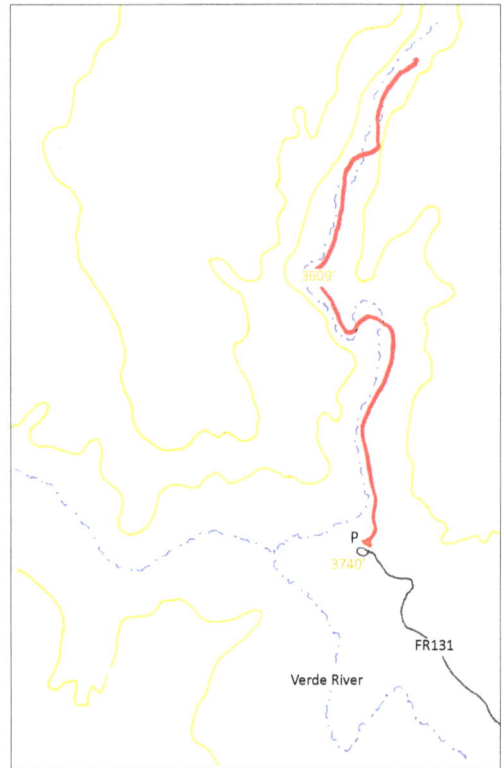

Driving Distance: 10.5 mile from Cottonwood.
Hiking Distance: 3.5 miles one way.
Rating: Moderate
Elevation: 3800' - 3650'
Best Season: Late spring and fall.
Precautions: Keep a sharp lookout for snakes.
       Debris from fire requires route finding.
Best Season: Early spring, the trail can be
       flooded.
Maps: USFS Prescott NFS map
Information: Red Rock Ranger District
       (928) 203-4119

Mingus Mountain & Woodchute

Most people who take the drive up Mingus Mountain are headed for the old mining town of Jerome. A visit to the McFarland Historical State Park is worthwhile to understand more of our state's history. A few pass through Jerome with only a glance at the gift shops and head for the summit. At the summit, hikers either turn *east* toward Mingus Mountain or turn *west* toward Potato Patch campground and the Wood Chute Trail.

The wood chute, for which the trail is named, was historically used to send logs skidding down to the mines. The trail is a nice walk through forest and meadows along the mountain side to a point overlooking the valley below. At a signed junction two miles in, stay right on trail #102. Some suggest that they feel as if they are being watched as they move through this historic area. Lots of friends and laughter help with that sense of uneasiness!

Those who turn *east* toward Mingus Mountain stay on FR104 as it winds along the terrain to a point where aerial gliders launch from a bluff overlooking the valley. Others follow the signs to the lookout tower that is manned during the warmer months.

I'm not a big fan of most of the trails on the eastern side of US89a. The forest is cluttered and populated by Mexican locust. Scrubby pinyon pine and juniper mix with the ponderosa pine. The trails often lack desirable destinations but the Woodchute trail is delightful. And the time outdoors give us a chance to stretch our legs and explore the woodland for an hour or two.

Driving Distance: 8.7 miles from
      Jerome, 27 miles from Prescott.
Hiking Distance: Wood Chute - 3.5 miles
      one way.
Rating: Easy
Elevation: 3,440'
Best Season: Late spring and fall.
Maps: USFS Prescott NFS map
Information: Verde Valley Ranger Station
      928-567-4121

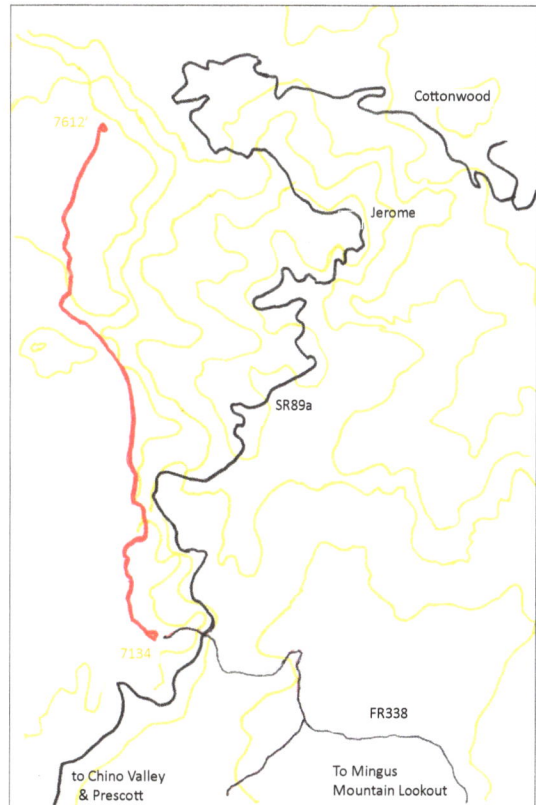

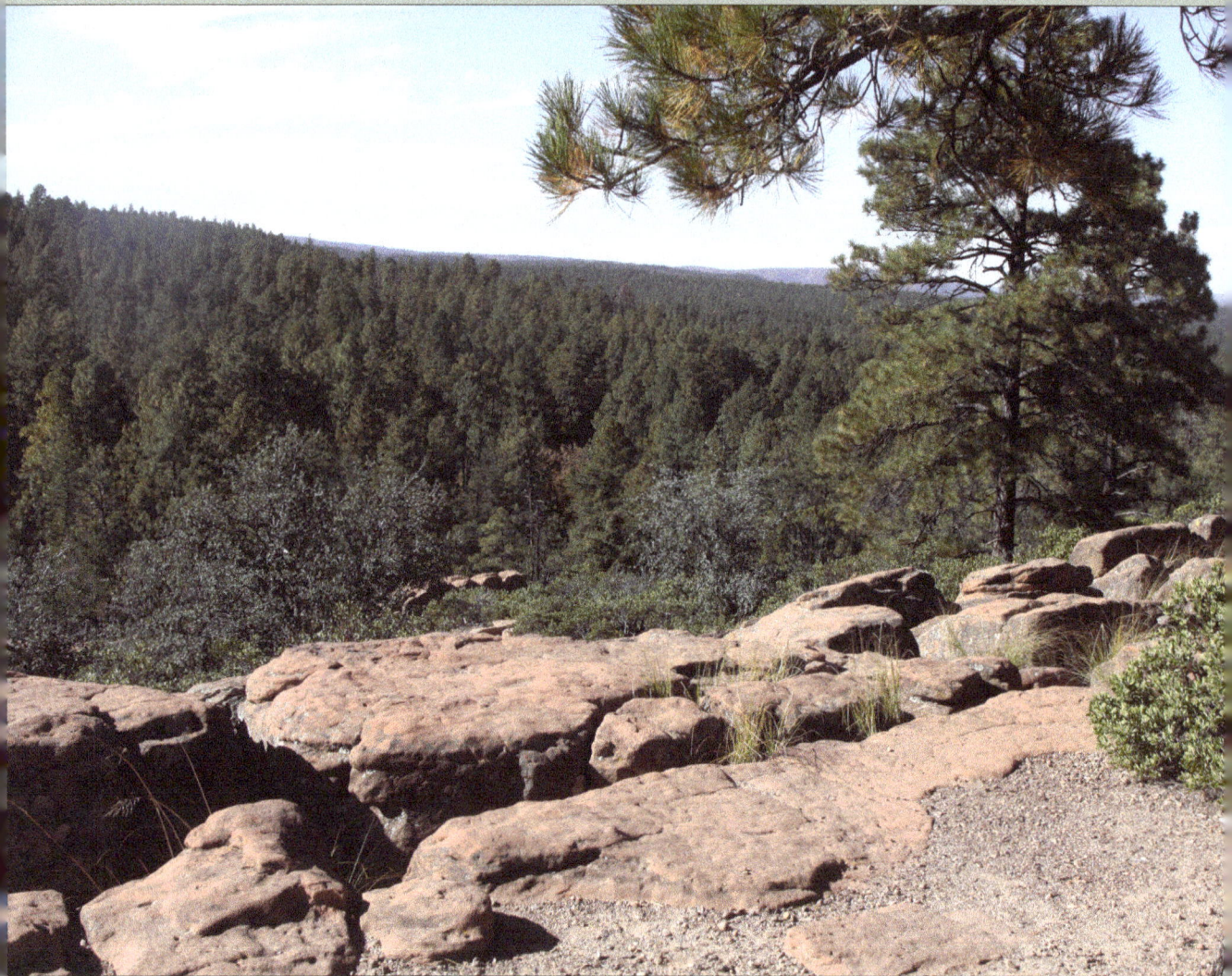

Payson is located in the transitional zone that sweeps in an arc from the southeast to the north-west across Arizona. Looking at the red rock along hillside cuts, we may think the area is dryer than further east along SR260.

Until recently, the region was still a hub for the many ranches that spread across the hills around Payson. Management for much of the land around Payson is under the authority of the United States government which has preserved the vast forest and kept the creeks open for public use.

Coming south from I-40 along SR87, the highway plunges over the Mogollon Rim in a series of switchbacks, passing through the litle towns of Strawberry and Pine. Countless cabins are hidden back in the forest around these small communities.

Arriving in Payson, visitors have the option of continuing south toward Phoenix or Roosevelt Lake. SR87 makes one last plunge toward the lower elevations as the primary vegetation changes from ponderosa pine to juniper and pinon pine.

Central Arizona - Payson

For drivers turning east out of Payson, SR260 crosses the Tonto Basin, historically one of the big ranching regions of the state. If visitors turn off SR260 to climb to the Diamond Point Lookout, they would gaze across many miles of lush green forest with meadows breaking the tree cover.

Above the Mogollow Rim, FR300 also designated as the Control Road, follows the rim with spectacular viewsacross the Tonto Basin. This dirt track follows the upper edge of the Mogollon Rim from SR87 to SR260. Campgrounds and hiking routes are scattered across the Basin, hardly seeming to make a dent in the vast forest of trees.

The Tonto Basin drains in the southwest toward Roosevelt Lake. SR288, one of only three state highways that is not paved, turns south off SR260 to trace a course behind Roosevelt Lake. Intersecting this long drive, the little town of Young remains a hub for ranches and the descendants of pioneering families.

Roosevelt Lake was created by building the Theodore Roosevelt Dam across the Salt River. This reservoir is the largest within Arizona.* SR88, east of the lake, follows the Apache Trail, a historic trade route along the Salt River to Apache Junction

The region is one of the most ecologically diverse areas in the state and recreation plays an important part in the economy of this region.

* Both Lakes Powell and Mead are shared with neighboring states.

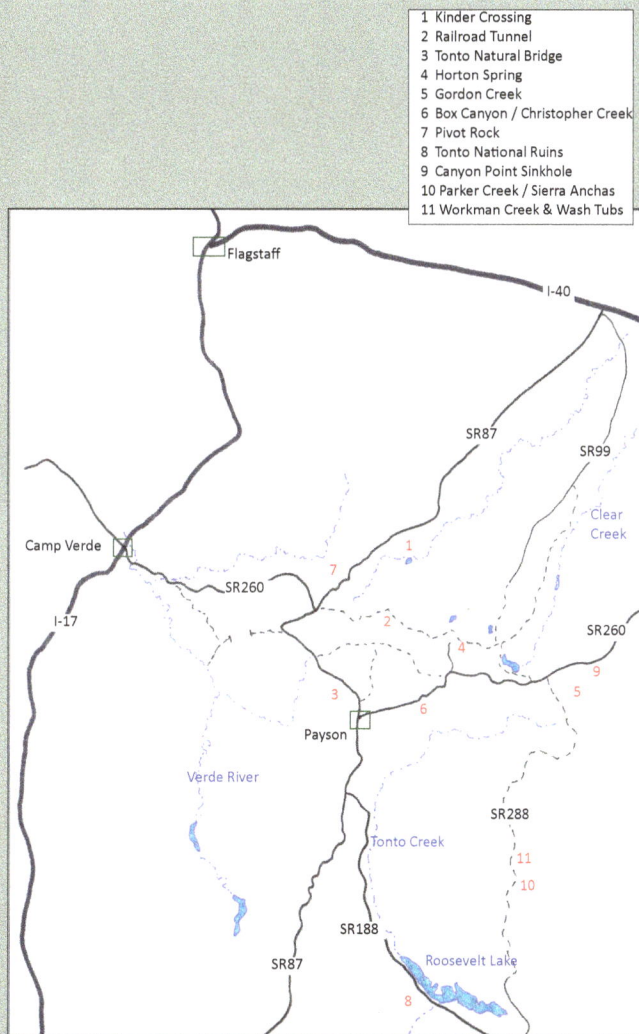

1	Kinder Crossing
2	Railroad Tunnel
3	Tonto Natural Bridge
4	Horton Spring
5	Gordon Creek
6	Box Canyon / Christopher Creek
7	Pivot Rock
8	Tonto National Ruins
9	Canyon Point Sinkhole
10	Parker Creek / Sierra Anchas
11	Workman Creek & Wash Tubs

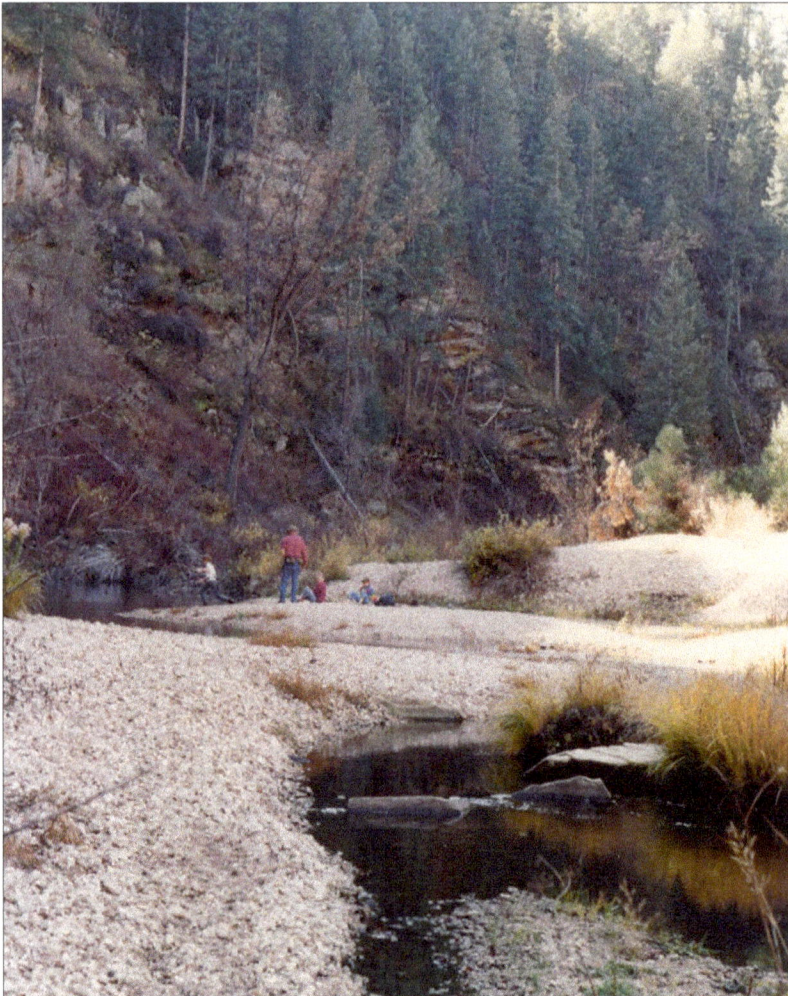

Kinder Crossing

As hikers reach the end of the ridge, the trail drops through switchbacks into East Clear Creek Canyon. The path is covered with loose rock, making footing a bit tricky. The view into the canyon is filled with red and white rock cliffs contrasting with the green ponderosa. The canyon's narrow bottom is creased by a rocky stream.

The canyon floor is wider than first anticipated from above. A sandy beach borders the stream with two large pools perfect for skipping rocks. Hiking downstream, the channel is choked with willows and brush. When hikers break through the brush on to a rocky point, they may find a large pool of water spreading across the canyon floor. The stream cascades over a rocky slope into the pool.

Depending on water levels, the trail downstream may require some route finding. Return along the Kinder trail, or for hikers wishing to do a loop with Horse Crossing, carry a good map and be prepared to shuttle between the two trailheads.

Hikers on the **Horse Crossing** trail also use FR95 to FR 513B. Both trail heads are well marked. Beyond the turnoff to Kinder Crossing, FR 95 crosses a branch of East Clear Creek with a swimming hole at the bridge.

Photo: Kinder Creek beach & pools

The beauty of East Clear Creek is awesome and harsh, making the jolting drive to the Kinder Crossing trailhead worth the visit. The **Kinder** trailhead is located off State Route 87, 30 miles north of Strawberry and 35 miles south of Winslow. From Flagstaff, hikers drive south on FH3 to Long Valley and turn north on SR 87 for 9.2 miles. Turn east onto FR95, just north of the Mogollon Rim Ranger Station. Drive southeast 4.1 miles to the signed turnoff. Turn left and drive .70 mile over a tire-crunching track to the parking area.

The trail into Kinder Crossing follows a narrow finger ridge with steep views on either side.

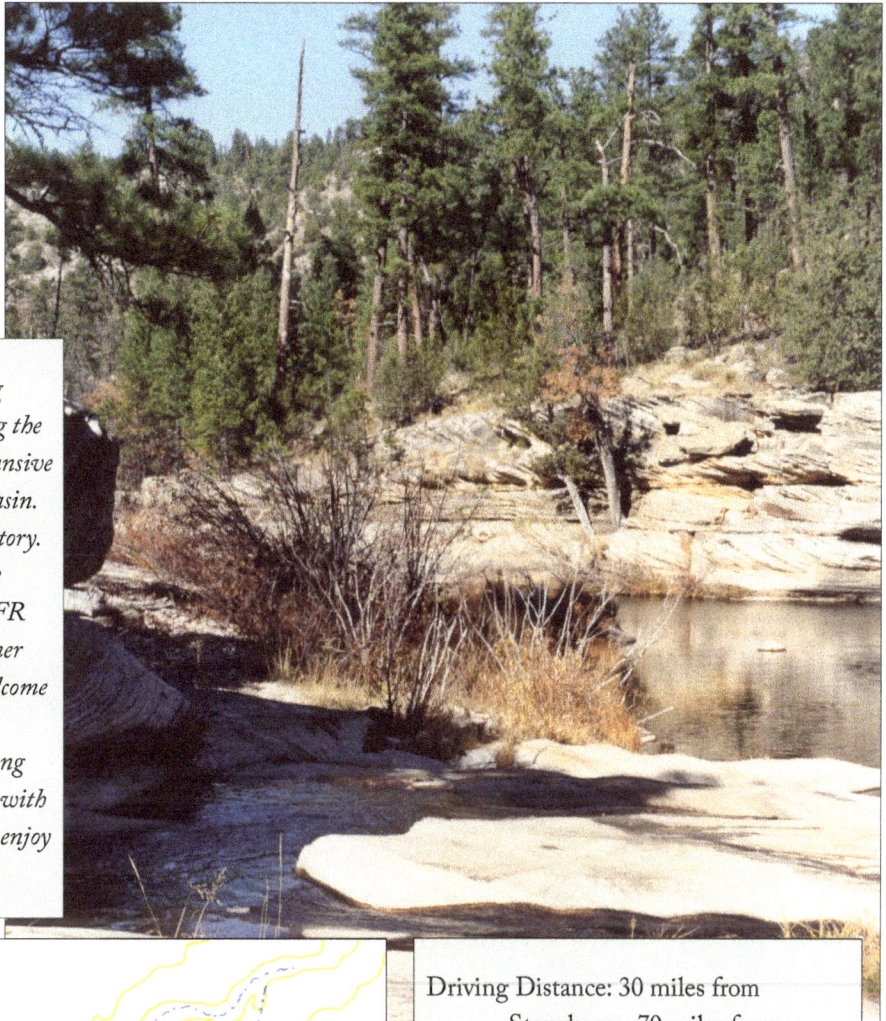

Forest Road 300 has long been the scenic route along the Mogollon Rim with expansive views across the Tonto Basin. This is an area rich in history.

Three of Arizona's fire towers are located along FR 300 and on a quiet summer day, the lookouts may welcome visitors.

The Rim Lakes lie along FR300 and are popular with fisherman and those who enjoy the outdoors.

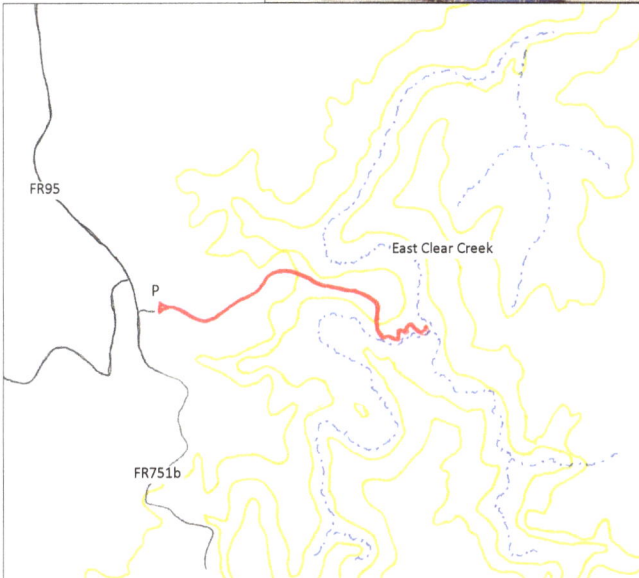

FR95

P

East Clear Creek

FR751b

Driving Distance: 30 miles from
    Strawberry, 70 miles from
    Flagstaff
Hiking Distance: 1.5 miles to the stream.
Rating: Moderate
Elevation: 7000'-6380'
Best Season: Summer & fall.
Special Features: Sandy beach with nice
    pools.
Precautions: Poison ivy.
Maps: USFS Coconino NFS map
Information:
    Mogollon Rim Ranger Station
        (928) 477-2255

Railroad Tunnel

Hidden along the Mogollon Rim is a piece of Arizona's mining history - a tunnel leading to nowhere. In 1881, as mining expanded in the Globe area, eastern investors saw an opportunity to ship ore to the Atlantic & Pacific Railroad in Flagstaff. Gandy men employed by the Mineral Belt Railroad soon began to lay tracks north from Globe. They planned to tunnel through the rim rather than taking a steeper route over the escarpment. The company ran out of money with the tunnel only partially uncompleted. Today, the tunnel is mostly quiet except when visitors bounce echoes against the rock walls. Water collects on the rocky floor, providing a quiet watering spot for wildlife. On one visit, as we stepped out of the tunnel we startled a large elk coming down for a drink.

There are two approaches to the tunnel. The longer of the two starts at the base of the rim, coming north from Washington Park along a pipeline road. This route is nearly four miles of steady ascent with little shade. I prefer the northern approach along Forest Road 300 off State Route 87. Drive about 12 miles from the turnoff on SR87 and look for the Monument to the Battle of Big Dry Wash on the left (north) side of the road. The monument commemorates a battle between the Apaches and the US Cavalry. The trailhead is located on the *south* side of the road with the trail dropping steeply over the rim. In just over a half mile, the turn off to the tunnel is marked by mega-cairns along the trail. Follow the footpath up several short switchbacks to the tunnel entrance.

The ruin of a rock building used for storing explosive black powder stands near the tunnel. The explosives were used to blast a passage into the rock wall.

During warm weather, the cool tunnel is a nice retreat. After examining the tunnel, hikers may imagine the construction crew shaking their heads as they walked away, wondering at such a futile investment.

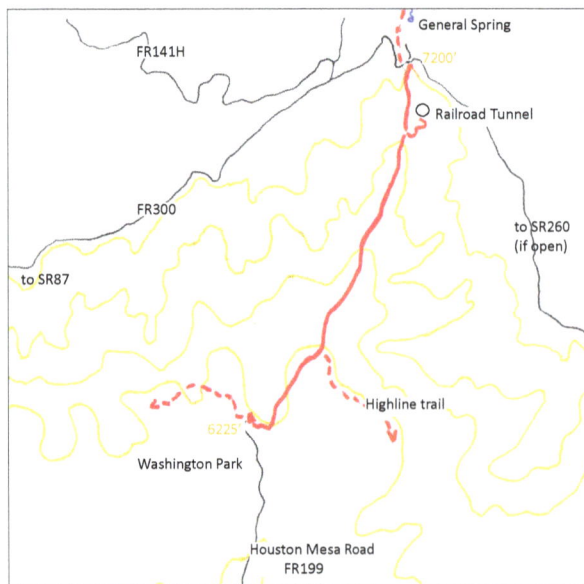

Driving Distance: Approx. 12.5 miles from SR 87 on FR 64, 14.5 from SR 260 on FR 64 or 12 miles from SR 87 along FR 300

Hiking Distance: 2.25 miles from Washington Park (southern trailhead) or .75 miles from FR300 (northern trailhead)

Rating: Moderate   Elevation: 7200'

Best Season: May through October.

Special Features: Old railroad tunnel. Beautiful forest around Washington Park.

Precautions: Watch carefully for cairns marking trail #390. Loose rock under foot can be hazardous last quarter mile.

Maps: Tonto NFS map

Information: Payson Ranger Station (928) 474-7900

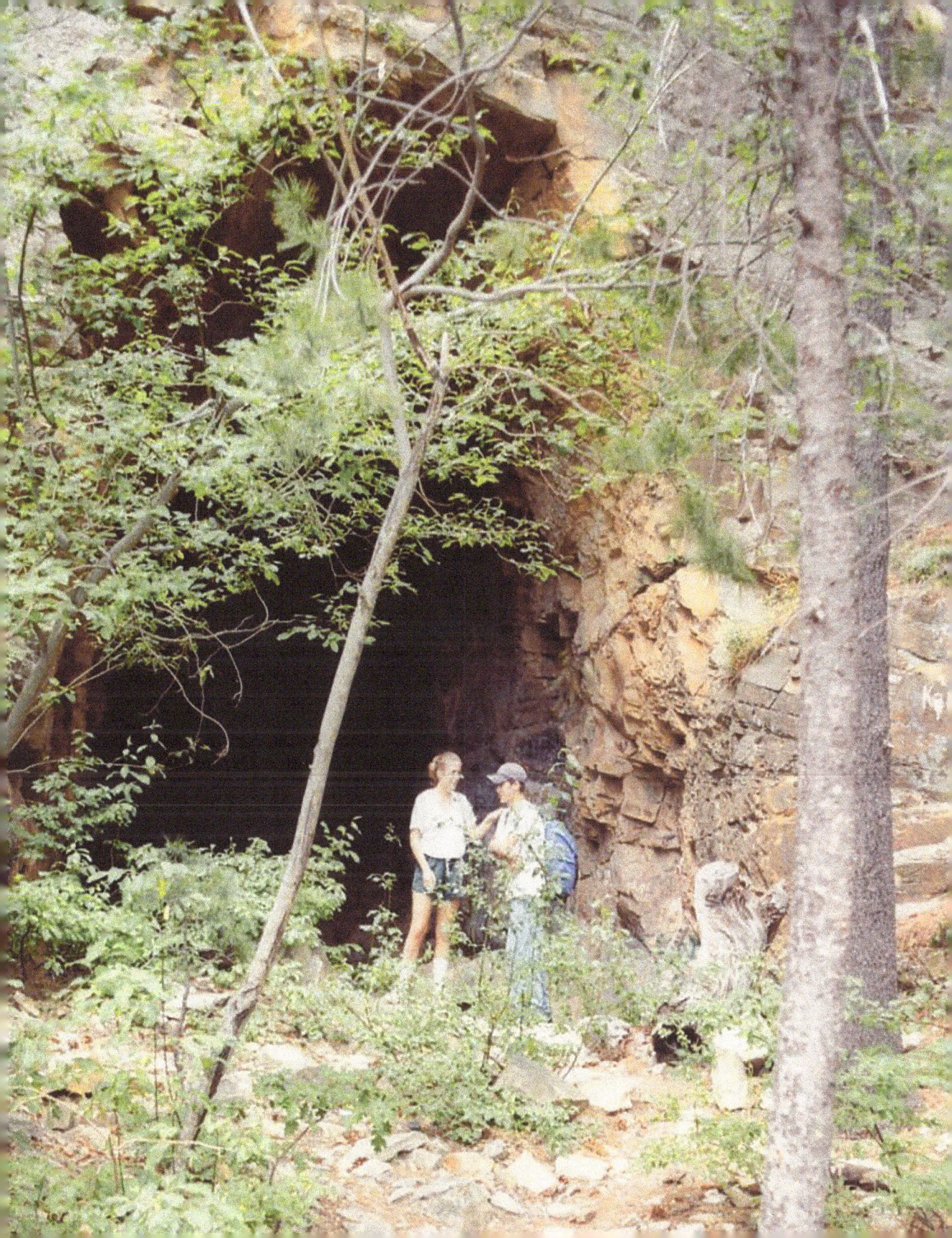

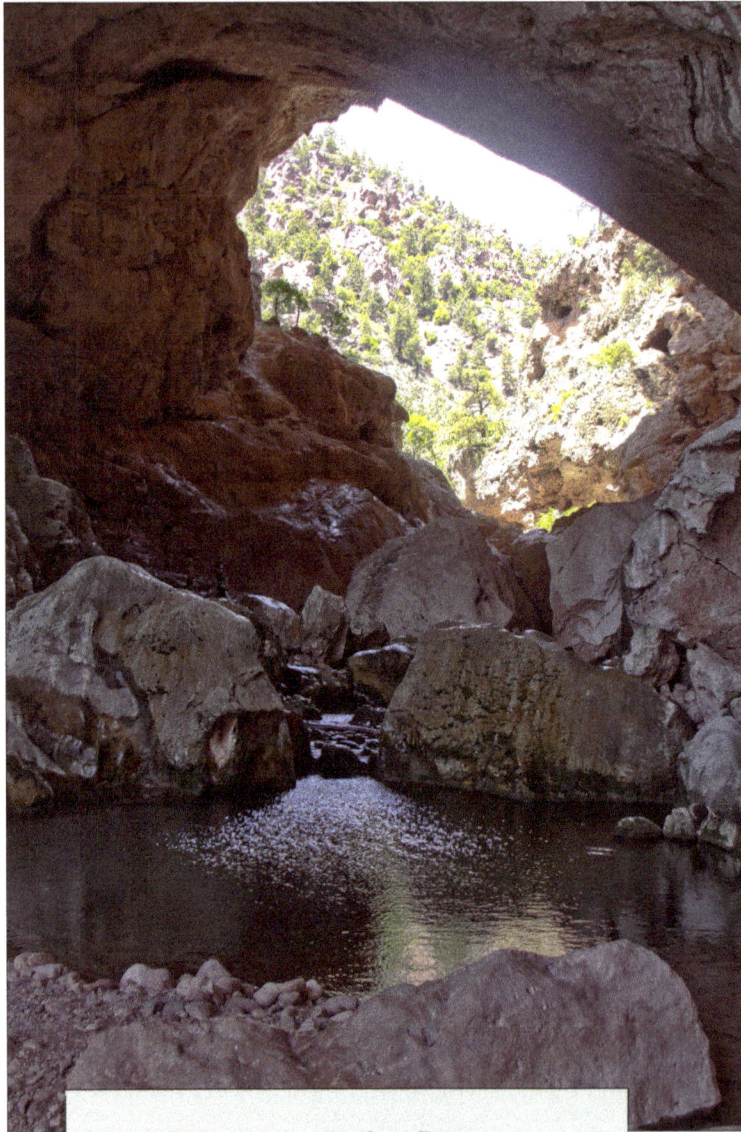

Tonto Natural Bridge

Tonto Natural Bridge State Park features a travertine bridge arching over Pine Creek, creating a rock-jumbled grotto, a perfect place to explore on a warm afternoon. The natural bridge was first discovered by prospector Dave Gowan in 1877. He returned in 1898, with a nephew from Scotland, to build a homestead. The men lowered their possessions by rope 500 feet into the canyon. The first road and lodge were built in the early 1900s. The present lodge, now used as park headquarters, was built in 1927 and is listed on the National Register of Historic Buildings.

To reach the State Park from Payson, drive north on SR 87 for 9 miles to mp 263.1 and turn west. The road descends steeply 3 miles to the entrance of the park where visitors pay a day use fee. Wide green lawns invite visitors to play and enjoy a picnic lunch after exploring the cavern.

Most visitors walk the trail descending into the grotto. Be careful! The rocks are very slick and it is easy to take a bad fall. The travertine bridge stands 183 feet at its highest point with a tunnel 400 feet in length and 150 feet at the widest point. While the creek water may look clear, it carries a load of minerals. The minerals form the deposits called travertine. Most visitors, enthralled by the bridge, miss a small natural spring located between the lodge and the bridge. The spring's water has been partly diverted for used by the park. As you explore, keep an eye out for snakes.

Driving Distance: 13 miles from Payson
Hiking Distance: .5 mile+
Rating: Moderate   Elevation: 5150' - 5000'
Best Season: Spring, summer, fall.
Special Features: Travertine bridge, historic lodge.
Precautions: Travertine is slick, proceed off the
        trail with great care.
Maps: Arizona Highways, Park map
Information: Tonto Natural Bridge State Park
        (928) 476-4202

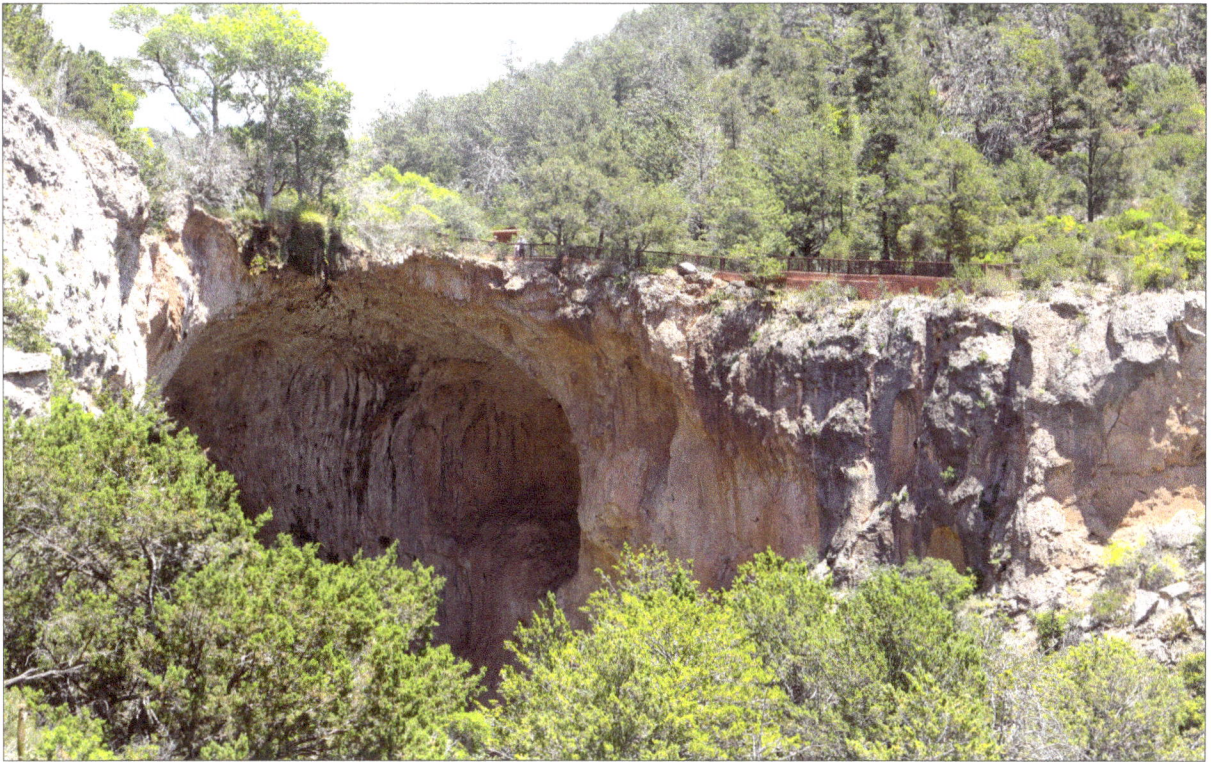

Tonto Natural Bridge

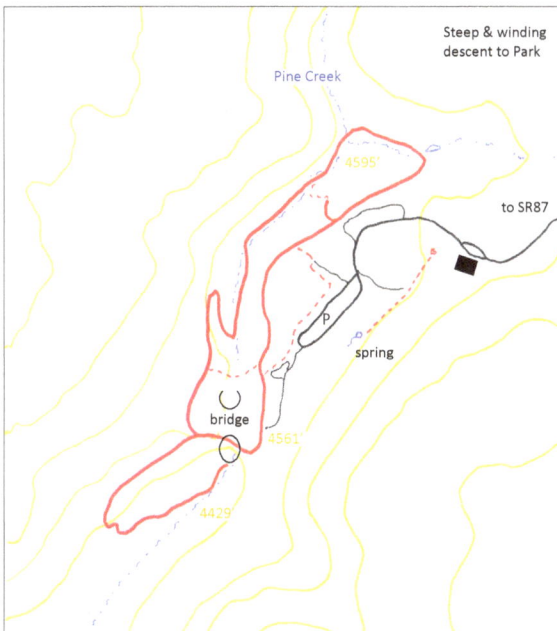

Ellison Creek / Verde River

Many of the creeks in this region drain into the East Verde River. There are several campgrounds along the East Verde. **Wagon Wheel campground** is located just below the confluence of **Ellison Creek** and the East Verde on Forest Road 199. To reach the campground turn east off of State Route 87 / Houston Mesa Road at mp 254.4. Drive just over 10 miles to the campground. Approaching the campground, there is a wet crossing - do not attempt to cross if the water is high. Beyond Water Wheel campground, are two more wet crossings.

From the campground, hikers can climb to the confluence with Ellison Creek and beyond. If rain is forecast along the rim, be aware that flash floods can sweep down the watercourse, carrying timber and other debris - a danger to those remaining in the river bed.

Horton Spring

Horton Spring pumps millions of gallons out of a hillside spring on the Mogollon Rim. The upper portion of the stream has beautiful little pools, perfect for a lazy afternoon. The creek disappears into the rocky streambed long before it reaches Tonto Creek.

Drive east from Payson on SR 260. Turn north at mp 268.7 and follow FR 289 to the bridge across Tonto Creek. If the small parking area is full there are some wide spots along the road. From the bridge, climb the east bank and follow the trail along the streambed. After the first mile, hikers catch glimpses of the creek. Social trails lead off to small pools. In the last mile, the trail leaves the creek and begins to switchback up a steep slope toward the spring.

Hikers top out on the hillside above the spring. The approach shows signs of overuse as vegetation is trampled into the dirt. The water flows from rock fractures in a shadowy glen with moss-covered rocks and pale yellow columbine bending toward the water. The cliffside path to the spring can be hazardous due to erosion.

Above the spring is a small primitive campground, popular with the Boy Scout Troops. Wandering along the stream on our return, we found a number of lovely spots among tall pines with wild flowers bending toward the water and photo-perfect icy pools. I jumped into a pool and the shock of the icy water seemed to rip the breath right out of my lungs. Refreshing!

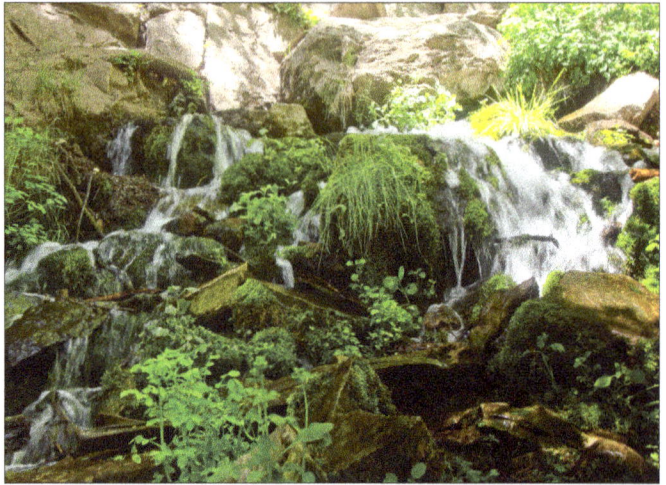

Photo: Horton Spring & Horton Creek

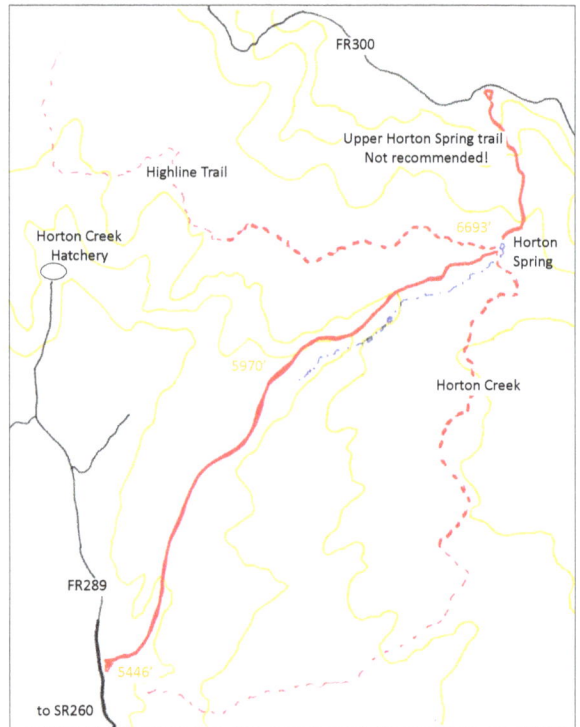

Driving Distance: 17 miles from Payson	thousands of gallons of water daily.
Hiking Distance: 4 miles one way	Precautions: Watch footing over loose trail rocks and
Rating: Moderate Elevation: 5480'	slippery rocks near spring.
Best Season: Late spring, summer, fall.	Maps: Tonto NFS map
Special Features: Natural spring producing	Information: Payson Ranger District (928) 474-7900

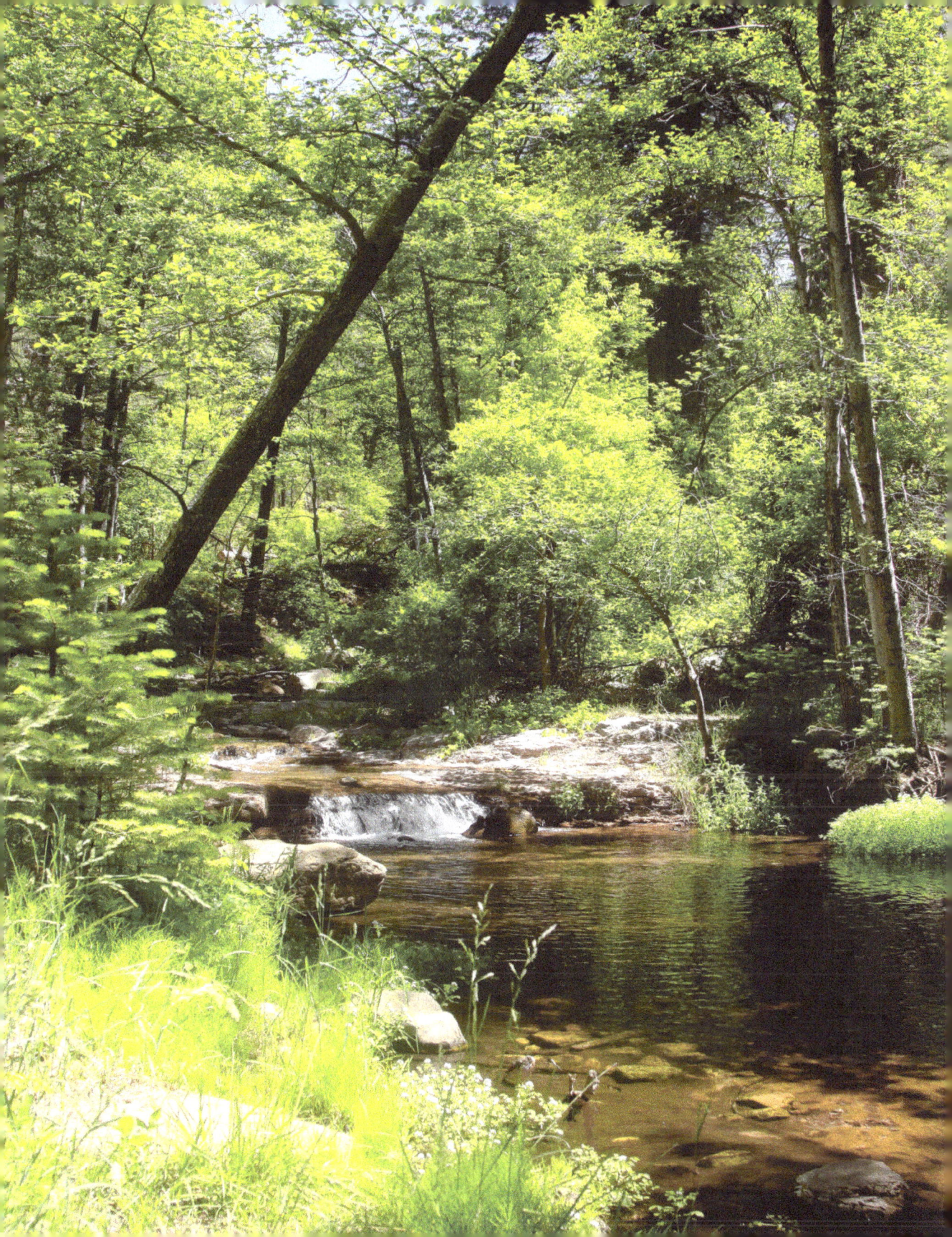

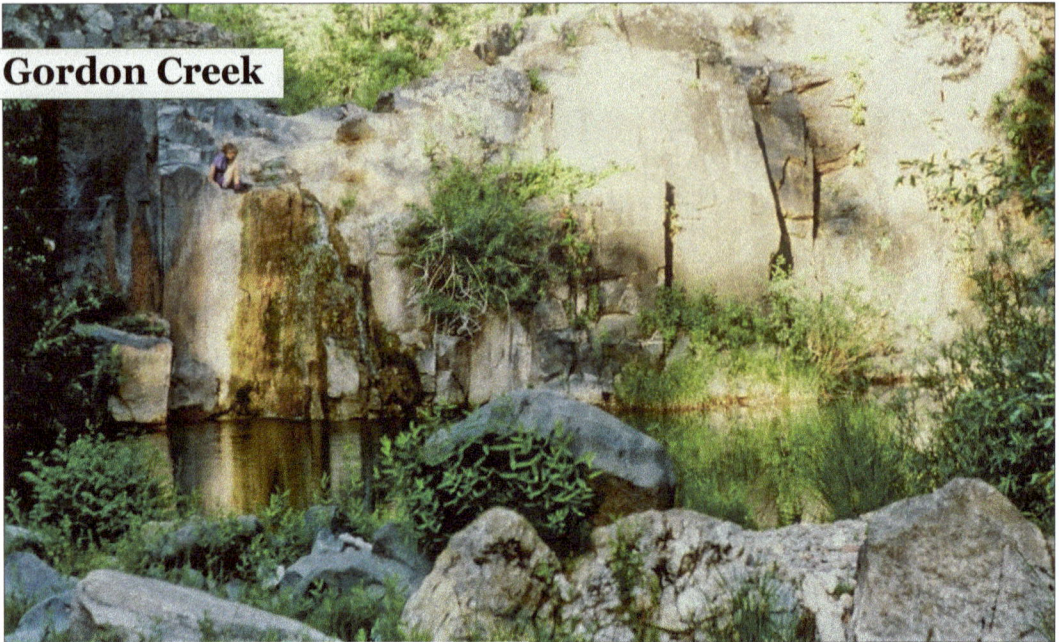

Gordon Creek

Gordon Creek is one of those incidental hikes that you either look for or stumble across. Turn south off SR260 at mp 277.2, drive 1.4 miles to the power line. Fifty yards beyond the power line is a dirt road. Park off the road but don't park in front of the metal gate as this is an access point to a ranch!

Follow the dirt road (not the power line) to a second metal gate and swing left. As you reach a pasture, direct your steps off to the right toward the entrance to a shallow canyon. This all takes a bit of route finding - no signs.

On years with more rainfall, small pools appear along the canyon floor. Hikers eventually reach a pour-over overlooking a large pool that spreads across the canyon bottom. We managed to work our way down below the pool but it was difficult. Below the pool the canyon is rough and hikers should turn back at the cliff edge without proceeding much further.

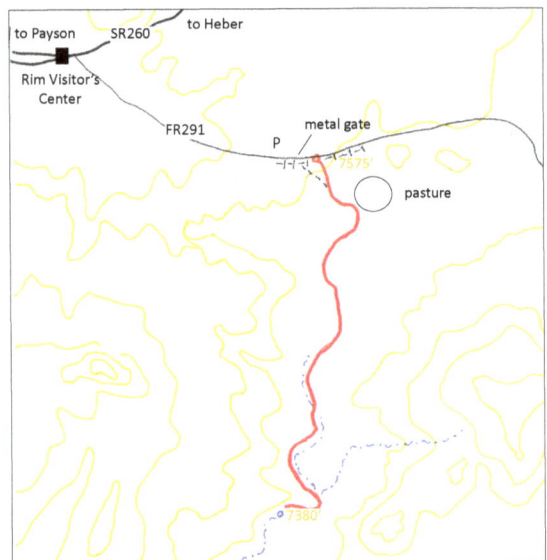

Driving Distance: 28 miles from Payson
Hiking Distance: 1.3 miles one way
Rating: Moderate   Elevation: 7,575- 7,380'

Best Season: Summer
Special Features: Beautiful creek with small water
     fall and green pool.
Precautions: Watch for flash floods during summer
     rainy season. Be careful when climbing
     around pool - a long way to medical help.
Maps: Tonto NFS map

Box Canyon / Christopher Creek

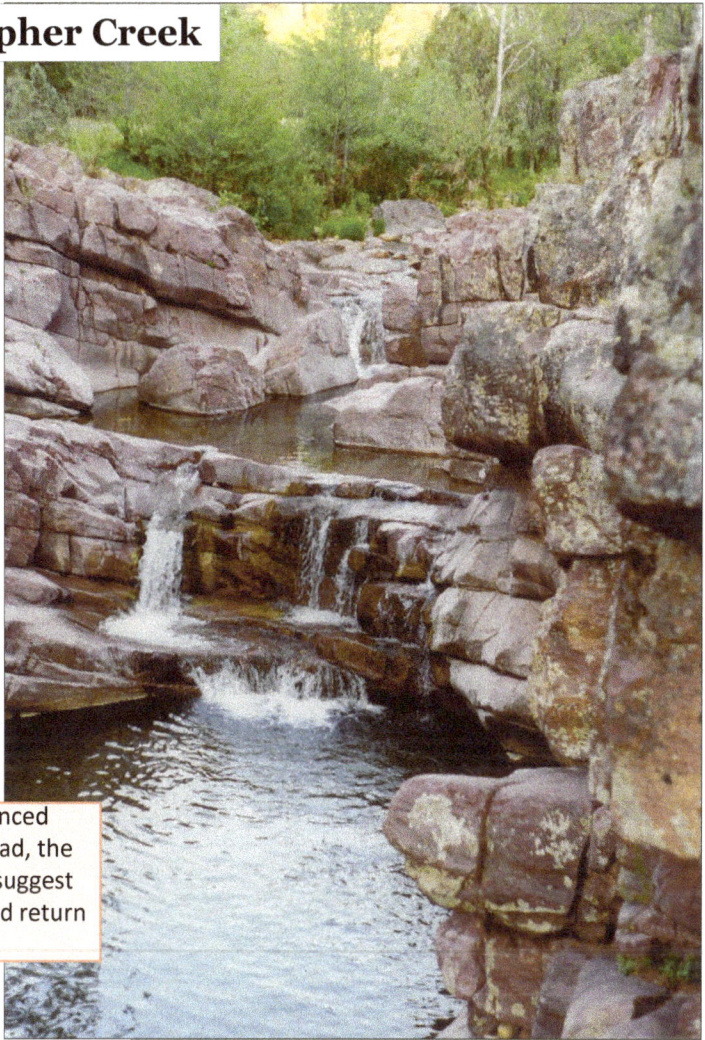

One of the most striking spots on the Rim near Payson has to be **Christopher Creek** as it runs through **Box Canyon.** Fractured rhyolite cliffs tower over deep green pools and streaks of falling water. Photographers find dramatic shots, using a wide angle lens, to capture this rocky canyon. It is also a great spot for a serious accident for the careless. This is not a good place for those averse to risk.

Drive 20 miles east from Payson on SR 260 to mp 271.3. This is just west of the Christopher Creek Campground. The trailhead is not easy to spot at 5o+ miles per hour. When SR 260 was widened, no room was left for parking and the trailhead was wiped out, making access along the road dangerous due to the speed of the traffic.

Warning: This hike is for more experienced hikers. Due to no parking at the trailhead, the only access is along the roadway. We suggest having a driver drop off passengers and return at a pre-arranged time.

A footpath proceeds south through the forest to the edge of the cliffs. At one point, the trails splits with the left fork descending a gentle slope toward the back of a Boy Scout facility. The camp is enclosed by a barb wire fence. Follow the streambed dowstream to Box canyon.

The right fork approaches the canyon rim and descends to the creek - the rock along the rim can be slick when wet - use caution! Hikers descend to the pools, climbing down the waterfalls.

Driving Distance: 19 miles from Payson.
Hiking Distance: .75 mile along cliff.
      1.25 mile by route behind Boy Scout camp.
Rating: Easy walk to the cliffs, steeper climb at falls.
Elevation: 5,400' - 5,650'
Best Season: Summer and fall.
Special Feature: Spectacular canyon, nice pools.
Precautions: Slick rock cliffs! Careful!
Maps: Tonto NFS map
Information: Payson Ranger Station
      (928)474-7900

Pivot Rock & Spring

Pivot Rock is located on the Mogollon Rim, north of the little town of Strawberry. The hike descends into a canyon to visit a small spring. The spring flows out of a dark recess in a limestone cliff. For those venturing deeper inside, the tunnel splits with the upper route revealing a glimpse of the streambed below. The lower route is a bit of a squeeze - not for those with claustrophobia!

Turn off SR87 onto FR616 and drive west about a mile to a parking area on the right side of the road. The trail head is located on the edge of the canyon but may not be signed.

Visitors who venture further down FR616 intersect FR149 in a small drainage. We turned into a primitive campground and began walking down the canyon to the first drainage on our right. This is the closest access to the rock formation known as Pivot Rock. Hikers can follow the canyon from the spring down to Pivot Rock but the canyon trail can be a bit overgrown.

This is a lovely area to explore with a trail leading north from the campground.

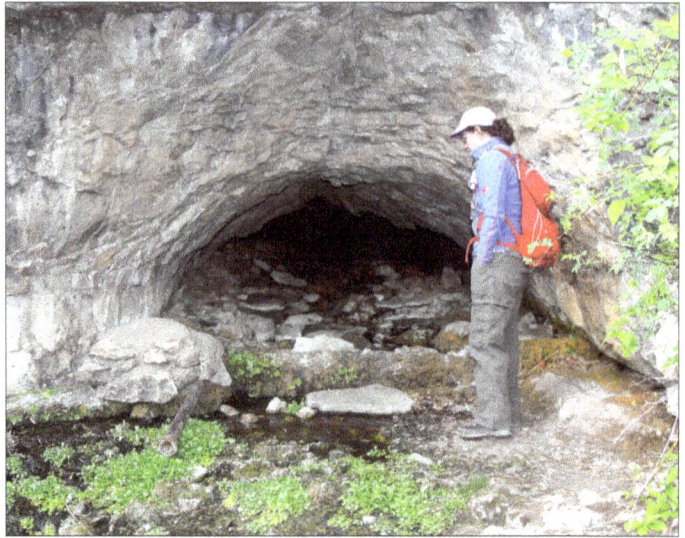

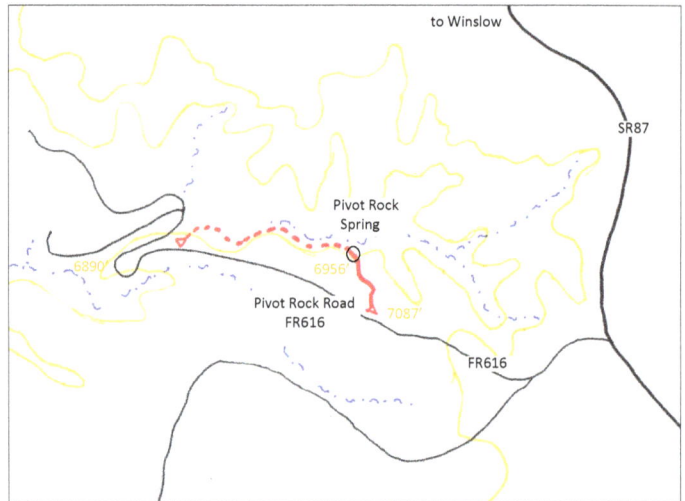

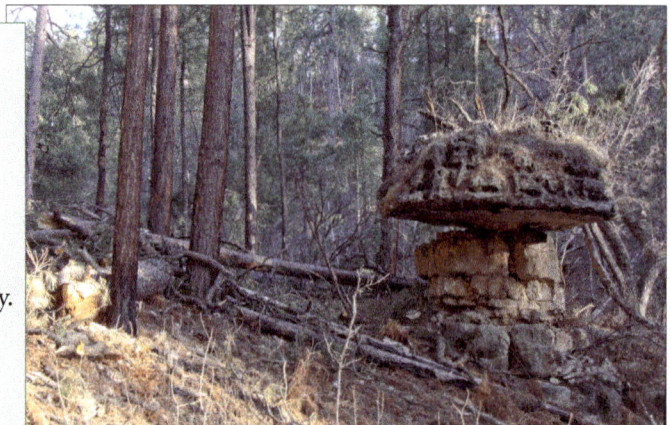

Driving Distance: 35 miles from Payson.
Hiking Distance: .75 mile
        1 mile from campground
Rating: Moderately easy.
Elevation: 7,087' - 6,890'
Best Season: Summer and fall.
Special Feature: Cave Spring, unique rock
Precautions: Route finding may be necessary.
Maps: Tonto NFS map
Information: Payson Ranger Station
        (928)474-7900

Tonto National Ruin

The region around Roosevelt Lake is home to a number of pueblo ruins, left by the ancient people who later assimilated into our modern day tribes. Early on, **Tonto National Ruin** was recognized as a pristine example of a pueblo despite the predation of pot hunters. In 1907, President Theodore Roosevelt sent a bill to Congress creating the Tonto National Ruin. Visitors are welcome to hike up the steep slope along a paved trail to the ruin where a docent is stationed to answer questions about the history and geology of the site. The paved path may take on a semblance of civilization but don't be fooled - this hike is a breath-stealer!

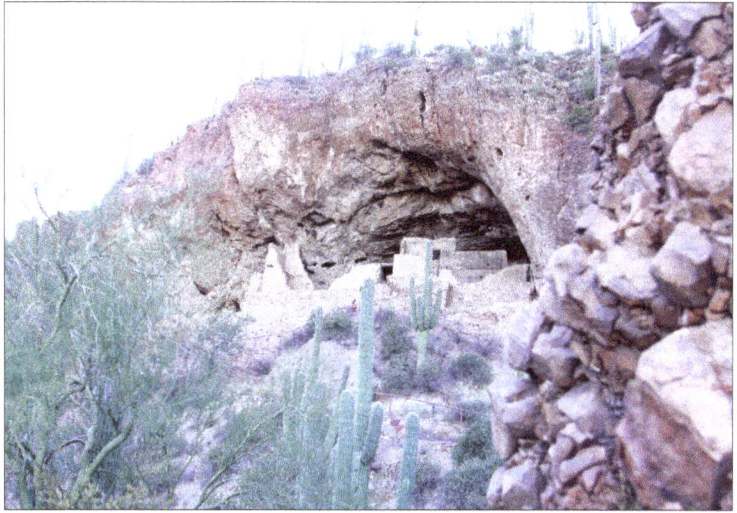

Top photo:
Tonto cliff Ruins

Bottom photo:
Canyon Point

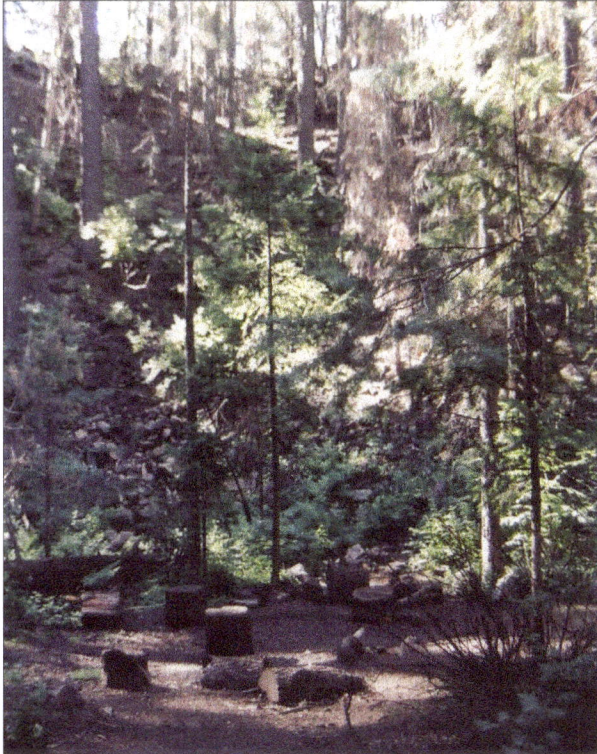

Canyon Point Sink Hole

This sink hole is one of the largest in Arizona and certainly the most accessible. The sinkhole is located just off State Route 260, south of Canyon Point Campground. Park at the campground's designated day use parking near the entrance station and follow the signs along the southern edge of the campground into the forest. An old dirt road guides hikers about a quarter mile to the sink hole. The route should be well marked but if not, ask for directions.

Sink holes give us a picture of the layers of rock and dirt beneath our feet. Unlike fine-grain volcanic rock, sandstone is porous. Water seeps through the rock and begins dissolving the minerals that fused the grains of sands together, creating fractures and caverns in the rock layers. When the weight of the earth can no longer be supported above a cavern, the roof collapses and a sink hole is formed. We know this sink hole happened long ago as we look at the mature trees growing in the depression. A short trail leads through the vegetation to the bottom of the pit.

Sierra Anchas / Parker Creek

The Tonto Basin once drew cattlemen and sheep herders to the meadows under the Mogollon Rim. Today, the residents of the community of Young drive a long way to shop in an urban area.

The southern approach, begins with an iron bridge over the Salt River, south of Roosevelt Lake. After miles of two-lane asphalt dipping and rising with the terrain, the road turns away from the lake and begins climbing into the Sierra Ancha Mountains.

On several occasions I've stopped to look out from the cliffs as range after range of purple mountains extend into the distance. The cliffs have been riven by powerful subterreanean forces, exposing vertical cracks of red rock that glow with the last rays of the setting sun. This is ranch land and drivers should be wary of coming across a cow sidling down the middle of the road, oblivious to the recreational driver. SR288 climbs into the ponderosa pine, crossing several major watersheds. We would suggest exploring along two creeks.

One, the **Parker Creek trail**, #160, is found 19 miles from the junction of 88/288 at the Parker Experimental Station. There is no established parking for day use visitors. The trailhead is located on the Station.

Hikers follow the trail, climbing along Parker Creek, under large sycamore and pine. Silvery streams of water trace a route from red-rock ledges. A water gauge is located about a half mile from the trail head. The path climbs four and a half miles to FR487, passing through three vegetation zones. Two decades ago, a wildfire swept through the higher peaks above the Station. Vegetation has reclaimed the steep slopes and the risk of flash flooding has diminished. However, the trail still shows a bit of debris and fallen logs.

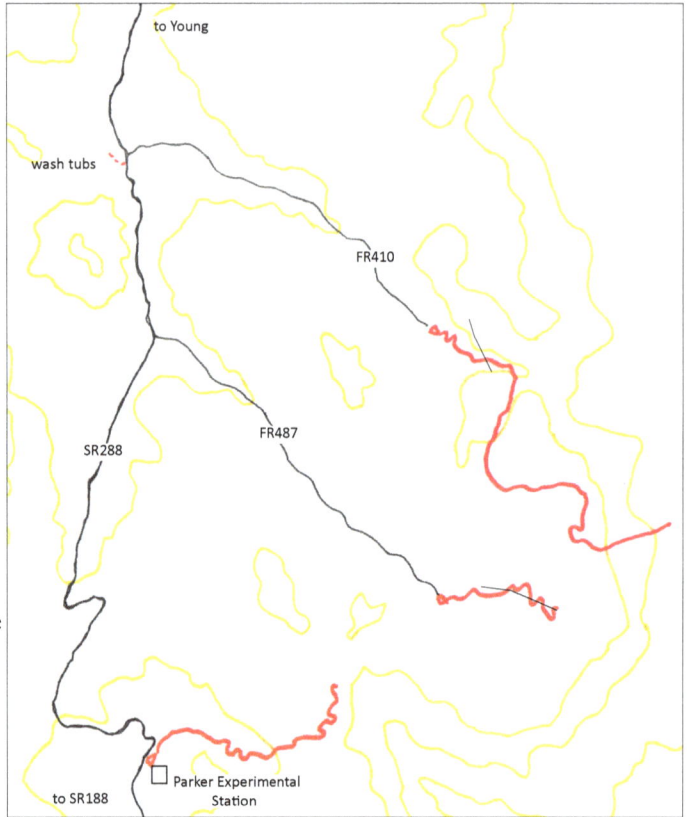

Parker Creek:
Driving Distance:
19 miles from Jct. 88/288
Hiking Distance:
4.5 miles one way, or any distance one chooses.
Rating: Moderately difficult
Elevation: 5,090 - 7,100
Special Features: Old Experimental Station
Precautions: Loose rock underfoot, rattlesnakes
Information: Tonto Visitors Center at Roosevelt Lake (928) 467-2236

Workman Creek Falls & the Wash Tubs

Five miles past the Experimental Station is another favorite stop at Workman Creek. A few yards downstream, visitors can find a set of descending pools along the creekbed called the **Wash Tubs**. Hollowed out of gray basalt, the pools do resemble old fashioned galvanized tubs. A small foot path cuts through heavy brush and tall grass to this site though some hikers prefer to bushwhack along the creek.

Turning east along the north bank of the creek, a dirt road follows the terrain, climbing up Aztec Peak. This is a popular route as the road crosses **Workman Creek** above one of the tallest waterfalls in Arizona. During snowmelt, the creek may leave the road impassable. As the flow diminishes, a spidery stream of water remains with the spray swept upward by the wind.

Visitors often park along the road and peer into the gorge below, gawking at the waterfall. Don't assume the rocks under your feet are secure! A few years ago, a Boy Scout was swept from the edge as the rocks collapsed into the gorge. Those who venture beyond the falls may continue on to Aztec Lookout tower, once the home of environmentalist Edward Abby. Camp sites and social trails are popular on the mesa above, giving hikers an opportunity to explore.

Further along SR 288, **Reynolds Creek** is another favorite stop with a foot path up the narrow canyon. The community is mostly private residences, some of which serve as bed & breakfast enterprises. The area is popular with hunters and all-terrain vehicle operators. From Young, many miles remain before visitors arrive at State Route 260 between Heber and Payson.

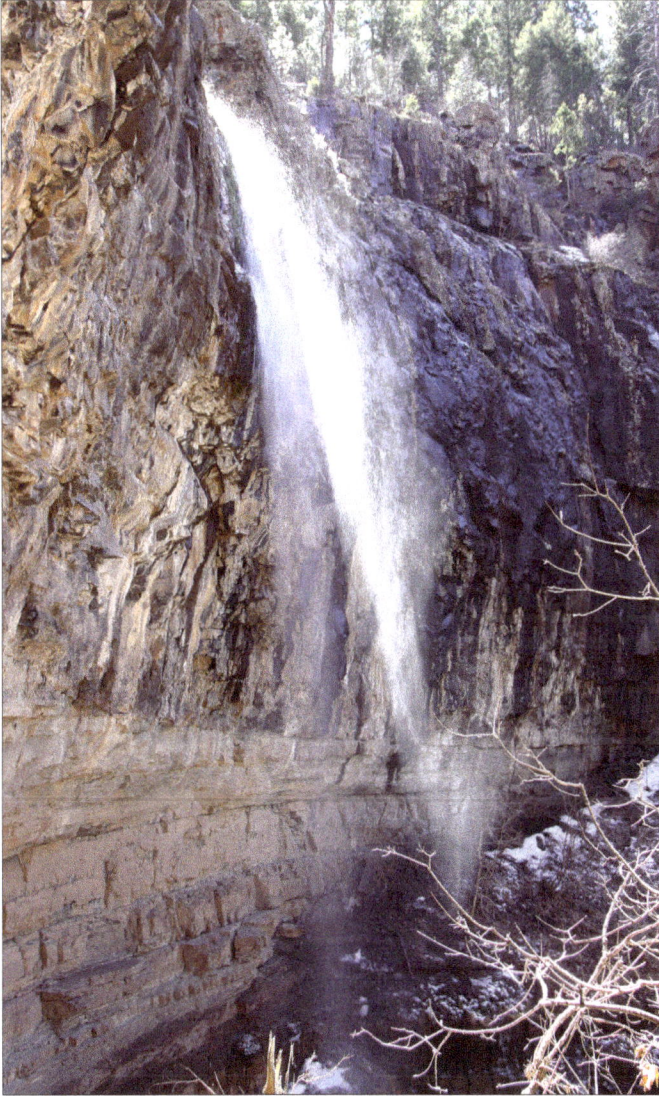

Workman Creek Falls on Aztec Peak

Why I avoid Camelback Mountain and the Urban Landscape.

How many million people live in the Valley of the Sun? Some weekends it seems as if at least a quarter of the population have come to the trails of the Valley and many fail to be courteous to other hikers. Firefighters are called to rescue those unprepared for hiking in the heat or those who get in trouble off the trail. Trail etiquette goes a long way toward sharing the trail and allowing everyone to enjoy their time outdoors. Here are some tips for trail etiquette:

1) Pick up your trash and take it out with you!

2) Uphill hikers have the right of way. Please be considerate and move to one side to allow them to pass, unless they indicate otherwise.

3) Do not create your own shortcuts or use existing shortcuts as this creates erosion and can cause confusion for those less experienced in hiking.

4) If you see someone in trouble, take a moment to stop and offer help.

5) Loud conversation and rude comments are verbal trash. Talk quietly and enjoy the silence that will flood your soul.

6) Like any dog owner, I would prefer to let my dog off the leash to enjoy a great run. However, this may prove to be a problem for other hikers. When coming up on another hiker, please bring your dog under your physical control until the other hiker is well past your location.

7) In hot climates, either leave the dog at home or take a considerable amount of water for the dog to drink! Too many dogs are dying on Valley trails due to the heat and the ignorance of their owners!

Camelback Mountain

This trail was once a premier urban trail experience. Now it has become a race track for exercise enthusiasts and scores of hikers. Parking is difficult with a long line of cars waiting for an open spot at the entrance. The trail is located off McDonald on Echo Canyon Place, just east of Tatum Blvd. Gates to the parking lot are closed from sunset to sunrise.
Hiking Distance: approx. 1.75 miles one way
Rating: moderate
Elevation: 1350 - 2050'

Piestewa Peak #300

The trail is located on Piestewa Peak Drive just off Lincoln Drive between 22nd & 24th Street. Look for the parking lot on the left.
The Mesquite trail circles the mountain. The Summit trail rises above the parking lot, turning northeast to follow a ridge before swinging to the back side of the peak in its final ascent.
Hiking distance: 1.2 miles one way
                     Nature Trail 1.52 miles
Rating: Moderate
Elevation: 1400' - 2080'

Tom's Thumb

This prominant rock formation is located on the north side of the McDowell Mountains. From Interstate 101, turn north onto Pima Road. Drive east on Happy Valley Road to Ranch Gate Road. Turn south onto 128th Street. Drive south to Paraiso Drive and turn east to the parking area. From the trailhead, the trail switchbacks up a ridge and into a small valley before the final ascent to the base of the 'thumb'.
Hiking Distance: 4.8 miles
Rating: Moderately Difficult
Elevation Gain: 1350 '

Central Arizona - Phoenix

At 1,100 feet elevation, Phoenix is definitely in the arid zone we think of as desert. Once a farming community with fields of cotton and citrus groves, now asphalt and tract homes seemseem to multiply month by month.

The saguaro and barrel cacti are iconic symbols of the Valley of the Sun. But as the Desert Botanical Gardens will witness, there is so much more to desert than cacti. Some of our most amazing creatures live in the arid climate and give us a demonstration of how they have adapted to a climate with heat and scarce moisture. We would be wise to pay attention and appreciate the diversity.

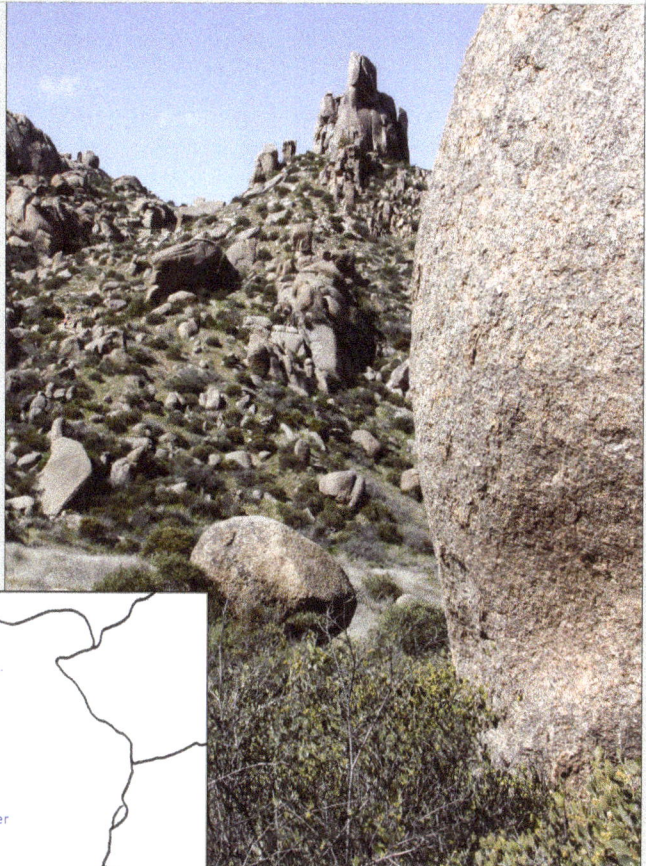

1 Camelback/Piestewa/Tom Thumb
2 Ash Creek at Dugas
3 Badger Spring Wash
4 Agua Fria at Black Canyon
5 Jewel of the Creek & Dragonfly
6 Hassayampa River Preserve
7 Waterfall trail & White Tanks
8 Fatman's Pass & Hidden Valley
9 Peralta Canyon
10 Hieroglyphic trail
11 Boulder & LaBarge Canyons
12 Fish Creek
13 Wind Cave & Usery State Park
14 Desert Botanical Garden
       & Papago Buttes

Along the trail to Tom's Thumb

Communities throughout the valley have made an effort to preserve a portion of the basin and range landscape for future generations. Green space is important within such a large urban center. However, as noted on the opposite page, many of the desert preserves are being over-run. We need to carefully think more about how we manage our open space so that all can have the opportunity to enjoy the outdoors.

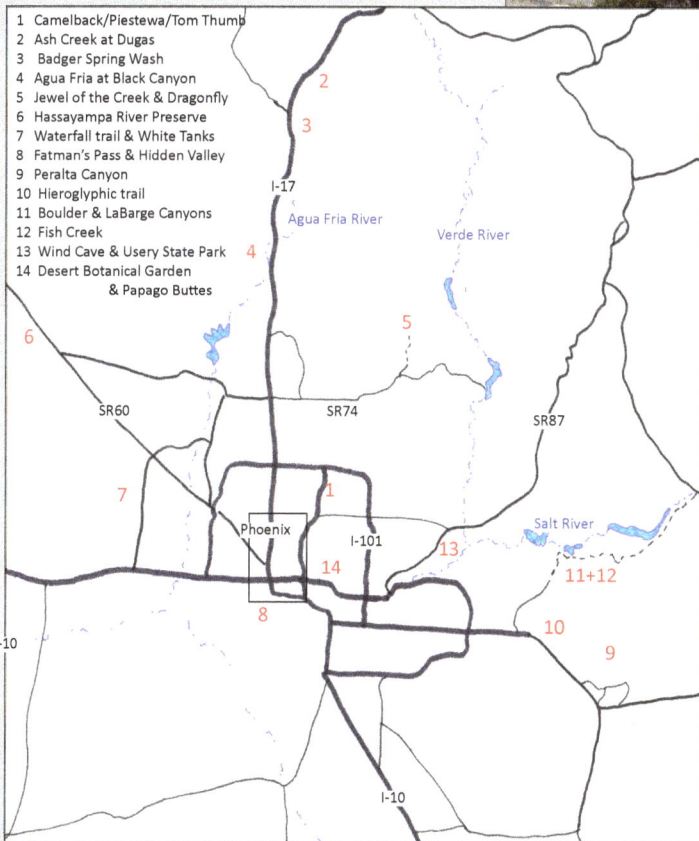

121

The I-17 Corridor

Interstate 17 between Phoenix and Flagstaff is a busy corridor with drivers either racing toward our largest urban metropolis or those racing north to our smaller communities in the high country. Traffic back-ups are frequent and frustrating. Drivers looking out over the hills of dried brush may wonder what lies beyond their line-of-sight from the freeway. We highlight three areas as little pockets of quiet away from the raceway.

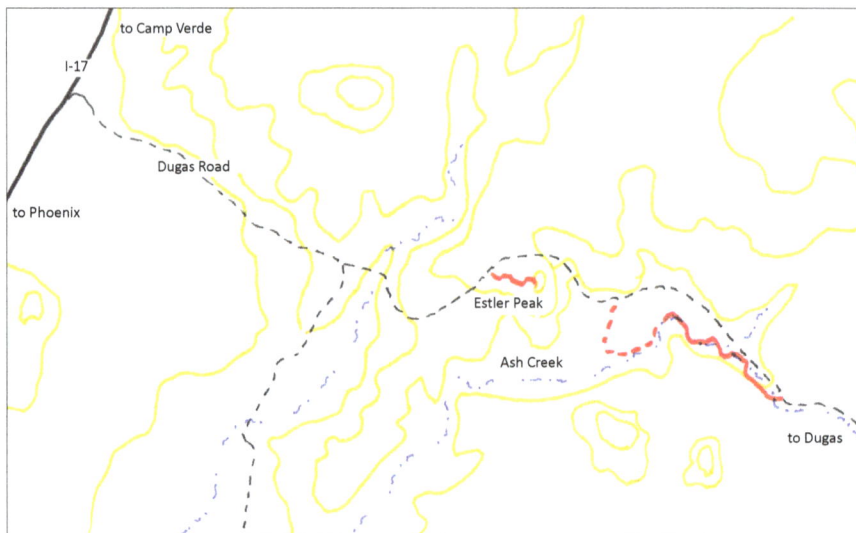

Ash Creek off Dugas Road

Dugas Road takes motorists back to an old ranching community. All that remains of the little community are a couple of private residences in the shadow of an old wind mill. A section of this road parallels Ash Creek. In the spring, this little stream can be a great place to sit and read in the shade of giant cottonwood and do a little boulder hopping as long as the creek isn't flooding with run-off.

From I-17, turn east onto Dugas Road and drive past Estler Peak to a point where the road dips down to within a few yards of the watercourse. Find a good place to pull to the side of the road and make your way through the brush down into the streambed.

We've found trees with the roots exposed four feet high. The erosion speaks to the volume of water that can course along this channel. In the spring, small pools remain with the water trickling through the rock-studded creek. We boulder-hopped along the creek bed, looking to see what small treasures we could find.

Badger Spring Wash / Agua Fria Monument

For motorists along I-17, Sunset Point Rest Aea sends out a siren call to stretch our legs or use the facilities. Take a closer look at exit 256 exit just north of Sunset Point. A barren dirt lot lies below the level of the freeway with a dirt track tracing a route east into the sun-scarred hills. A sign on I-17 identifies this as the Agua Fria National Monument; with not a building in sight.

Parking below the freeway, follow the dirt track east as it drops into the Agua Fria River watercourse. In just under a mile the trail comes to a rocky wash. After a good year of snowmelt, there will be run-off in the river bed. Other times of the year, the wash is mostly dry. Badger Spring doesn't release much water from the aquifer these days as the increase in population is slowly dropping the water table.

During the summer this hike is a bit warm. In the spring and late fall, hikers should watch for rattlesnakes along the trail. They prefer the shade of a bush or large rock on a warm day - if you take a break, look closely at the ground around your feet to ensure that you're not straying into their territory.

Agua Fria River Trail at Black Canyon

Many motorists notice the sign for Rock Springs Pies and Cafe as they drive south through Black Canyon City. Most don't notice the trail down to the Agua Fria River below Rock Springs.

The river descends from the high country, passing under I-17, through this small community and on to Lake Pleasant. This short section of the Black Canyon trail drops into a green riparian zone along the Agua Fria. Take exit 242 to the west side of the freeway. Turn north onto the frontage road, then west onto Warner Road. In a quarter mile a large parking area and trailhead are on the right side of the dirt road.

The trail descends over three quarters of a mile to the riverbed and most of the trail is exposed - this is not a trail to do in the heat of summer. However, in the spring months a nice pool remains, created by winter runoff and a natural spring. Local residents enjoy a little time off in this oasis.

This hike is part of a longer trail stretching from Cordes Junction down to SR74, just east of Lake Pleasant.

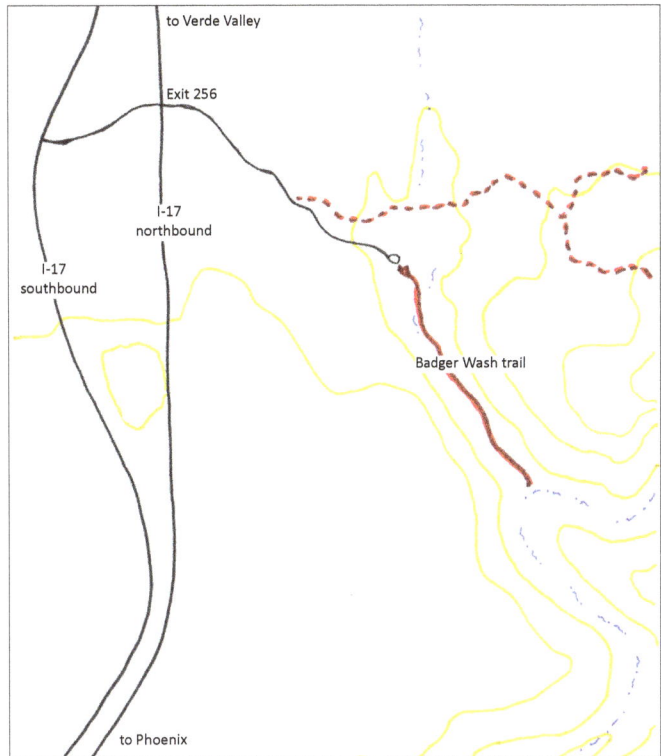

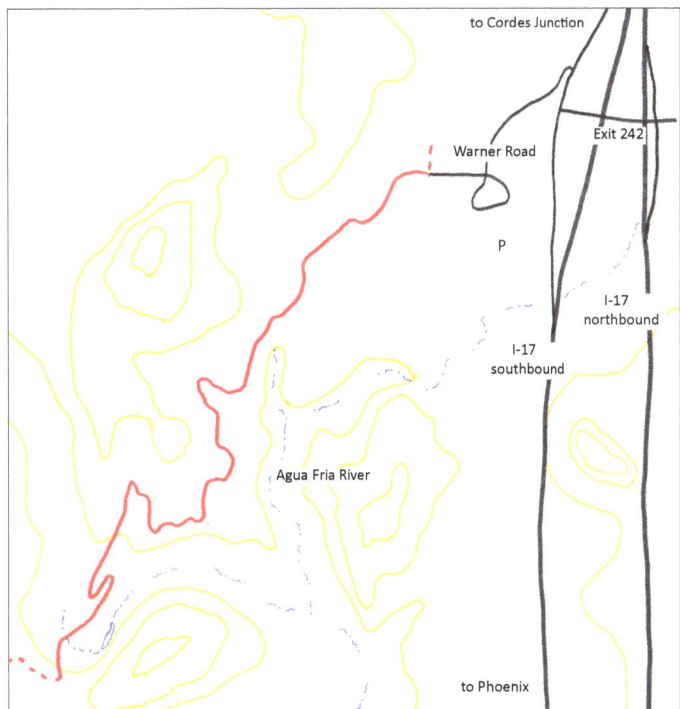

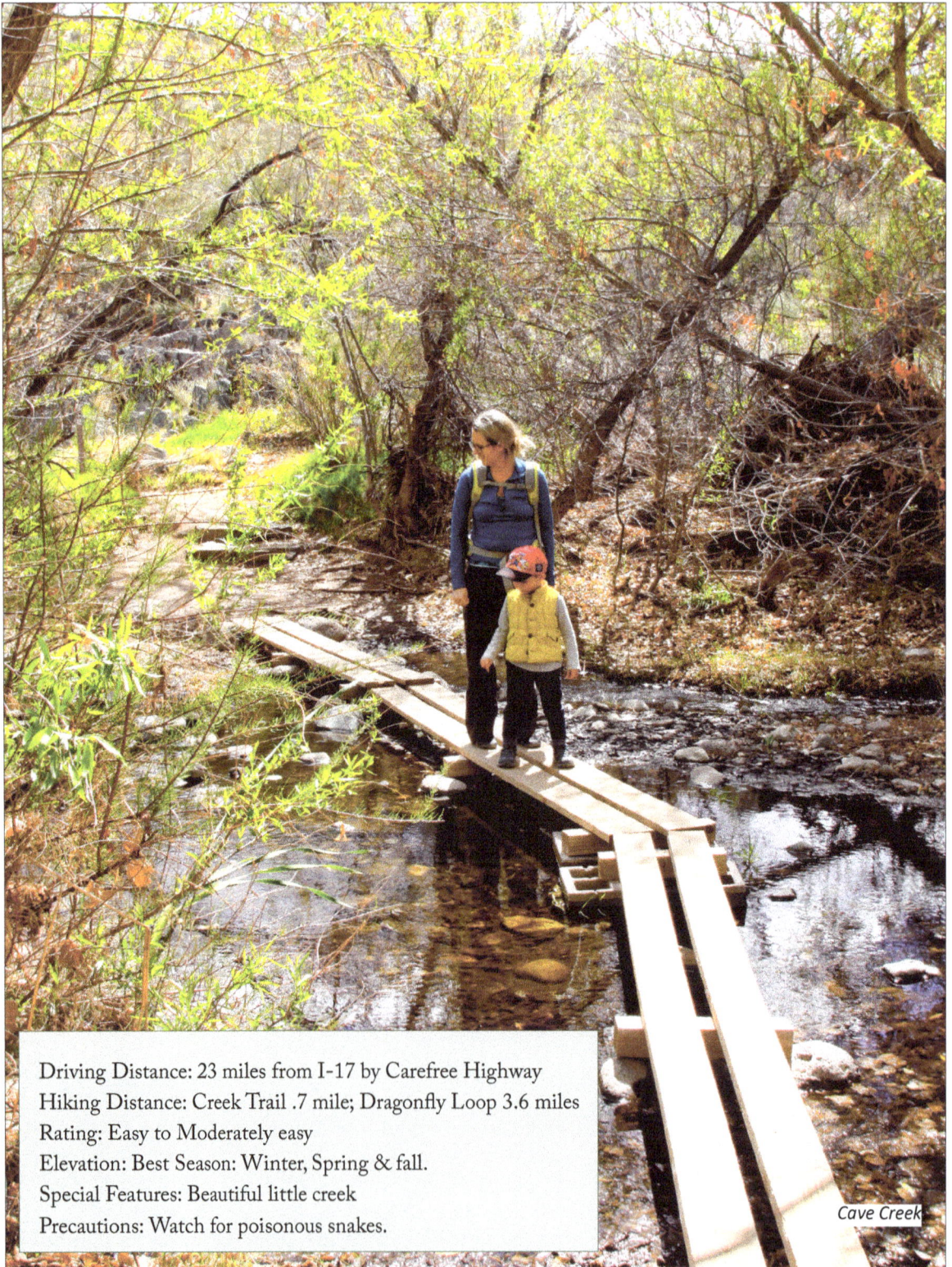

Driving Distance: 23 miles from I-17 by Carefree Highway
Hiking Distance: Creek Trail .7 mile; Dragonfly Loop 3.6 miles
Rating: Easy to Moderately easy
Elevation: Best Season: Winter, Spring & fall.
Special Features: Beautiful little creek
Precautions: Watch for poisonous snakes.

Cave Creek

Cave Creek / Jewel of the Creek and the Dragonfly Loop

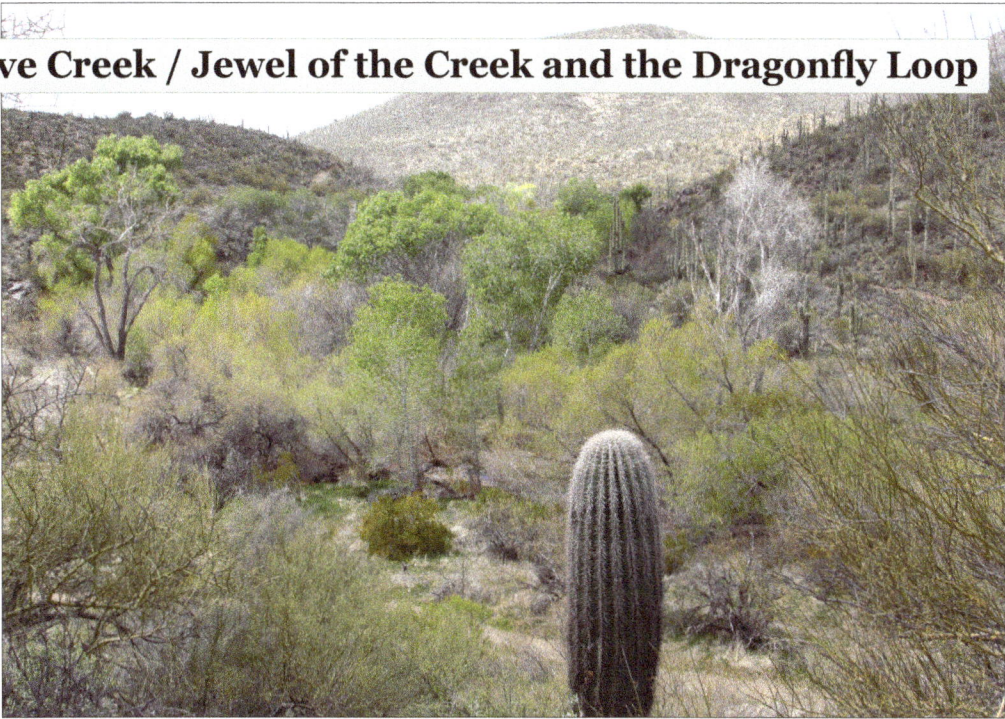

This little trail, part of a larger network of trails, is aptly named a Jewel. Springs contribute to the flow of the creek which nurtures a lovely riparian area along the watercourse.

To reach this section of Cave Creek, drive I-17 to exit #223 and turn east onto the Cave Creek Highway. Drive 26 miles and turn north onto Spur Cross Road. Drive through a small neighborhood as the route twists and turns, staying on Spur Cross as the pavement turns to dirt. Just over 7 miles from the Carefree Highway, turn into one of two parking areas.

The trail descends into a large wash and follows the wash south to a footbridge. After about a half mile, the trail splits and hikers can turn left to cross the creek again, returning to the parking lot.

This route is also part of the Dragonfly loop trail. Many hikers turn right and ascend the hillside to top out on the mesa. Dragonfly dips through a couple of washes before descending right toward the parking areas for a total of 3.9 miles.

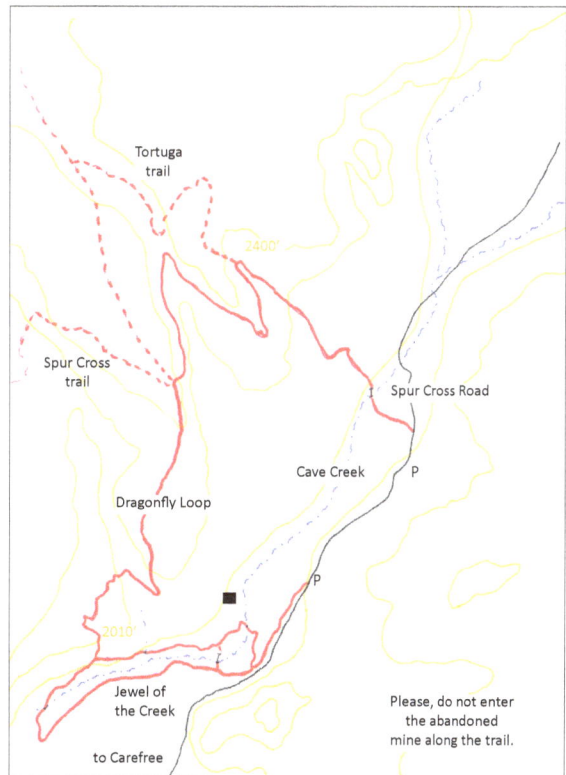

Tortuga trail

Spur Cross trail

Spur Cross Road

Cave Creek

P

Dragonfly Loop

P

Jewel of the Creek

to Carefree

Please, do not enter the abandoned mine along the trail.

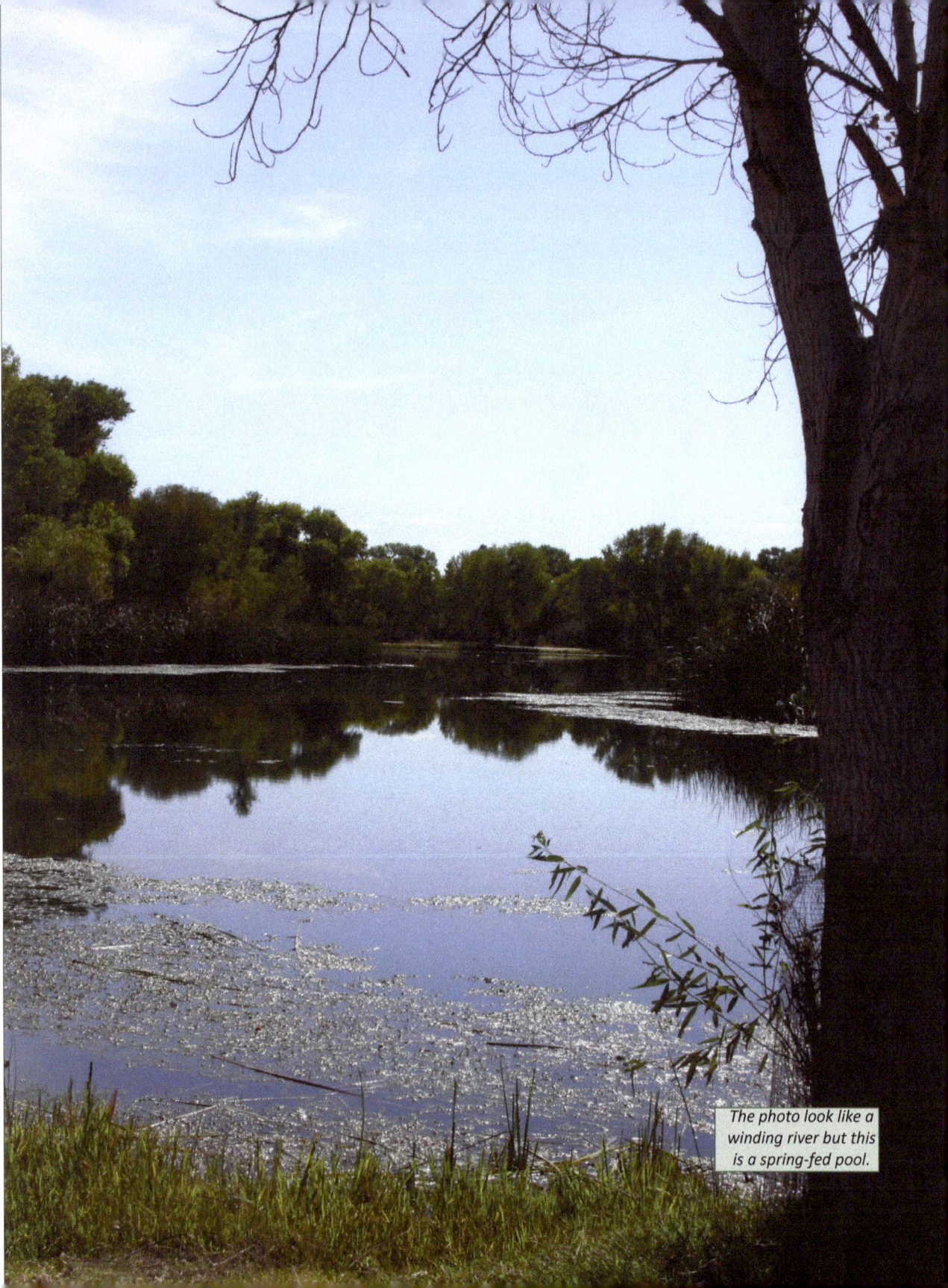

The photo look like a winding river but this is a spring-fed pool.

Hassayampa River Preserve

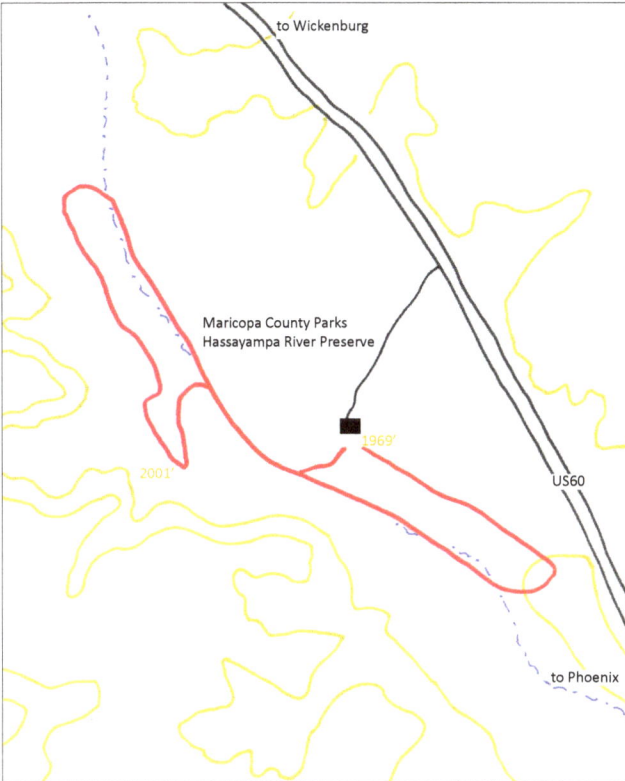

In the late 1800's, small gold strikes lured prospectors to the banks of the Hassayampa River. As stories were traded about mining prospects, the legend began that anyone who drank the water of the Hassayampa could never tell the truth again.

As mining petered out, private investors established a country club in the wetlands along US 60. A marsh was partly drained and a small lake created for members to enjoy.

The Nature Conservancy eventually purchased the site with 770 acres around the lake, creating the Hassayampa River Preserve. The property includes tall palms, a mesquite bosque with willow and old cottonwood trees. The lake was retained, part of it as an algae-covered marsh. The wetlands are supported by 26 springs, along the Hassayampa River.

Hikers follow the trail around the lake to a large open pool. Other trails descend to the Hassayampa River and a network of trails in the riverbed. Visitors may catch a glimpse of racoons, javelina, coyotes and mule deer along the hiking trails and streambed. Ducks nest is the reeds along the shoreline of the pool. We also met a couple of cows.

The Preserve is now a Maricopa County Regional Park. The Visitors Center is open Wednesday through Sunday, 8:00-5:00. The entrance is located off US 60 at mp 114, three miles south of Wickenburg. Turn west through the gate and park in the lot. Check in at the Visitors' Center. There is a fee to enter the park and use the trails.

Driving Distance: 3 miles from Wickenburg,
        55 miles from central Phoenix.
Hiking Distance: Palm Lake - .5 mile,
        River loop - 1.5 mile
Rating: Easy   Elevation: 1969 - 2001'
Best Season: Winter, spring & fall.
Special Features: Small Lake and wildlife.
Precautions: Be careful to leave only footprints
        as this area is important to wildlife.
Maps: Visitors' guide booklet
Information: Hassayampa River Preserve
                (928) 684-2772

The **White Tank Mountains** rise along the western edge of the Valley of the Sun. Once the home of the Hohokam, the area must have been popular due to the Hassayampa River to the north and the Agua Fria River a little further east. Both rivers brought water to the Hohokam canals. Petroglyphs dot the volcanic rock of the range as a fingerprint of the ancient tribe.

As metropolitan Phoenix has spread west, the range has become a popular area for hikers, horse owners and campers. To reach the White Tanks from Interstate 303, take the Dunlap/Olive exit, driving west. Olive Avenue ends at the park entrance. A gatehouse overlooks the entrance to the park with the gate locked at 10:00 pm. An entry fee may be charged either at the gatehouse or Visitors Center. Follow the main road as it swings right or north along the base of the mountain range. Most of the trails begin on the left side of the road and trailheads are signed.

Waterfall Trail

One of the most popular trails each spring is the **Waterfall trail** leading to a thin stream of water flowing over a rock face and into a shallow pool in a rocky cleft.

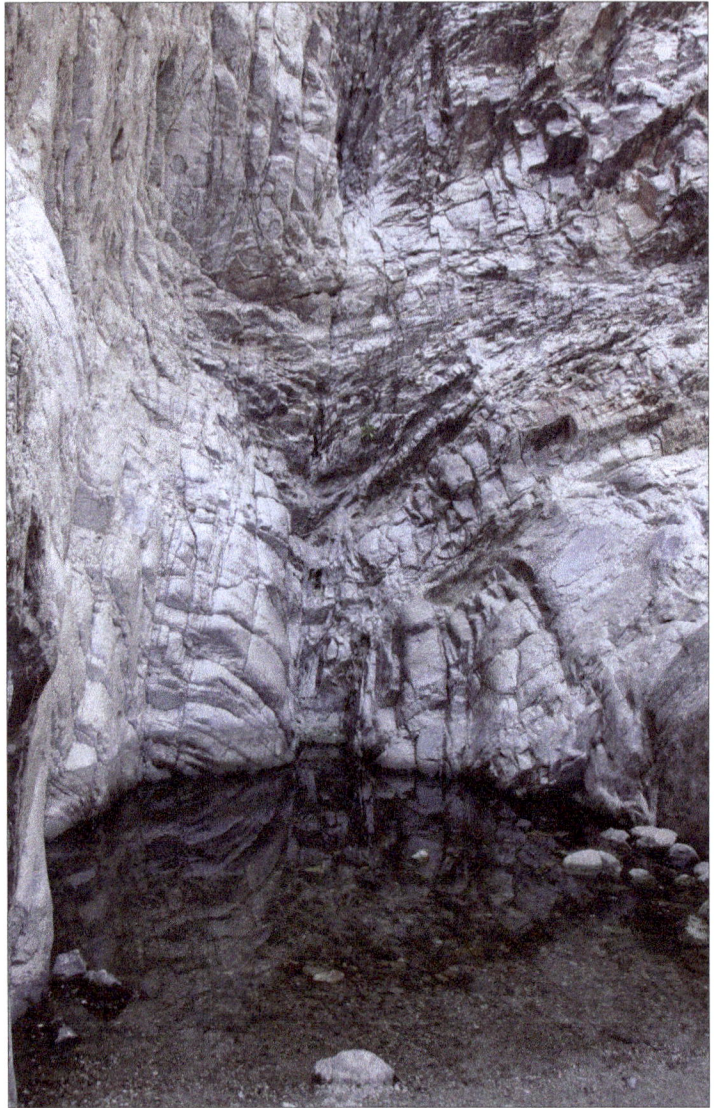

Waterfall pool

Driving into the park, turn into Use Area #6 and park in the large lot. The trailhead is at the west end of the parking lot. Early risers appreciate the desert sunrise before visitors crowd the trail.

For the first three quarters of a mile the trail is relatively flat. Look for flowering cactus and petroglyphs. At .75 of a mile, the trail passes a water storage tank on the right. A rock face behind the tank has a panel of petroglyphs. The final quarter mile is a rocky scramble to the foot of the waterfall. The time to see the waterfall is after a rain or during the winter; otherwise it may be dry. Hikers can feel a distinct change in the air when water falls through the crevice, leaving the canyon a cool refuge in the warmer months.

Waterfall Trail and White Tank Mountain Regional Park

Waterfall Trail
Driving Distance: 10-plus miles
Hiking Distance: 1 mile
Rating: Easy
Elevation: 1560'-2480'
Best Season: Winter & spring
Special Features: Waterfall
Precautions: Watch for poisonous
    reptiles.
Maps: Maricopa Parks &
    Recreation map
Information: (602) 506-2930

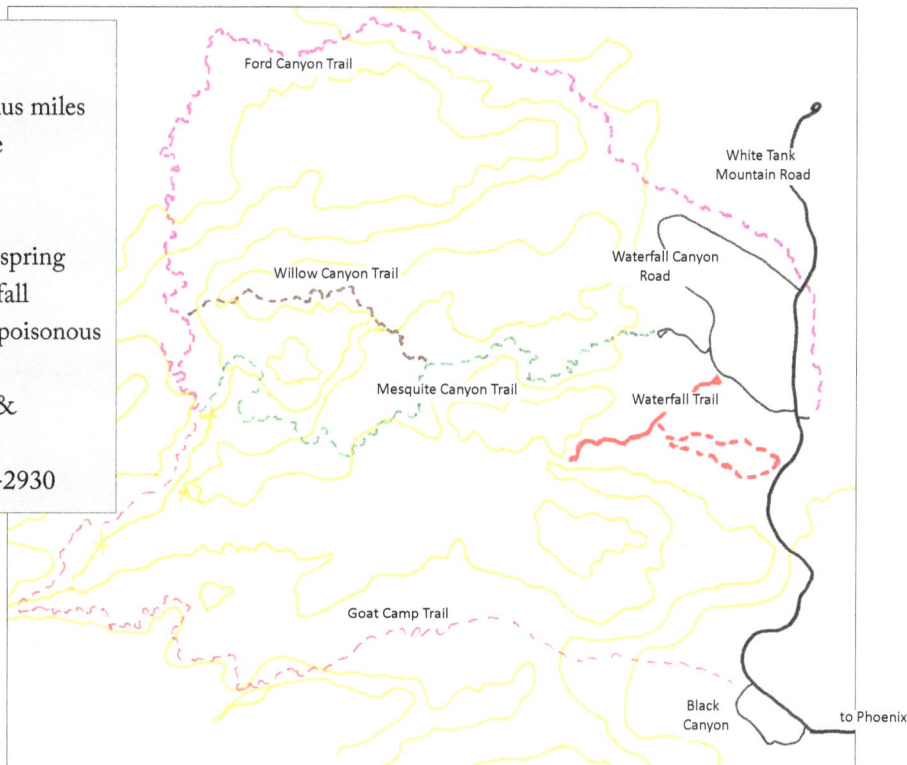

Ford Canyon Trail

White Tank
Mountain Road

Willow Canyon Trail

Waterfall Canyon
Road

Mesquite Canyon Trail

Waterfall Trail

Goat Camp Trail

Black
Canyon

to Phoenix

A well disguised desert toad near the pool on the Waterfall trail.

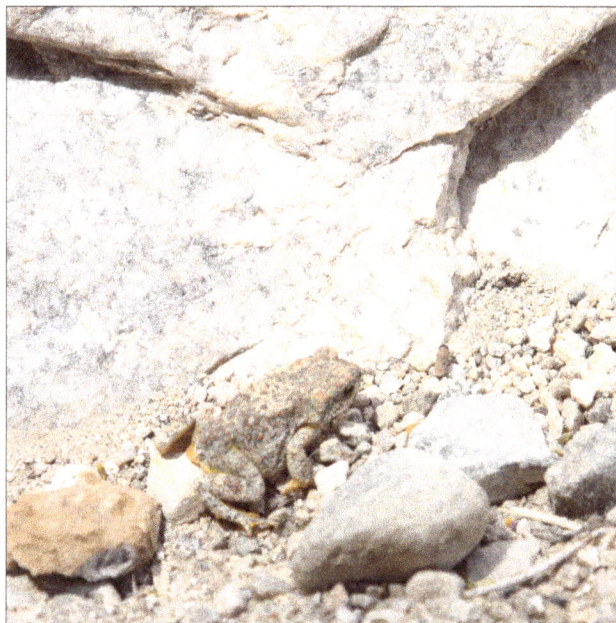

As the population of Phoenix expands toward the White Tank Mountains, the Waterfall Trail has been overwhelmed with people. Hikers seeking a less social outing may want to hike other trails in the White Tanks. We recommend obtaining a park map at either the Visitors Center. A topo map might also be helpful.

Hiking Distance:	
Goat Camp trail	6.3 miles
Goat Camp to Willow Springs	.7 mile
Willow Canyon trail	1.6 miles
Mesquite Canyon	5 miles
Ford Canyon to Willow Springs	7.4 miles

Fat Man's Pass & Hidden Valley in South Mountain Park

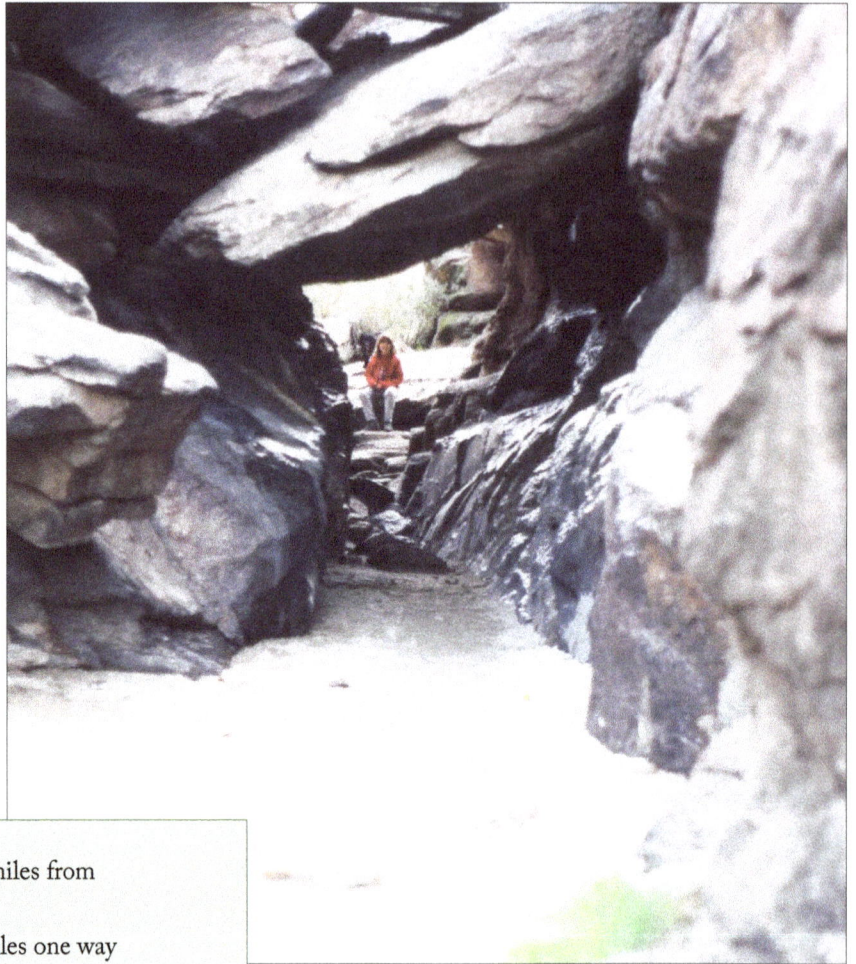

Natural Rock Tunnel in Hidden Valley.

Driving Distance: 20+ miles from
    central Phoenix
Hiking Distance: 1.8 miles one way
Rating: Moderate
Elevation: 1500' - 2330'
Best Season: Early spring, fall & winter.
Special Features: Unique tunnel in hidden
    valley.
Precautions: Watch for 'kamikaze' mountain
    bikers.
Maps: City of Phoenix Parks & Recreation
    map.
Information: City of Phoenix Parks &
    Recreation   (602) 495-5458

Can I say it again?
Arizona's summers are hot! As I write this, two hikers have died on desert trails in the last week. One death happened on a reasonably short trail in the Phoenix area. We recommend against hiking in mid-day temperatures during the summer. It is just too hot! Early morning or evening hours with sufficient water are the best times to be out. Don't push your luck. I've hiked all my adult life and yet on two different occasions we were in real trouble due to poor decisions and lack of water.

South Mountain Park has long been a favorite location to look down on the urban sprawl across the Valley of the Sun. On a warm summer night, visitors to South Mountain absorb the beauty of the marvelous light show at their feet. Hikers and mountain bikers also love this area and a popular trail descends through **Hidden Valley, Fat Man's Pass** and the **natural rock tunnel**. We recommend picking up a Park map to get an overview of the trail network.

There are two trailheads, hikers might consider if interested in hiking into Hidden Valley. Buena Vista is located near the summit of the range. Visitors drive south along Central Avenue into the Park and follow the signage along the main road to the parking area.

The Mormon trailhead is accessible from 24th Street with a small parking lot at the base of the range. There are other trailheads and we strongly recommend becoming familiar with the

trail map before setting off.

I personally like the **Mormon trail** as the ascent seemed less demanding. Whether you're ascending or descending the Buena Vista, be aware that you share the trail with mountain bikes who may come skidding over the rocky hillside. Most riders try to be polite but be prepared to move off the path quickly.

Hidden Valley, true to its name, is hidden between two high ridges. We think two features give the trail a fun twist. Fatmans Pass is a narrow slot between large boulders - this one is not for the portly hiker. Another section of the trail passes through a natural tunnel formed by huge slabs of rock, forcing adult hikers to bend low as they scurry through the passage. Follow the signage to both locations.

A two car shuttle allows hikers to complete the route without doubling back but it is a long drive between the two trail heads.

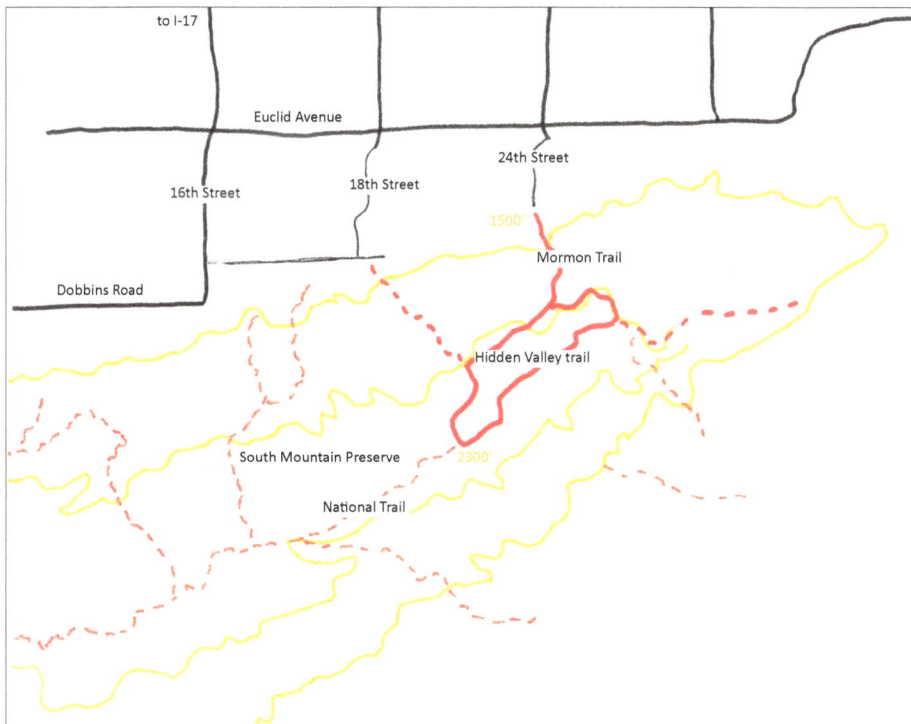

Peralta Canyon Trail

The Superstition Mountains have long been a landmark for those traveling US 60. During the cooler months, the trails in this range are drawing more hikers. One popular hike follows Peralta Canyon up to Fremont Pass with its awesome view of the Weaver's Needle.

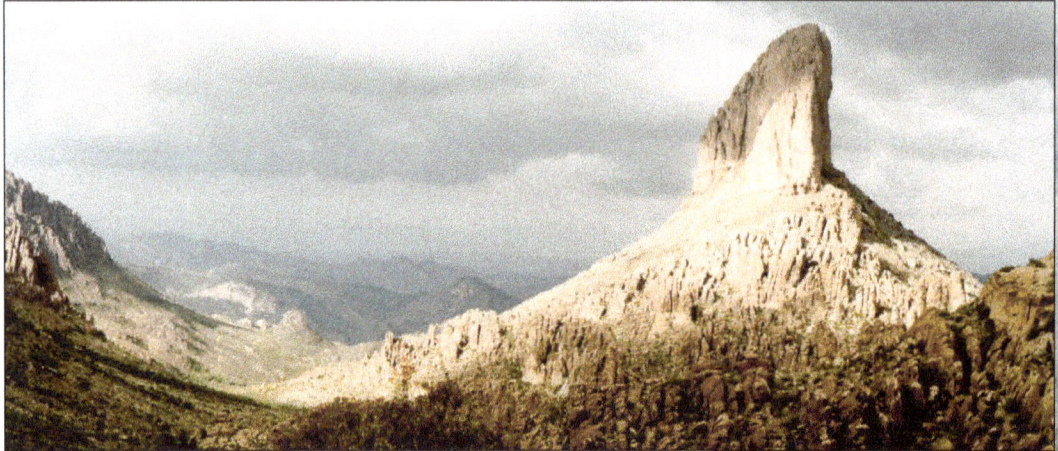

Photo: Weaver's Needle

To reach Peralta Canyon, drive east from Apache Junction on US 60. At mp 204.2, turn onto Peralta Road. Follow Peralta Road (FR 77) northeast 7 miles to the parking lot. At 5.5 miles, stay left at a fork in the road.

Three trails branch out from this trailhead. The Dutchman Trail #104 and #235 are on the right, Peralta Canyon Trail on the left.

Peralta Canyon trail follows a seasonal creek. After a recent rain, hikers enjoy the sound of little waterfalls and the trickle of running water. As the trail ascends, toward Fremont Saddle, it crosses the creek several times. Hikers cannot see the saddle until about half way up the canyon. Nearing the top, rock cairns guide hikers over the rock ledges. Looking back, hikers find spectacular views to the south and east with range after range of purple mountains and hazy plains.

Topping out on the saddle, Weaver's Needle seems just a short distance further. The size of the monument makes the distance deceiving. Beyond the saddle, the trail turns northwest toward a junction with Trail #104. The saddle is a popular spot for hikers to snap a few photos and turn back to the parking lot.

Driving Distance: 12.6 miles from Jct. US 60 and SR 88.
Hiking Distance: 2.3 miles
Rating: Moderate
Elevation: 1350-1800'
Best Season: Winter, spring & fall.
Special Features: Seasonal stream, spectacular views, old mining legend.
Precautions: During wet weather, caution crossing rock ledges.
Maps: Tonto NFS map
Information: Tonto NFS District Office (602) 255-5200

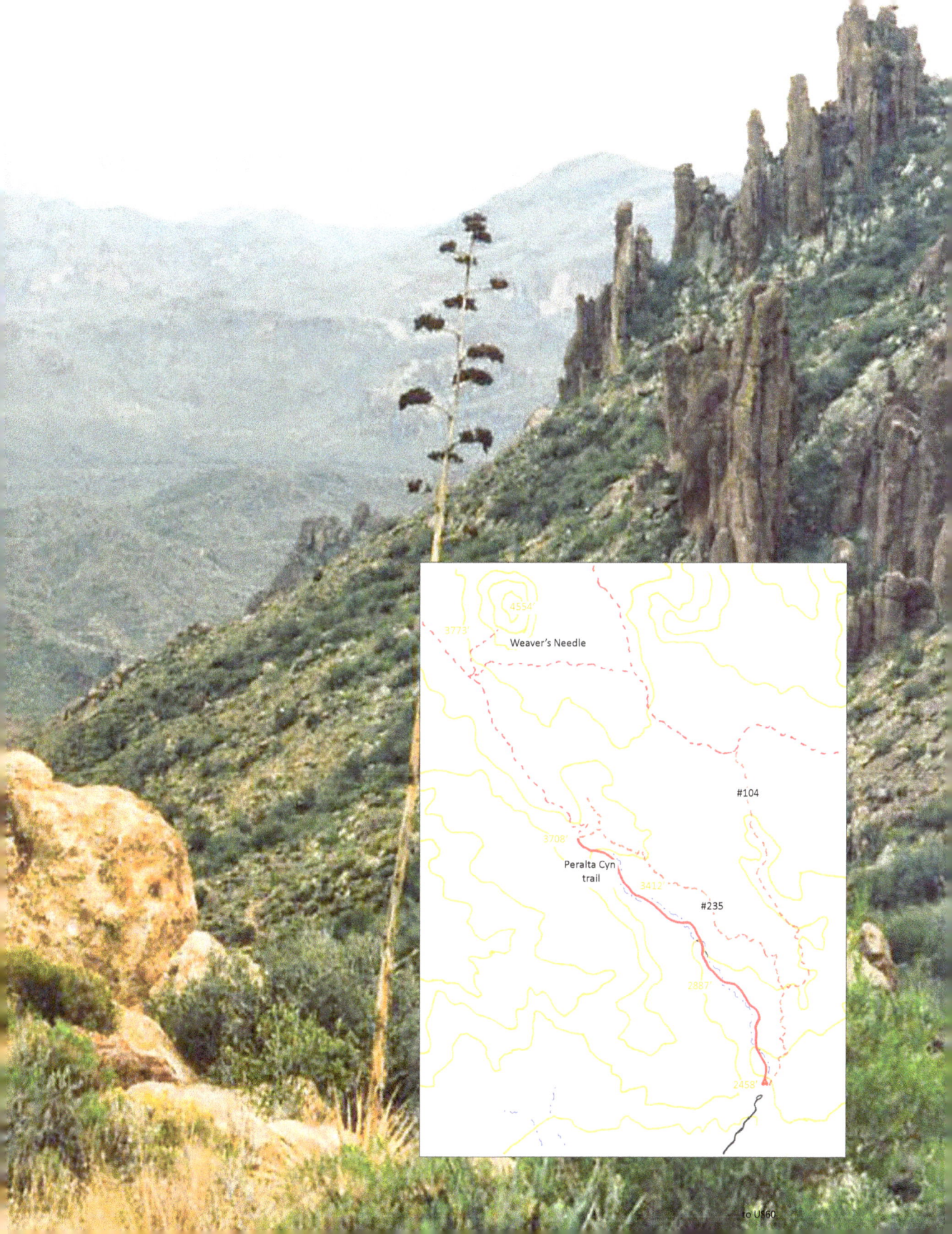

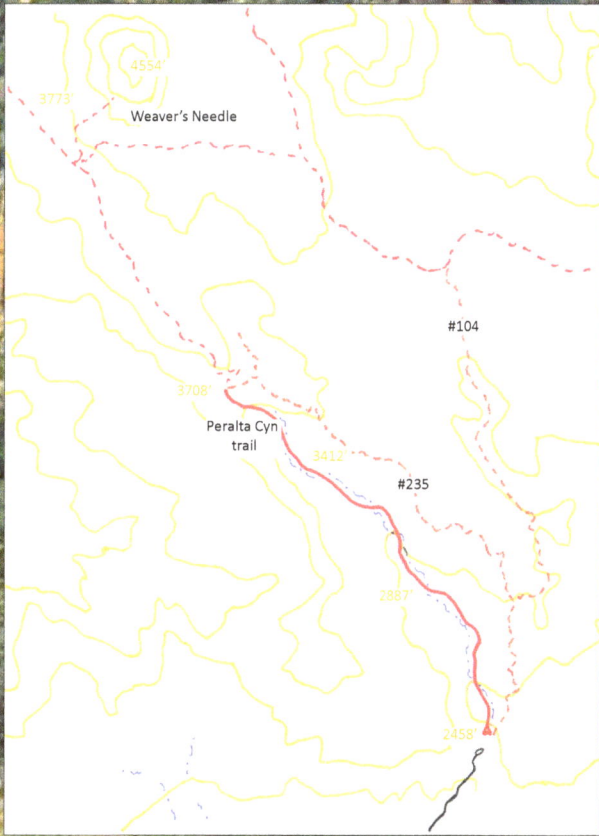

4554'

3773'

Weaver's Needle

#104

3708'

Peralta Cyn
trail

3412'

#235

2887'

2458'

to US60

Hieroglyphic Trail

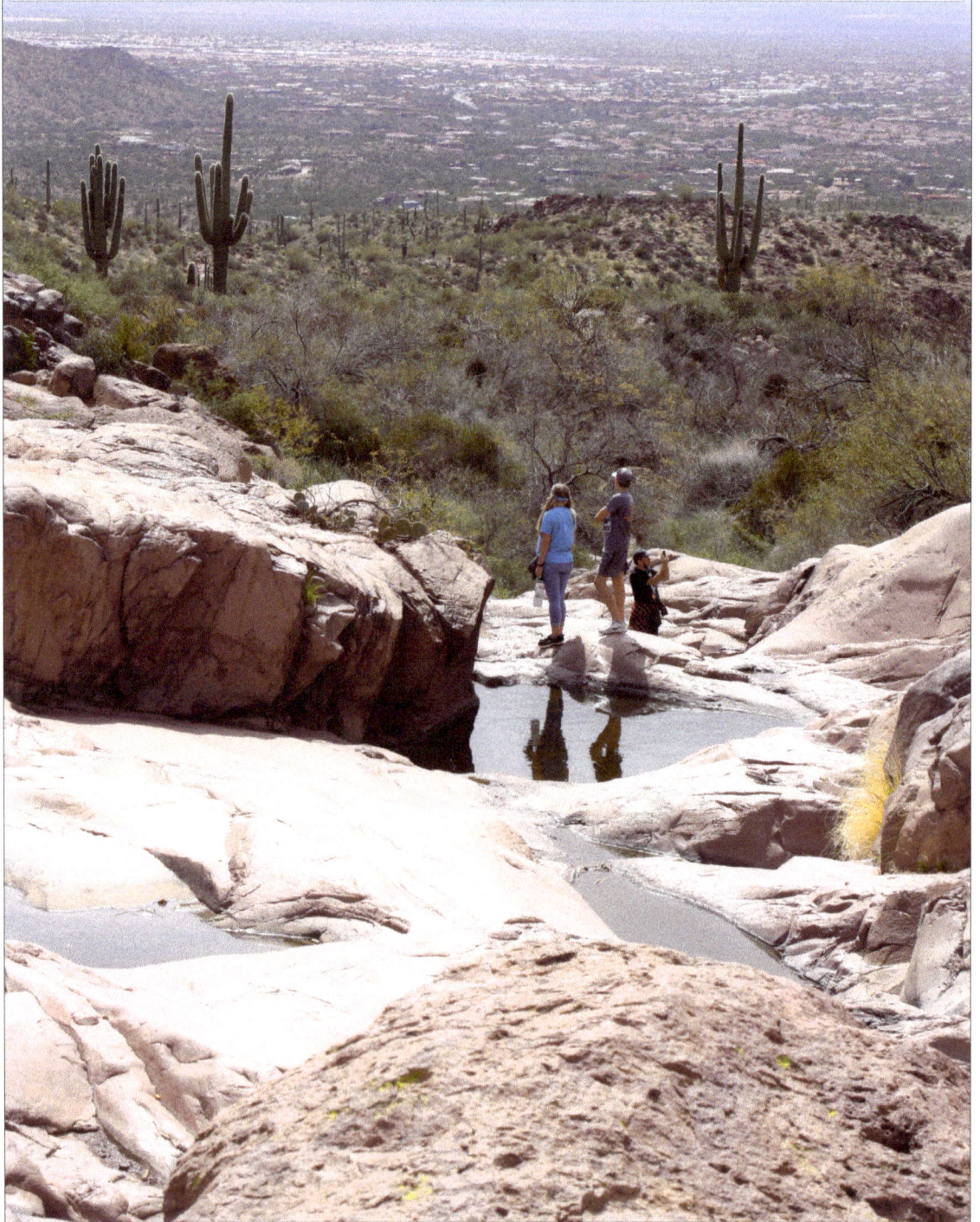

The **Hieroglypic Trail** became popular the last few years as a fairly easy trail at the edge of the Superstition Mountains. The trailhead is located on the upper end of a neighborhood off the Apache Trail/State Route 60. This is not a trail for the summer months as there is no shade.

From the parking area, the trail passes through a gate and then climbs steadily along a ridge for about a mile. Approaching the mountain, hikers navigate around large boulders to arrive at two or three basins hollowed out of the granite bedrock. These were known to Spanish explorers as tinajas, rocky depressions that held water well into the warmer months. Looking closer, it is easy to see how the rocky hillside sheds a torrent of rain into the gulch between two rocky hillsides.

The tinajas were an important source of water to wildlife and to the ancient people hunting in the Superstition Mountains. Take a moment to examine the petroglyphs carved into the rocks overlooking the pools. One petroglyph shows a wavy line as if indicating a stream. Another shows a mountain sheep within a cave, possibly indicating that this is a site frequented by the animals. The symbols tell us this was an important site to the people who noted the location as a place they could find water in a desert land.

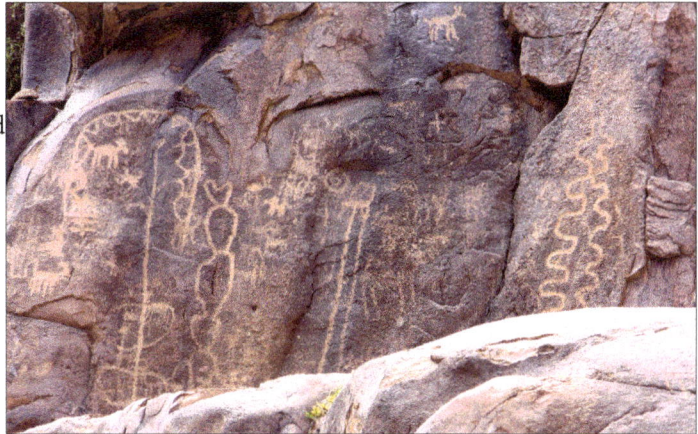

To reach the site from Phoenix, drive east along US 60 to Kings Ranch Road, turn north. Drive to Baseline, turning right, then left onto Mohican, followed by a left on Valley View. Take one last right turn onto Cloudview, driving east to the parking area which may be crowded.

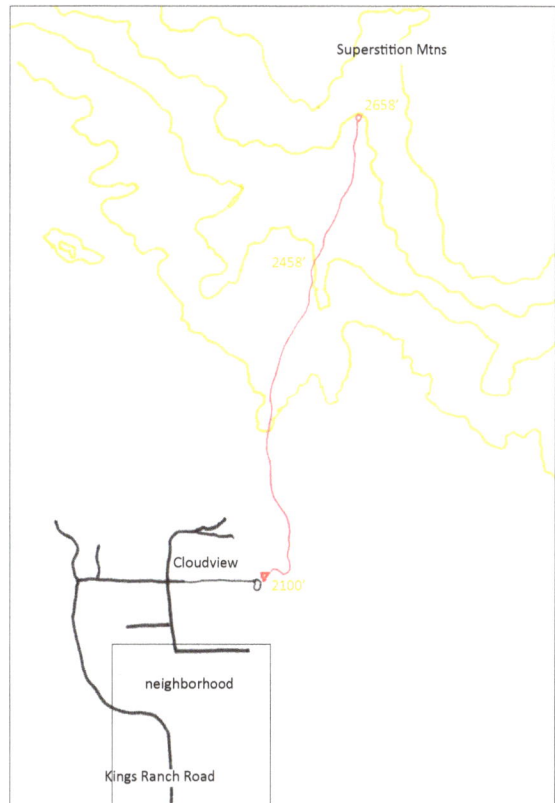

Hiking Distance: 1.5 miles
Rating: Moderate   Elevation: 2093-2649'
Best Season: Winter, spring & fall.
Special Features: Tinajas, petroglyphs
Precautions: Be careful on slick rock.
Maps: Tonto NFS map
Information: Tonto NFS District Office
(602) 255-5200

Boulder Canyon

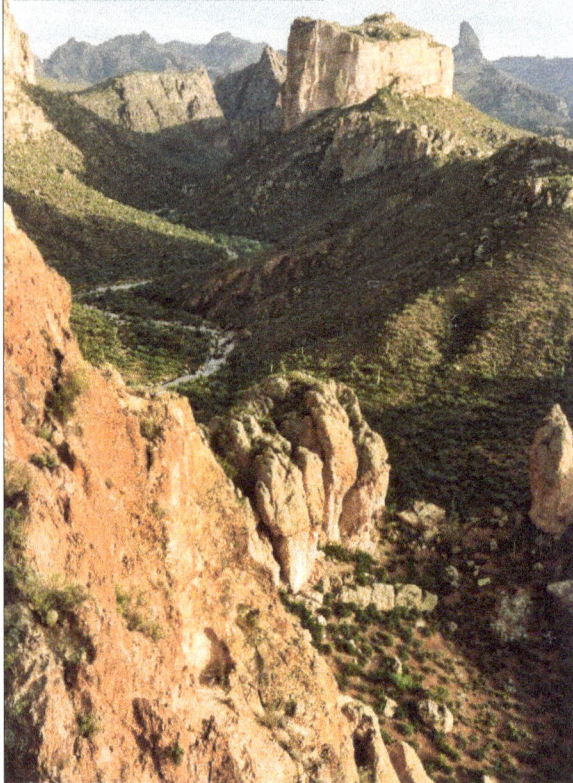

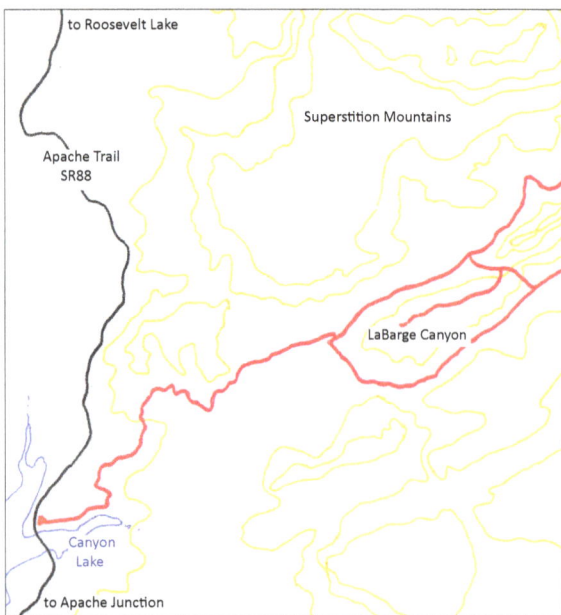

From **Canyon Lake** to **LaBarge Canyon**, the **Boulder Canyon** trail gives wide-open views across the top of the Superstitions. Follow State Route 88 from either Apache Junction or Roosevelt Lake to the Canyon Lake Marina. For those unfamiliar with the Apache Trail, part of this state highway is a narrow 2-lane dirt road with few guardrails. Park at the marina and cross the highway to the trailhead.

From the trailhead, the trail heads east, then south to switchback up a hill, giving hikers spectacular views of Canyon Lake. After the initial ascent, the trail dips and climbs with the terrain to a small saddle. Passing onto the back side of the ridge, hikers peer across the Superstitions and into LaBarge Canyon. The green strip along the canyon bottom seems to indicate a stream but surface water is present only during the winter and early spring. From this enticing viewpoint, the trail drops .75 mile through a series of switchbacks to a fork.

The right branch of the fork descends to LaBarge Creek while the left climbs to the Indian Paint Mine. When in doubt about side trails, stay with the heavily traveled route. Hikers return by the same route or choose to backpack across the Superstitions. A good map of the Superstitions is helpful.

Driving Distance: 16 miles from Apache Jct.
to Canyon Lake
Hiking Distance: 1.75 miles to La Barge Canyon,
3.5 miles to Boulder Canyon
Rating: Moderate
Best Season: Winter, early spring.
Special Features: Historic area with pretty canyon.
Precautions: Rattlesnakes; take adequate water,
note landmarks along trail for return trip.
Maps: Tonto NFS map
Information: Tonto District Office
(602) 255-5200

Fish Creek

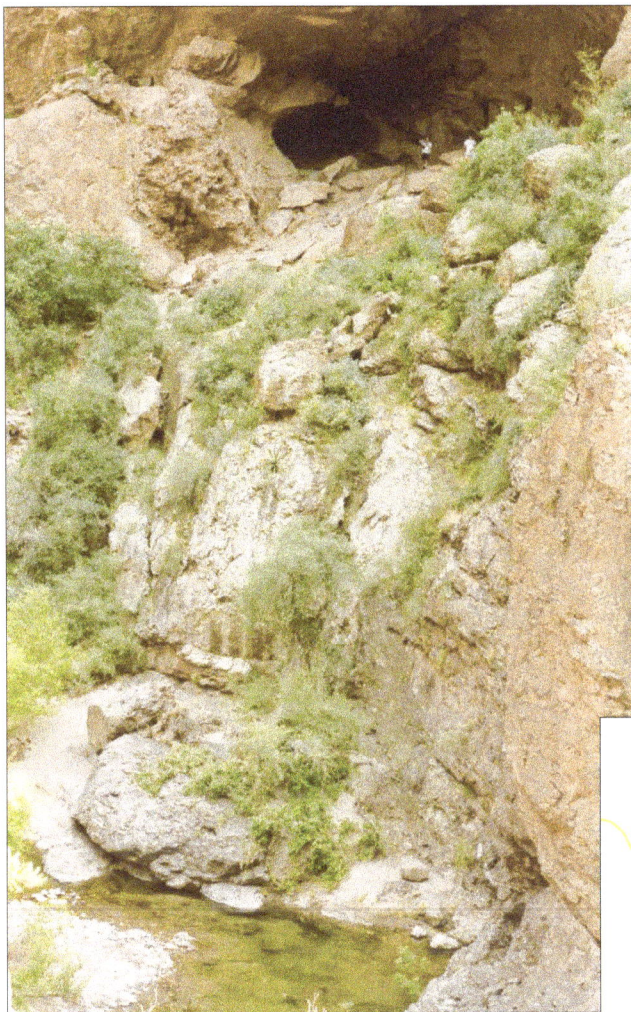

The Apache Trail / SR88 follows an old trade route across the Superstitions Mountains, from Roosevelt Lake to Apache Junction. Prehaps the most treacherous location along the Apache Trail is the descent into **Fish Creek Canyon**. Drivers rounding a blind curve suddenly face a single lane descent on the cliff face. Do not attempt to pass - the edge of the road is not stable. Drivers ascending the hill should expect to back down if they meet another car.

At the bottom of the hill, a bridge crosses the creek bed with several parking spaces at one end. A short climb from the bridge reaches a shallow cave overlooking the canyon. A footpath descends from the cave to the canyon bottom where hikers may choose to explore either upstream or down. If it looks likes rain, stay out of the canyon due to the danger of flash floods!

Driving Distance: 16 miles from Apache Jct.
                to Canyon Lake
Hiking Distance: 1.75 miles to La Barge Canyon,
                3.5 miles to Boulder Canyon
Rating: Moderate
Best Season: Winter, early spring.
Special Features: Historic area with pretty canyon.
Precautions: Rattlesnakes; take adequate water,
        note landmarks along trail for return trip.
Maps: Tonto NFS map
Information: Tonto District Office

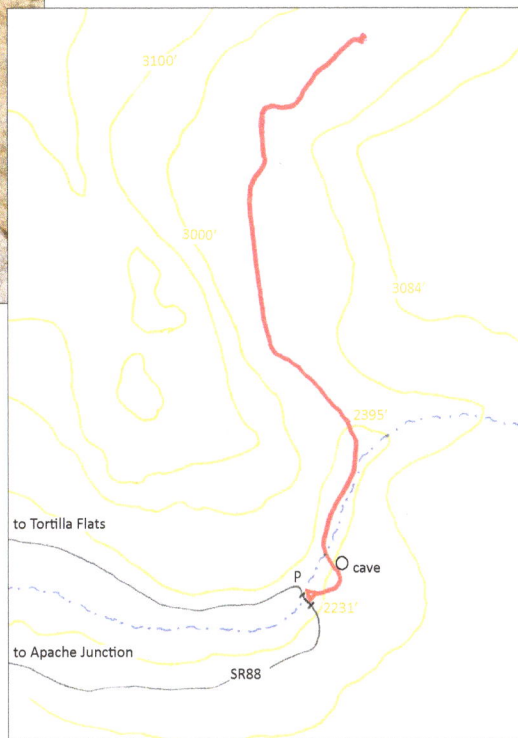

Usery Mountain Regional Park and the Wind Cave

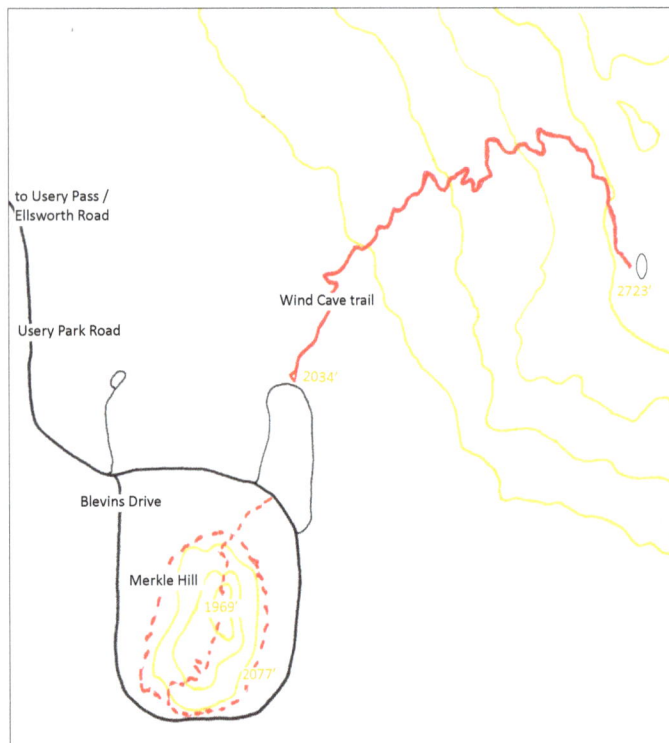

to Usery Pass /
Ellsworth Road

Usery Park Road

Wind Cave trail

2723'

2034'

Blevins Drive

Merkle Hill

1969'

2077'

Driving Distance: 12 miles from central Mesa.
Hiking Distance: Wind Cave 1.6 miles one way.
Rating: Moderate   Best Season: Winter, spring, or fall.
Special Features: Natural overhang with water seeps &
    wild bee hives.
Precautions: Sit quietly and do not disturb the bees.
Information: Maricopa Parks & Recreation Dept.
                    (602) 506-2930

One hiker described an incident where he was surrounded by a swarm of bees in migration to a new nesting site. He crouched down, covering his face with his hands. The bees' beating wings created a pitch black, icy cold environment around his head. After hovering briefly around him, they moved on, leaving him unharmed.

Hollowed from a ridge by wind and water, the Wind Cave is fanned by cool breezes on warm afternoons. Hikers may find a healthy bee population investigating each new arrival. Their hives are hidden from view in fractures in the rocky surface. The cave is found high on a ridge in **Usery Mountain Regional Park,** one of a series of mountain preserves on the perimeter of the Valley of the Sun. To reach the park, drive east on US 60 toward Apache Junction. Turn north onto Ellsworth Road which becomes Usery Mountain Road at the Park boundary. It is 6 miles to the park entrance from US 60. An entrance fee may be charged.

A large sign on Wind Cave Drive, at the day use area, marks the trailhead. The trail turns northeast, crossing a plain toward the Usery Mountain Range. Hikers begin with a gradual ascent. As elevation increases the trail switchbacks up a steeper portion of the ridge. The last half mile is follows the ridge to a broad ledge in the shadow of an overhanging rock face. During the cooler months of the year water seeps from the rocks. The moisture attracts hummingbirds and wild bees. Do not swat at the bees as they buzz nearby. If they seem irritated, leave quickly.

Beyong the ledge, the trail climbs the peak to the summit. The ascent, is rough and steep, not for novice hikers.

The **Desert Botanical Gardens** in Papago Park offer two unique trails featuring cacti, succulents, beautiful wildflowers and structures friendly to the desert environment. This institution is dedicated to preserving rare and endangered plant species found in arid climates. While not part of the wild back country that many prefer for hiking, this public garden allows us to stretch our legs and learn more about the desert

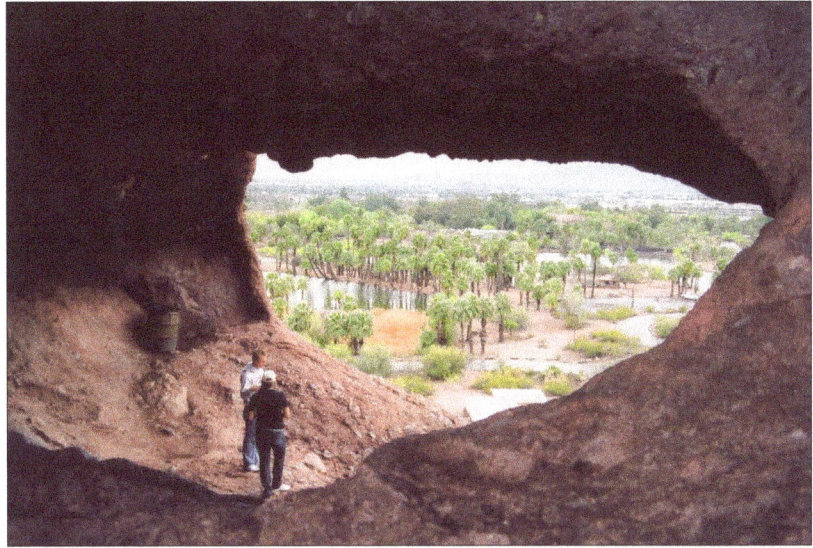

Hole in the Rock: A unique view of the Phoenix Zoo from City of Phoenix Papago Park. The park is adjacent to the Botanical Gardens.

environment. Perhaps the best time to visit is in the spring when so many of the plants are blooming and temperatures are moderately warm.

The **Desert Discovery Trail**, a loop trail through the facility, is paved with brick to distinguish it from other paths branching off to special areas. Among the exhibits are a special cacti house and a succulent house. About one third of the cacti and plants are from the Sonoran Desert while the remaining two thirds are from arid regions all over the world.

We think of the desert as an inhospitable place, defying us to survive its rugged environment. Yet, for thousands of years, people have survived in a region where water is scarce and summer temperatures very hot. A second trail, named the **Plants and People of the Sonoran Desert**, provides great hands-on exhibits. The guide booklet at the entrance of the trail is very helpful.

This unique park is located between Van Buren Street and McDowell Road off the Papago Parkway (an extension of 64th St.). The Botanical Gardens are part of the larger area known as Papago Park, which also contains the Phoenix Zoo and a rock formation known as Hole in the Rock. Hikers frequently follow the short trail to the cave at the top of the butte.

Desert Botanical Gardens and Papago Buttes

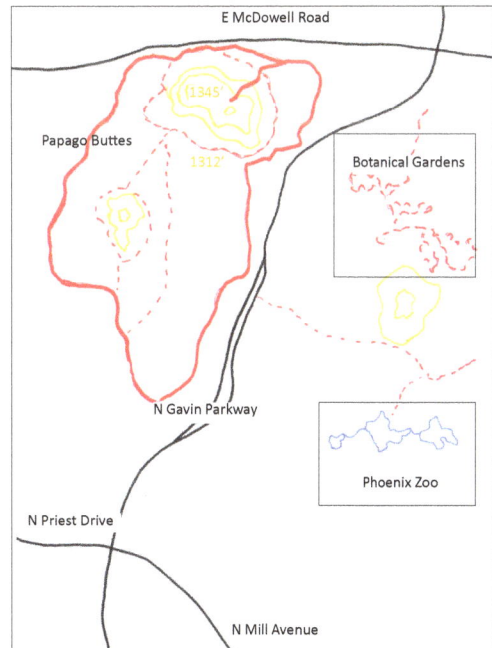

139

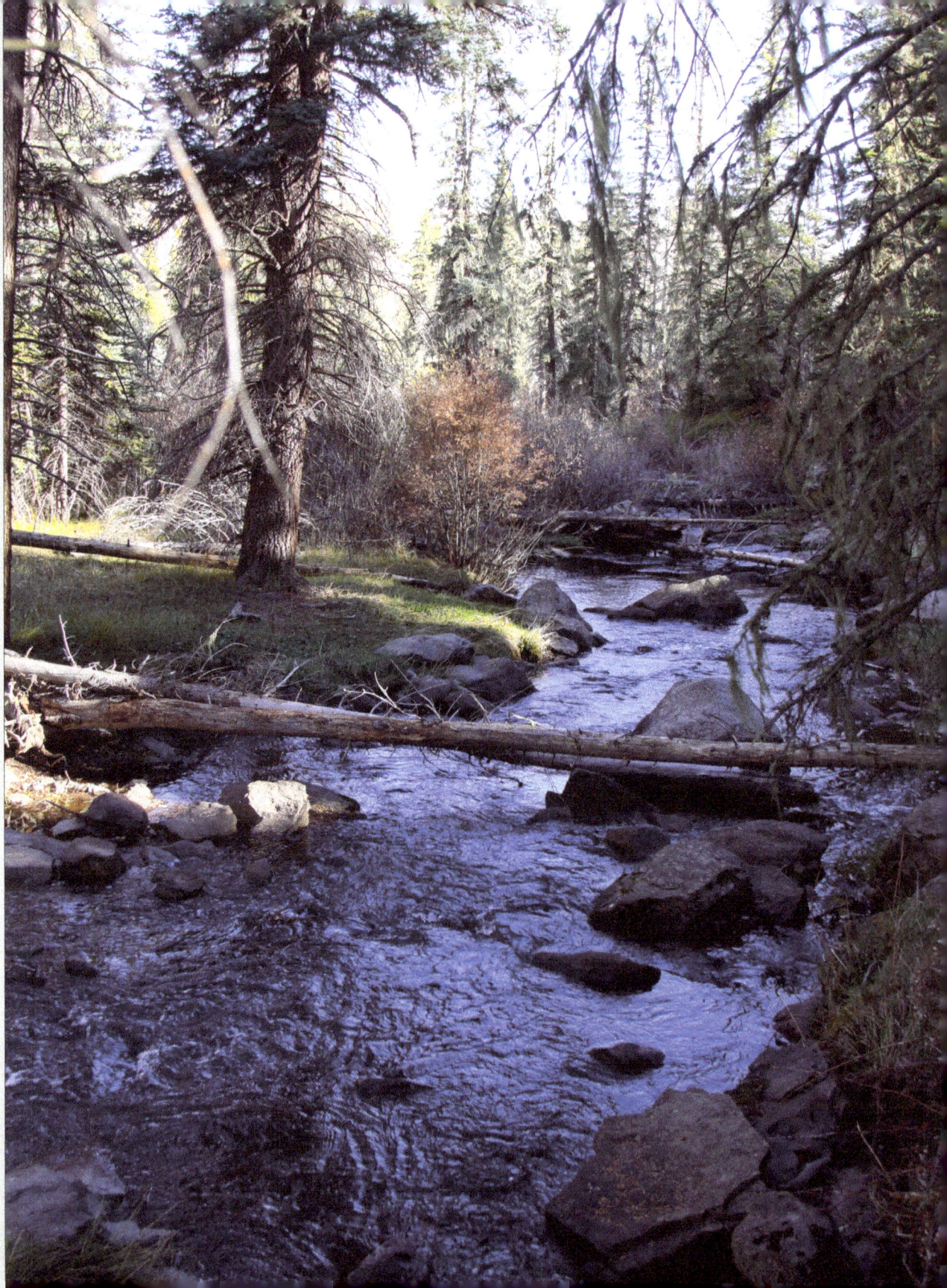

White Mountains and Eastern AZ

The high country of the White Mountains is covered with thick forests of spruce, fir and pine, intersected by clear mountain streams. The lush forests draw visitors to spend time fishing and dreaming along the creeks as hikers celebrate the stream-side trails.

Pinetop-Lakeside sees visitors during the summer for hiking and camping, snow play in the winter months and hunting in the fall. Many make their way to the small lakes south of SR260 and beyond to Alpine and Hannagan Meadow.

A smaller number of visitors venture along US191 as it swings through curve after curve following the ridges between the small towns of Alpine and Clifton. Even fewer visitors actually make the trek to the shallow pools along the Blue River where they may encounter cattle from local ranches.

The trails that descend from US191 are challenging. We've recommended a couple but as a rule, it is important when venturing off the beaten track to let someone know where you are going and when you will return.

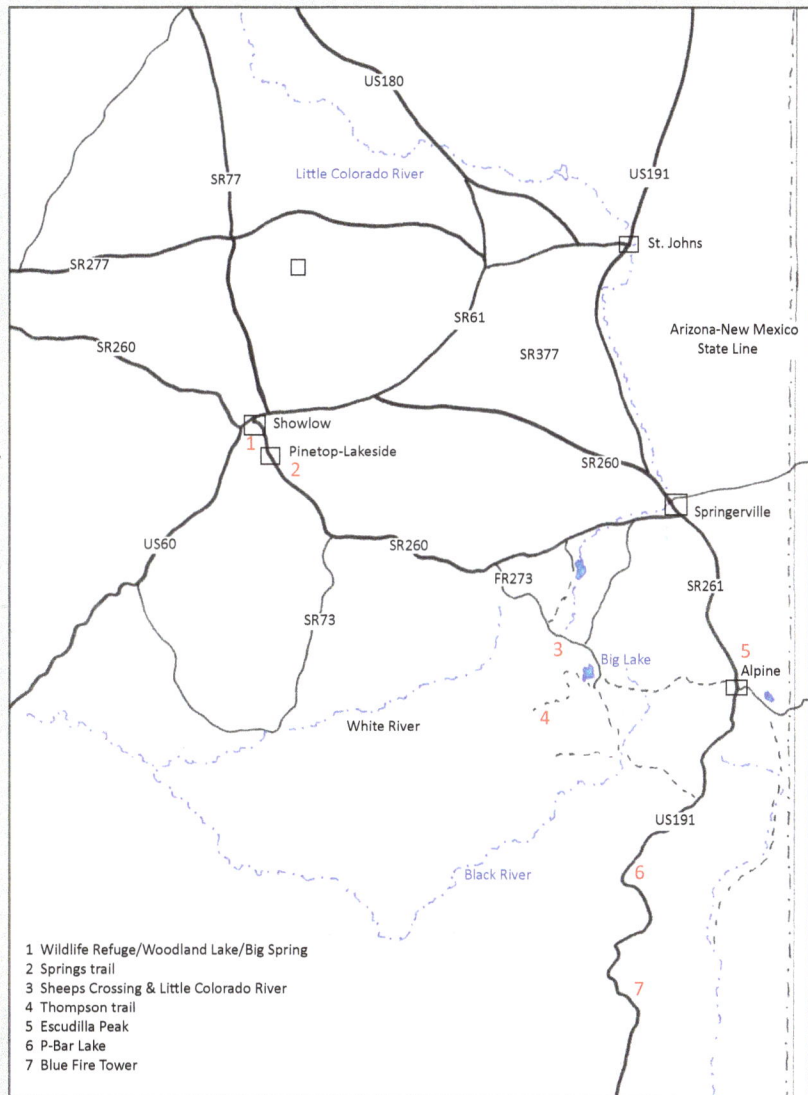

US180

Little Colorado River

SR77

US191

SR277

St. Johns

SR61

Arizona-New Mexico State Line

SR260

SR377

Showlow

1 Pinetop-Lakeside
2

SR260

Springerville

US60

SR260

FR273

SR261

SR73

3 Big Lake

5 Alpine

4

White River

US191

Black River

6

7

1 Wildlife Refuge/Woodland Lake/Big Spring
2 Springs trail
3 Sheeps Crossing & Little Colorado River
4 Thompson trail
5 Escudilla Peak
6 P-Bar Lake
7 Blue Fire Tower

The Black River along the Thompson Trail.

Pinetop-Lakeside Urban Trails

A network of trails spreads beyond the confines of Showlow and Pinetop-Lakeside, giving residents and visitors a wonderful opportunity to explore the hills and valleys around these communities.

Allen Severson Memorial Wildlife Refuge
Just north of Showlow on SR 77 is Pintail Lake located in the Allen Severson Memorial Wildlife Refuge. The lake serves as a wildlife refuge as well as recycling the effluent from the City of Show-Low. The turnoff is located at mp 345 on SR 77, just north of Showlow. A paved path leads from the parking lot about a third of a mile to the lake. Before reaching the lake, the trail splits with a cindered trail on the right leading to a small deck overlooking the water. The left branch is paved, leading down to a blind built of cement block. Open slots in the block walls allow visitors to look out over the water. Since the birds do not visitors as separate from the blind that they live with daily, people may get a close up of little mud hens, coots, egrets, and mallards. The marsh is also visited by raptors.

Big Springs
This riparian habitat is located northeast of Woodland Lake in Pinetop-Lakeside. To reach the trailhead, drive through the community along White Mountain Blvd to mp 351.5, turn onto Woodland Road, driving south to the Nature Center. The pond below the Center is spring-fed. A footpath circles the pond and crosses the shallow wash before returning to the Nature Center. Pick up a trail guide at the Nature Center to learn more about the area.

Woodland Lake Park Trail System
Further south, Woodland Reservoir is the focal point of an urban trail network. The entrance along Woodland Lake Road is just off White Mountain Blvd in Lakeside. After parking near the boat dock, hikers choose from several trails. The Woodland Lake Loop circles the reservoir while Meadowview drops below the dam. Turkey Track leads north, making a loop with the Walnut Creek trail. The Hitching Post Trail makes a loop northwest of the reservoir with a connector trail to the Big Springs trail.

Mogollon Rim Nature Trail
Following Hwy 260, drive 3 miles northwest of the Lakeside Ranger Station. Just north of the Camp Tatiyee entrance, a small sign directs hikers to a parking area west of the highway. Small signs along the paved trail reveal the geological formation of the Mogollon Rim and the history of the area with great views off the Rim.

Photo Opposite Page: *Big Spring*

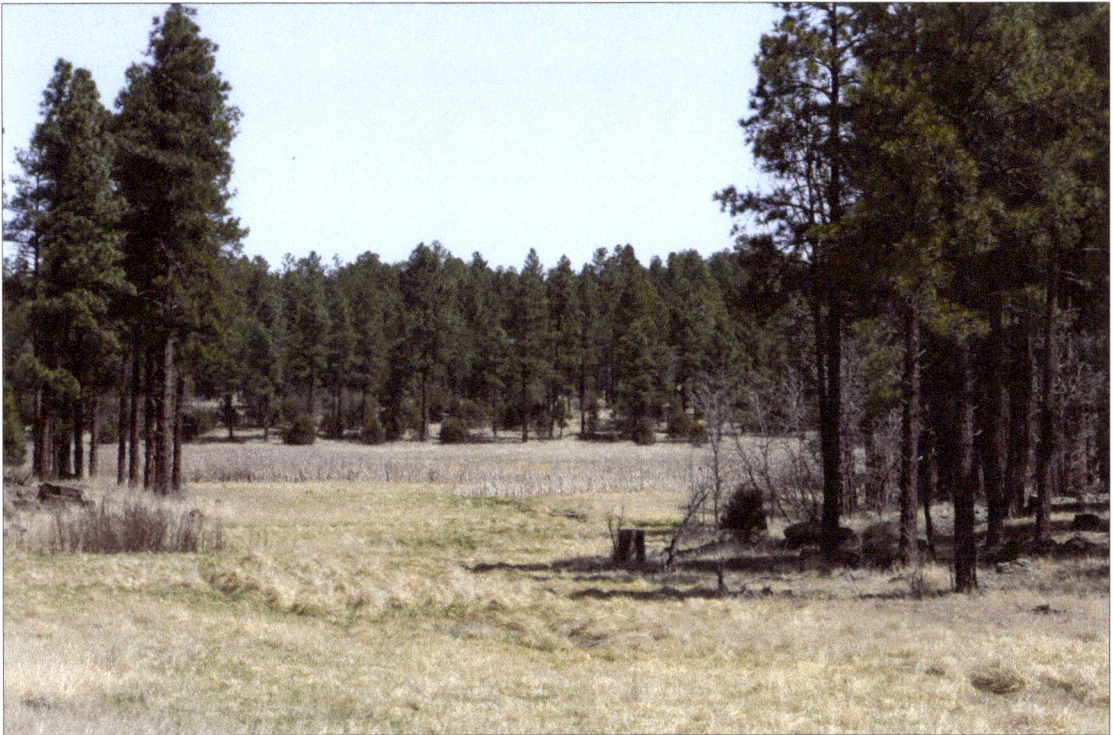

Trails & Mileage

Woodland Lake Loop	1.2	mile
Meadowview	.2	mile
Hitching Post Trail	3	miles
Turkey Track	1.4	mile
Walnut Creek	.7	mile
Big Springs	.75	mile
Nature Center	.6	mile
Mogollon Nature trail	.5	mile
Wildlife Refuge	.5 mile	

Rating: Easy

Best Season: Winter, spring or fall.

Special Features: Natural spring, small lakes

Information: White Mountain Nature Center (928) 368-2100

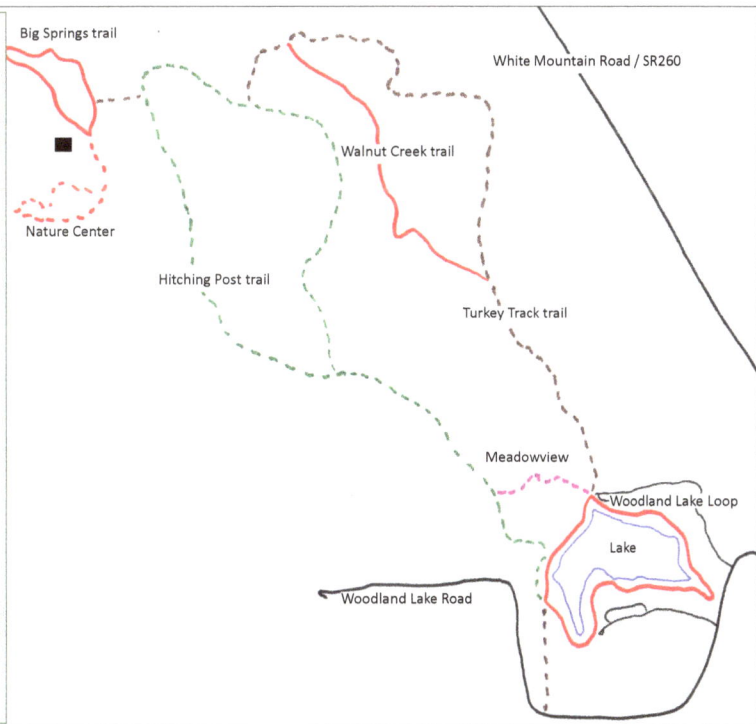

Springs Trail

The City of Pinetop-Lakeside has a network of trails in and around their small community. One of my favorites is the Springs trail for the small spring-fed pools along the north side of the loop.

Many hikers start the loop on the north side, turning right just a short distance beyond the trailhead. Notice that the surface of the ground has been displaced, forming a shallow canyon - this is a geologic fault that has allowed the water in a shallow aquifer to seep to the surface. The aquifer is fed by the snow that the region receives each winter.

During the warm month, the pools seem isolated one from another along the watercourse but in the spring a small stream flows between the pools.

As the trail turns southwest, hikers climb out of the creek bottom and pass through a dry forest toward SR260. The noise of the traffic becomes more prominant. There is a signed side trail that takes hikers to the site of an old fish hatchery, one of the first in the state.

The trail becomes more exposed and begins to climb again as it turns north, back to the trailhead. With the day warming, I longed to be back along the pools. Maybe we should have considered starting the loop on the left side, saving the cool streamside hiking for the last stretch - something to consider.

The trailhead for both the Springs trail and the Pat Mullen trail is located on Sky Hi Road. From SR260, turn east onto Buck Springs Road, driving through the small neighborhood. Turn left onto Sky Hi Road

as it opens into the forest, leaving the neighborhood behind. You'll still hear the traffic at the trailhead and along the west side of the trail. Look for the trailhead on the left side of the road.

Driving Distance: 6 miles from miles from Lakeside Ranger Station
Hiking Distance: 3.6 mile loop
Rating: Easy
Elevation: 7185 - 7120'
Best Season: Late spring, summer and fall.
Special Features: Spring-fed pools, urban trail.
Map: City of Pine-Lakeside Trail map
Information: Lakeside Ranger Station
(928) 368-2100

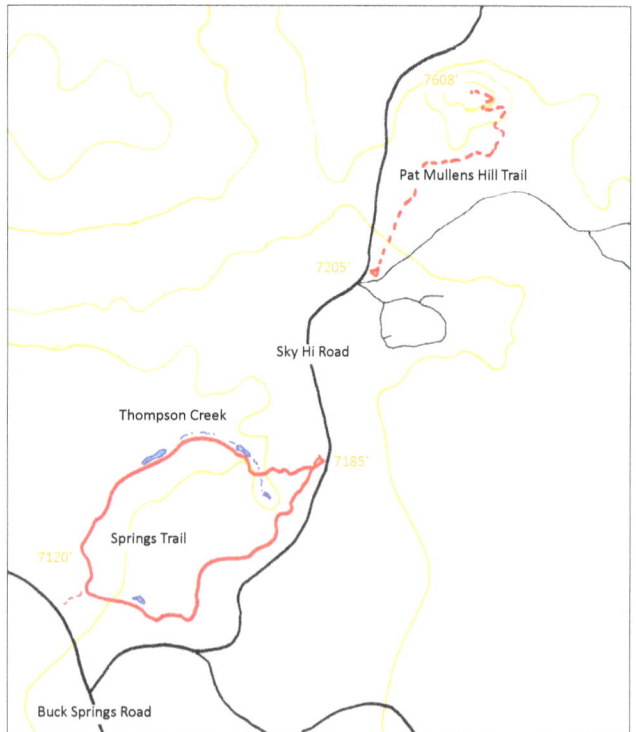

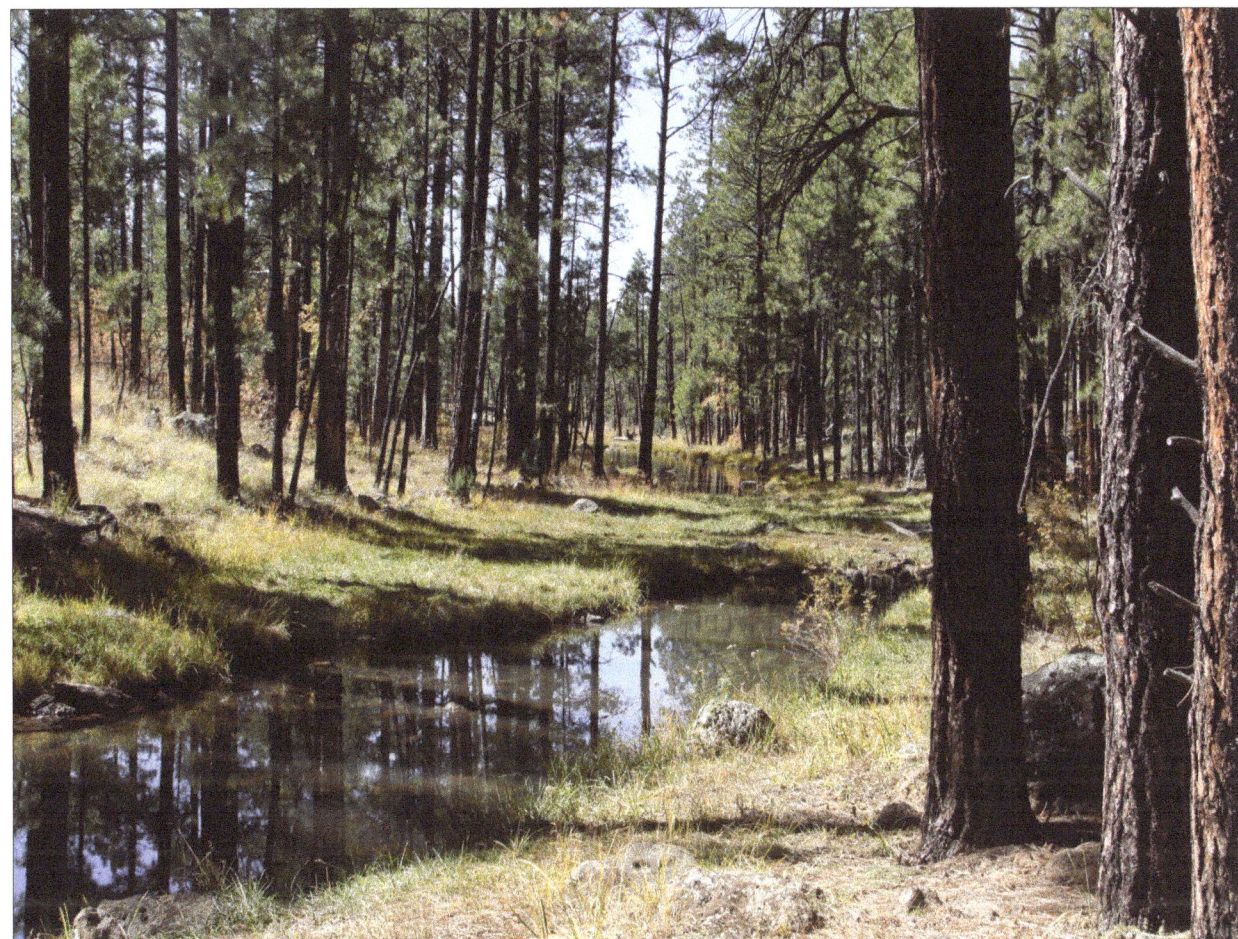

Along the Springs Trail

Pat Mullens Mountain

Just up the road from the Springs Trail, the popular Pat Mullens trail climbs a low hill, giving hikers a great view of the surrounding area.

Drive a short distance beyond the Springs trailhead to Sierra Spring Drive and turn east. Look for the trailhead on the east side of the road. The trail is popular with bicyclists and hikers due to the change in elevation, this is a good workout.

Return to the trailhead along the same trail used for the ascent.

Driving Distance: 6.5 miles from Ranger Station
Hiking Distance: 1.75 miles one way.
Rating: Moderate
Elevation: 7,205 - 7,608'
Beast Season: Summer and fall.
Special Features: Looking out over the town
        of Pinetop-Lakeside.
Map: City of Pine-Lakeside Trail map
Information: Lakeside Ranger Station
        928-333-6280

Sheep's Crossing
& the West Fork of the Little Colorado River

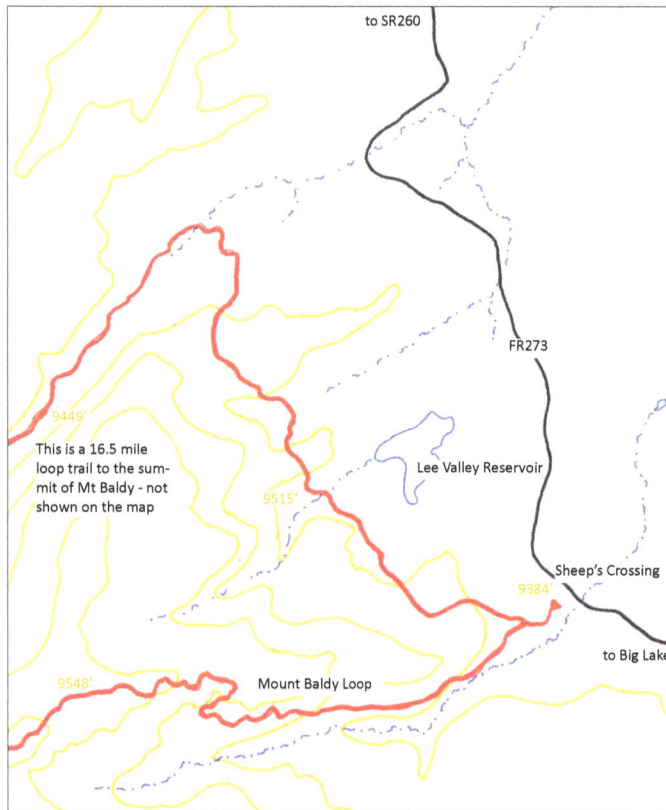

Map labels:
- to SR260
- FR273
- 9449'
- This is a 16.5 mile loop trail to the summit of Mt Baldy - not shown on the map
- Lee Valley Reservoir
- 9515'
- Sheep's Crossing
- 9384'
- to Big Lake
- 9548'
- Mount Baldy Loop

Mount Baldy is one of the highest peaks in Arizona. Sunrise Ski Area is located on its slopes. The snow crowning its summit each winter melts in the spring, running into the head waters of the west and east forks of the Little Colorado.

Sheep Crossing, at the base of Mount Baldy, is a favorite destination for both hikers and anglers for its clear stream and sunny alpine meadows.

To reach Sheep Crossing, turn off SR 260 west of Springerville onto SR 273, the route to Sunrise Ski Area. Driving south, the pavement turns to gravel and the road is signed as FR 113. In about eight miles, FR 113 crosses the west fork of the Little Colorado. The trailhead is on the west side of FR 113, a quarter mile above the crossing.

The Sheep Crossing Trail to the summit of Mt. Baldy is seven miles one way making it a popular backpacking trail. The summit is closed to hikers as the Apache Tribe regards the peak as sacred. Some geologists insist that the true summit lies on a neighboring peak which has not been fenced off.

For families and hikers who are not interested in an overnight backpack, the trail along the stream is a delight no matter where one chooses to turn back. In the first mile, the trail follows the west fork of the Little Colorado through lush meadows and dark spruce before it begins to climb away from the stream. Around each bend is a new view luring the hiker onward. As the trail climbs, hikers leave the forest behind, exposed to the winds raking the grasslands below tree-line.

Big Lake Fire Tower

A small fire tower once overlooked Big Lake, giving lookouts a bird's eye view of the forest and lakes in the region. The day came when flames from a wildfire crept up the slope and burned the tower. There are no plans to rebuild but the trail remains with a view out over the hills and valleys below. It can be a lovely walk.

Look for the signed trail head off FR249E, southwest of Big Lake. The trail climbs gently through the forest, around amazing rock outcroppings and encounters with chattering squirrels.
Hiking Distance: 1+ mile
Rating: Moderate

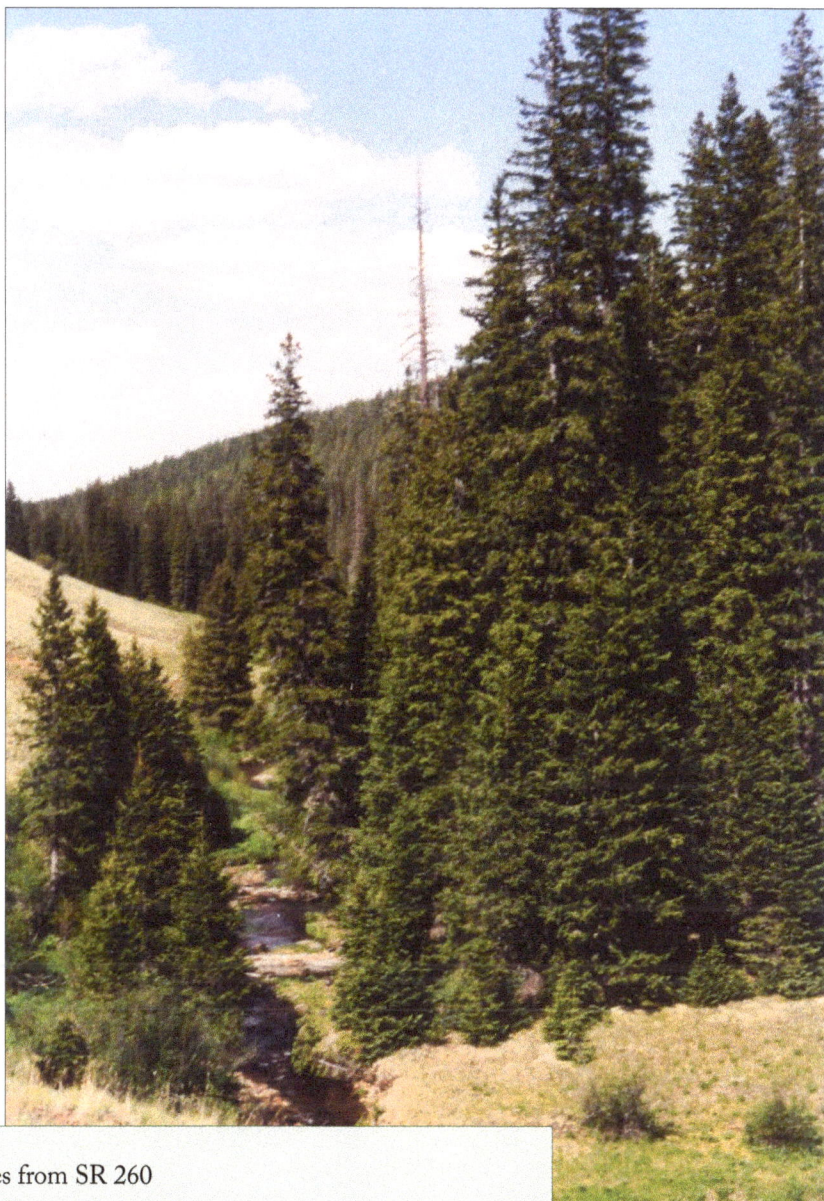

*Along the
Mount Baldy trail*

Driving Distance: 8.5 miles from SR 260

Hiking Distance: Summit 7 miles one way.

Rating: Moderate   Elevation: 7500'-11,403'

Best Season: Summer & early fall.

Special Features: Fishermen dot the stream while families play in the meadows.

Precautions: Don't let enthusiasm lure you further along than planned as nights get cold and the trail is long.

Maps: Apache-Sitgreaves NFS map

Info: Springerville Ranger Station (928) 333-6200

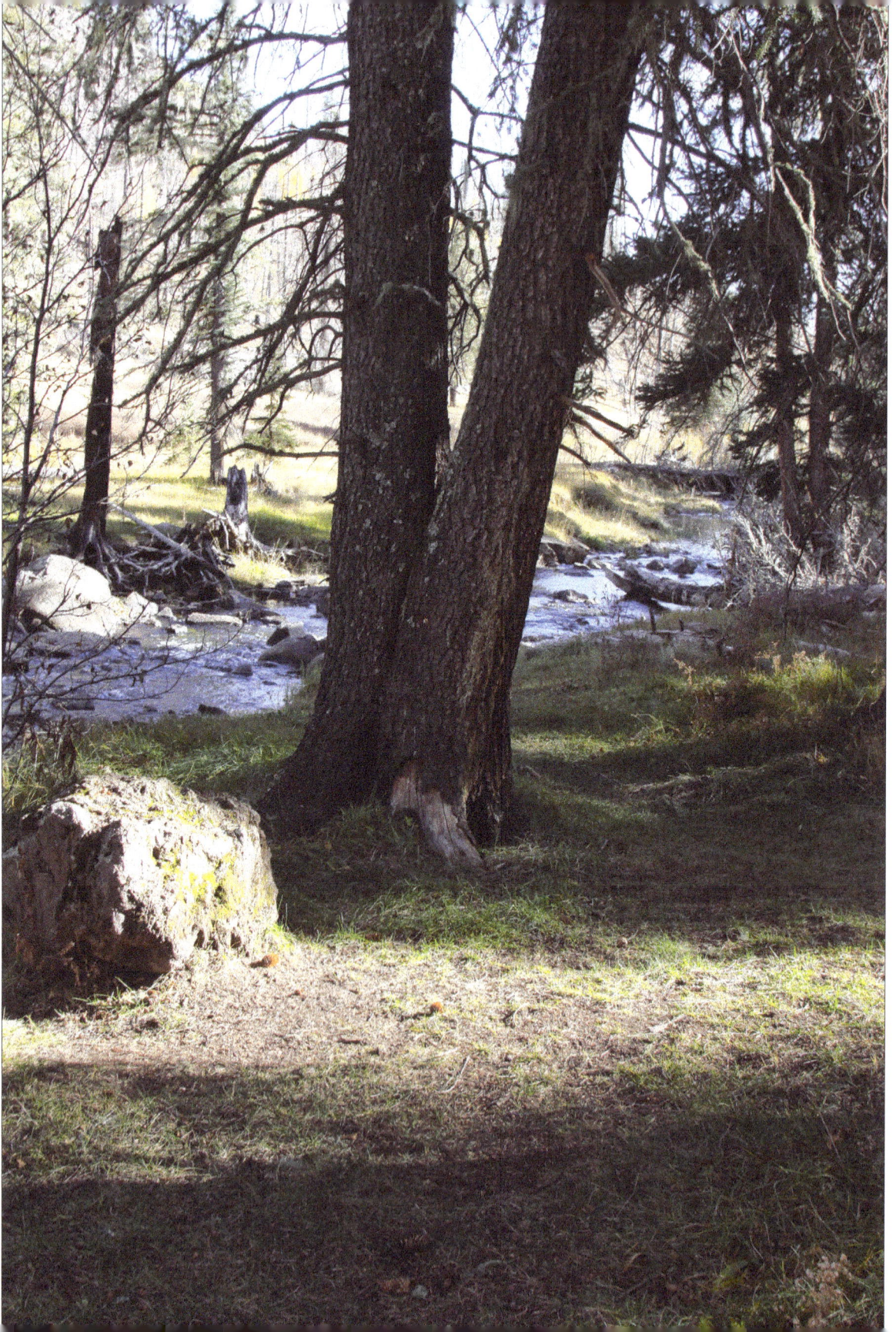

Thompson Trail at Big Lake

Arizona residents love water and that's no surprise living in an arid state. The Black River is a favorite for anglers and hikers alike. I've enjoyed a pleasant hike along the Black River on the **Thompson trail** near Big Lake as my wolfhound splashes in and out of the water or chases a squirrel around a tree. No worries, the squirrel wins!

From SR260, turn south on SR273 toward the Sunrise Ski Park. Drive past both Sunrise Lake and the White Mountain Reservoir, and the bridge over Sheep Crossing on the Little Colorado River. About four miles past the Crossing, look for FR116 on your right. If the road is open, it will save you the long drive around Big Lake on FR249E. Turn south onto FR 116, drive down to the junction with FR249E and turn right. FR116 runs parallel to the Black River to a bridge crossing the watercourse. Find a parking spot just beyond the bridge. Otherwise you'll need to park on a pull out above the river and hike down to the bridge.

The trail drops below the road and follows the stream south. A quarter mile down, visitors will see a fish trap across the river to keep predatory species away from the Apache or Gila Trout as part of a recovery program. Walk another half mile and you'll find a second fish trap across the stream.

Three miles downstream, hikers intersect a dirt track label 72M. This trail makes a loop that circles west and returns back to the Black River. We would suggest returning to the trailhead after taking time for a picnic and maybe a little time playing in the water.

Photo opposite page:
The Black River along the Thompson trail

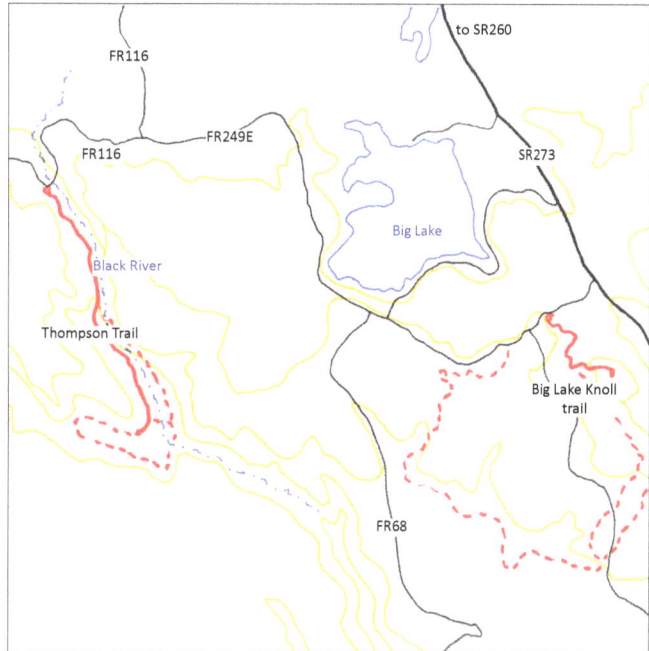

to SR260
FR116
FR249E
FR116
SR273
Black River
Big Lake
Thompson Trail
Big Lake Knoll trail
FR68

Driving Distance: about 18 miles from SR 260
Hiking Distance: 3 miles one way.
Rating: Easy
Elevation: 8,924'-8,725'
Best Season: Summer & early fall.
Special Features: A sparkling mountain stream with a fish trap.
Precautions:
Maps: Watch for flash flood is raining upstream.
Apache-Sitgreaves NFS map
Info: Springerville Ranger Station
(928) 333-6200

Escudilla Peak

The forests around Alpine and the Blue Range are beautiful but a time comes when hikers long to get above it all and see how the land spreads out below their feet. Towering above the Alpine Divide, **Escudilla Mountain** gives hikers that opportunity with a beautiful trail across grasslands and through aspen forests.

Follow US 666/191 north out of Alpine as it rises to the Divide enroute to Nutrioso. Just north of the Divide, turn right (east) onto FR56 and follow this steep gravel track for 6.32 miles to a small parking area at the trailhead. The dirt road goes beyond the trailhead.

Sadly, a number of years ago, fire destroyed the old forest that shrouded this peak. However, aspen trees respond well to fire and quickly repopulate once the flames are gone. The trail begins by climbing through quaking aspen groves up the side of the mountain. In some places the trail is an easy stroll, others stretches are breath stealers. Within a mile, the trail reaches the edge of a large meadow, offering gorgeous views of the slopes below and the Blue Range Wilderness area to the south. Beyond the meadows, the trail climbs steeply to the 55-foot fire tower.

From the base of the tower, hikers have excellent views into New Mexico and across the Blue Range. Gazing across the landscape, hikers gain a better understanding of how this region is a maze of high ridges and narrow canyons.

Photo opposite page: Escudilla Peak and Fire Tower

Driving Distance: 8 miles from Alpine
Hiking Distance: 3.3 miles one way
Rating: Moderately strenuous
Elevation: 9480'-10,875'
Best Season: Summer and fall.
	Special Features: Fire tower at summit.
	    Beautiful aspen groves.
	Maps: Apache-Sitgreaves NFS map
	Information: Alpine Ranger Station
	    (928) 339-4384

South Fork Canyon Trail

Hikers might regard the South Fork Trail as a good place to stretch their legs. The trail follows the South Fork of the Little Colorado River as it climbs toward Mexican Lake. In the dry years, this lake has been little more than a mud hole waiting for moisture.

The turnoff to **South Fork** is along State Route 260, four miles east of Eager. After turning south, the road crosses the Little Colorado and begins to climb. Look for a small sign along the road to South Fork Ranch. After passing the ranch and a small campground, the trailhead is on the right side of the road. A well used trail follows the stream. At three miles it joins the trail to Mexican Lake, a total of six miles one way. The canyon has an open mix of willows, deciduous trees and pine trees. For the first three miles, the stream remains a constant even as the trail varies in elevation.

Hiking Distance: 3-6 miles one way
Rating: Moderately Easy
Best Season: Late Spring, summer, early fall.
Special Features: Small stream
Maps: Apache- Sitgreaves NFS map.
Information: Springerville Ranger Station

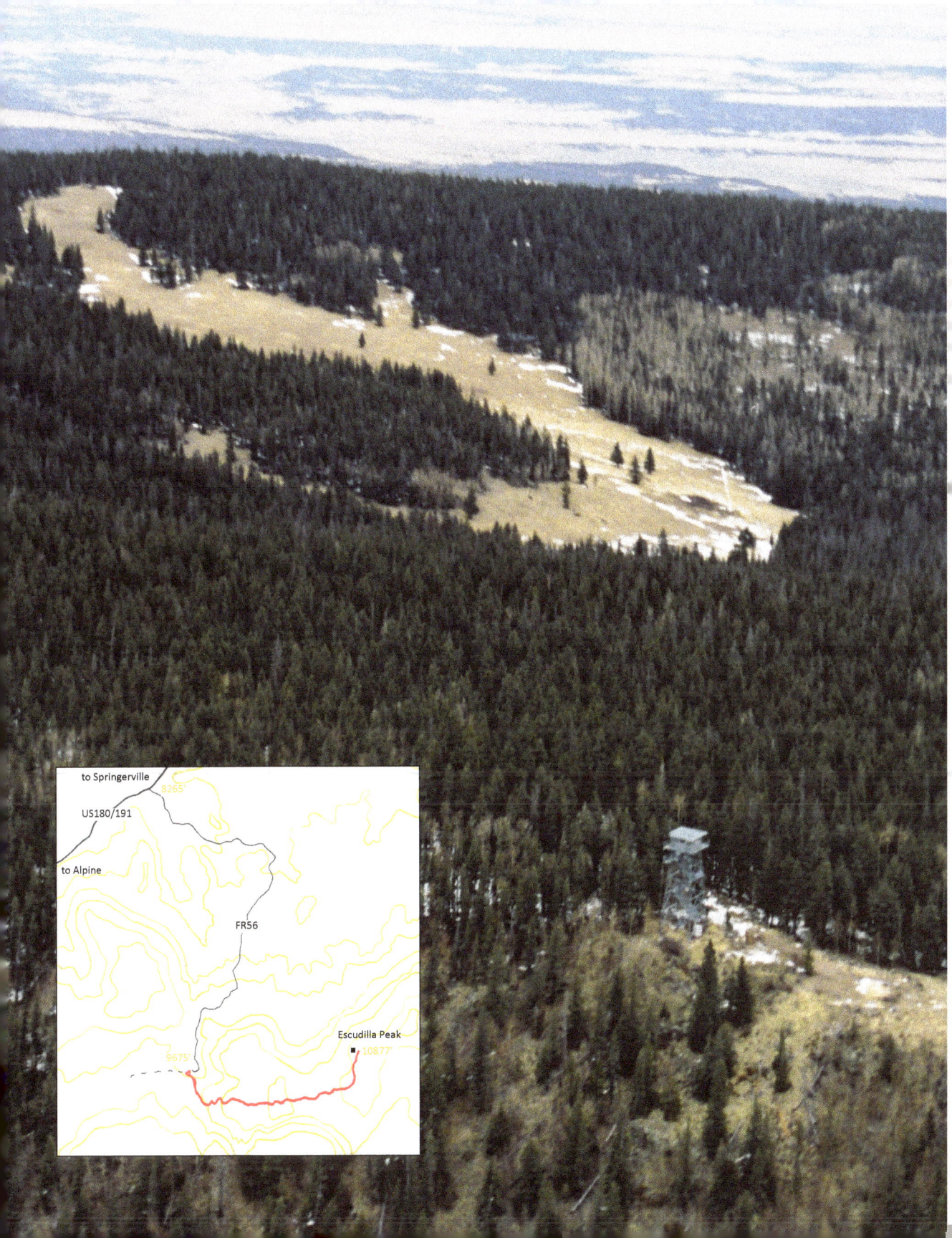

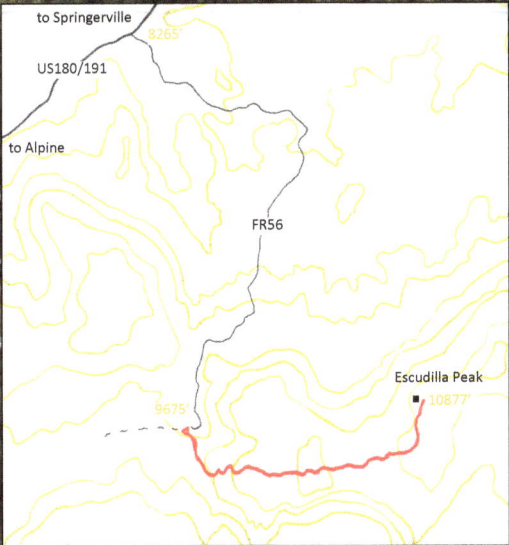

to Springerville
8265'
US180/191
to Alpine
FR56
Escudilla Peak
9675'
10877'

Hannagan Meadow and the Blue Range

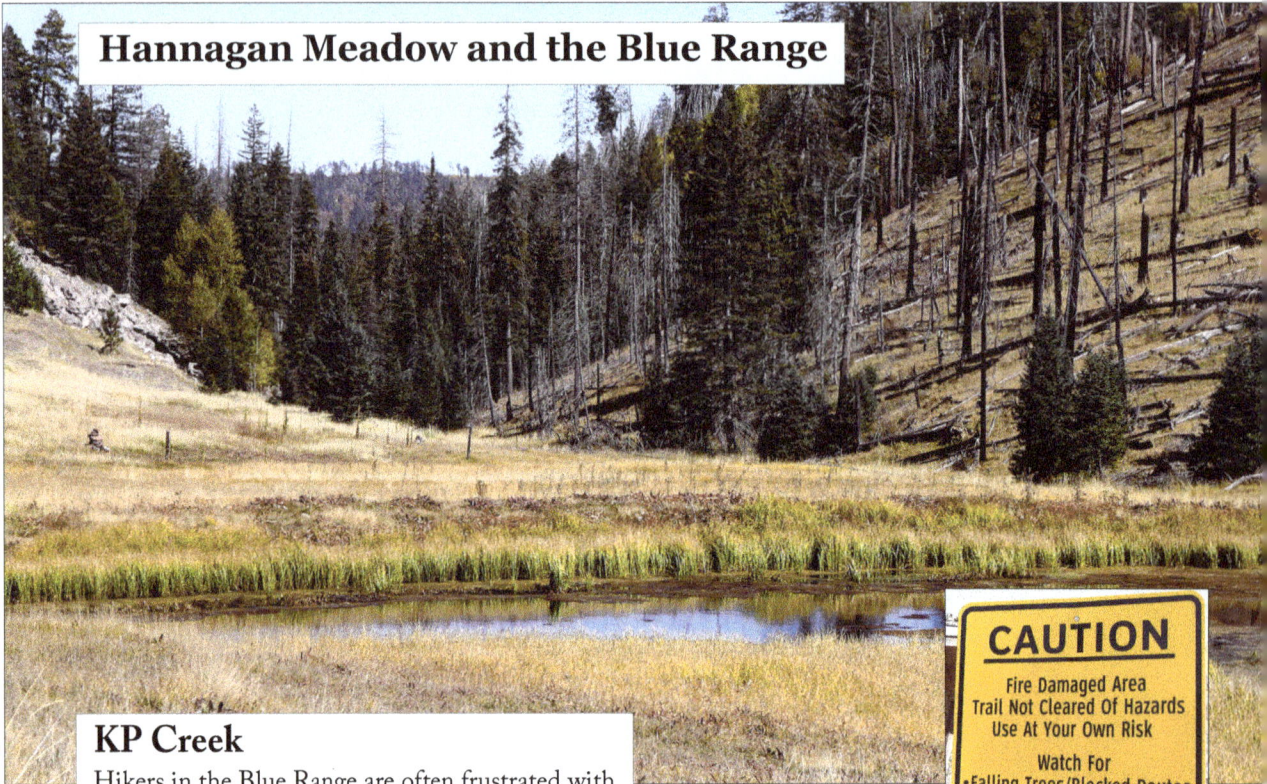

KP Creek

Hikers in the Blue Range are often frustrated with the lack of good information about the trails. For those who enjoy wandering through meadows and along a stream, try **KP Cienega Creek**. This area was burned over several years ago and the vegetation is recovering. A sign near the trailhead warns hikers that the trail has not been cleared so you are hiking at your own risk. Due to the fire there is little shade overhead. The trail is located above the creek and hikers intent on being near the water have a more demanding walk along the banks. The trailhead is located near the cienega as drivers approach the campground.

Driving Distance: 23 miles south of Alpine to campground.
Hiking Distance: 1 or more miles
Rating: Easy   Elevation: 8000'
Best Season: Late Spring, summer, early fall
Special Features: Beautiful meadows, water may be running.
Information: Alpine Ranger Station   (928) 339-4384

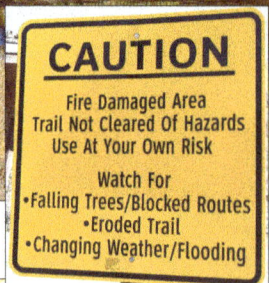

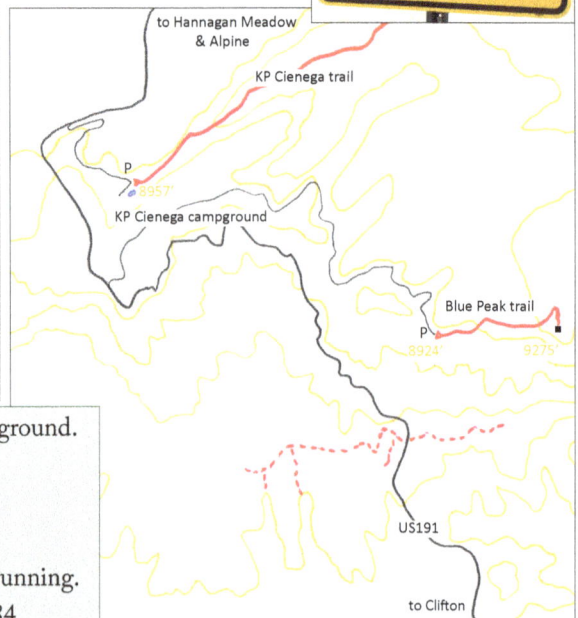

CAUTION

Fire Damaged Area
Trail Not Cleared Of Hazards
Use At Your Own Risk

Watch For
•Falling Trees/Blocked Routes
•Eroded Trail
•Changing Weather/Flooding

to Hannagan Meadow & Alpine

KP Cienega trail

P
8957'

KP Cienega campground

Blue Peak trail

P
8924'   9275'

US191

to Clifton

Blue Fire Tower

When writing Standing Watch: The Fire Towers of Arizona, I hiked into the decommissioned **Blue Fire Tower** and found it a pleasant hike. One problem - a fire had swept through the area, leaving a lot of dead snags creaking and swaying in the wind. I wondered if one would fall across the trail, striking me, as I climbed to the tower. Fifteen years later many of the dead trees have fallen, providing nutrients to the new vegetation.

Drive south along US 191 from Hannagan Meadow about 25 miles - this is one twisting roadway! After passing the turnoff to KP Cienega campground, watch for FR84 on the left. Turn onto FR84 and drive almost five miles to the end of the road and the trailhead. The path drops into a drainage and then begins to climb to the old tower.

Do not attempt to climb the tower. It has not been maintained and has been the residence of rodents possibly carrying the hantavirus. The trees are beginning to obscure the views across the Blue Range but the view remains beautiful. The tower was once critical to controlling wild fires. Today, only a few towers remain in operation and more modern methods are used to chart the progress of any fire.

Driving Distance: From Hannagan Meadow, around 30 miles.
Hiking distance: 1.5 miles one way
Rating: Moderate
Elevation: 9,000 - 9,354 feet
Best Season: Summer and fall
Special Feature: Old Fire Tower
Information: Alpine Ranger Station (928) 339-4384

Photo opposite page:
KP Cienega Spring

Foote Creek to P-Bar Lake

The Foote Creek trail can be accessed from two trailheads. Turning south onto US 191 from Hannagan Meadow, drive a quarter mile to the turnoff and another half mile to a small parking area. The trail follows an old road for a short distance before a foot path leads off to the right at a signed junction. The trail descends steadily through mixed aspen, fir and spruce. On the north side of the path is the Foote Creek drainage with thick meadows and good cover for wildlife. In the late afternoon it is common to see deer and elk feeding in the meadows.

After two miles a sign directs hikers to an old logging road. Another mile and the trail reaches the signed junction with trail #326 from US 191/666. P-Bar Lake is an additional half mile on the edge of a little meadow ringed with aspen and fir. This depression stores water for stock and wildlife in the area. It is not suitable for human consumption. Just past the lake is the junction of Foote Creek and Grant Creek trails.

Driving Distance: 22 miles south of Alpine
Hiking Distance: 3.5 miles one way
Rating: Moderately easy
Elevation: 8000'-7500'
Best Season: Summer, early fall
Special Features: Little pond & excellent
     opportunity to see deer and elk.
Precautions: Bear country.
Maps: Apache-Sitgreaves NFS map
Information: Alpine Ranger Station
     (928) 339-4384

Tucson and the Central Corridor

Tucson, once the site of a Spanish Presidio, has been transformed from its early history as a small Spanish town to an urban hub for commerce, education and one of the most wide-spread national forests.

The area around Tucson is rich in Spanish history that preceded the western expansion of a young country eagerly seeking new lands for its people.

The sky islands of southern Arizona offer a diverse range of zones stretching upward from grasslands to pine-shrouded peaks. Birds and animals rarely seen in the upper 48 states migrate into the sky islands giving residents a glimpse of wildlife.

Many of the trails across southern Arizona are dry and rocky. We've chosen to feature trails that have either interesting historical background or a geographical feature. There are so many interesting areas in south-central Arizona - we could not include all the trails we've enjoyed.

Unfortunately, in recent years the migration of people across the southern border without legal paperwork has created a challenge on trails along the border. We've featured both Organ Pipe and Slaughter's Ranch, knowing there are personnel who can advise visitors on trail access.

One of my favorite trails is Sycamore Canyon in the Pajarita Wilderness but this canyon has become an access point to illegal entrants. If the day comes when this area is again safe, we hope you take the time to visit the Pajarita Wilderness Area and this small canyon. *Photo: Anza Trail*

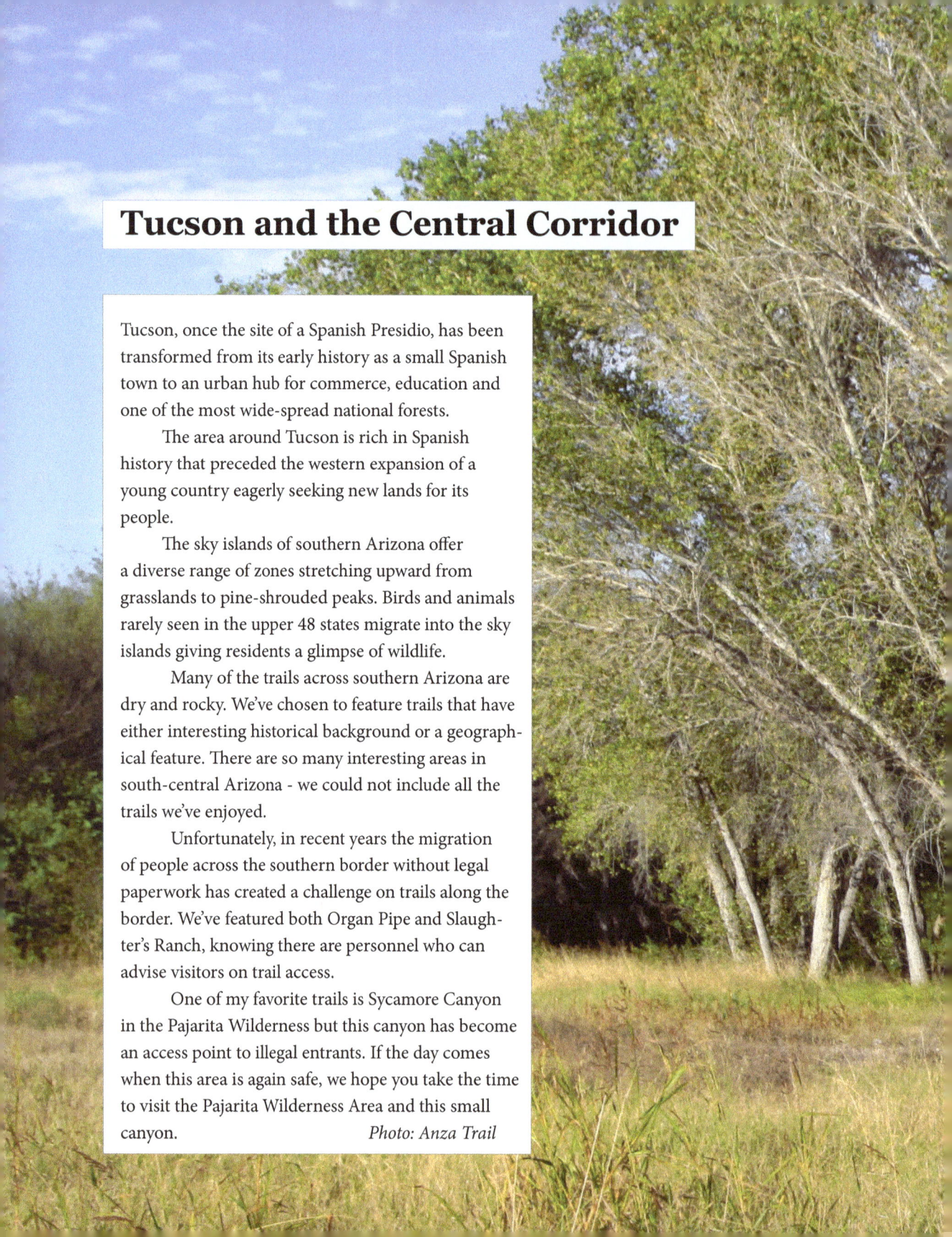

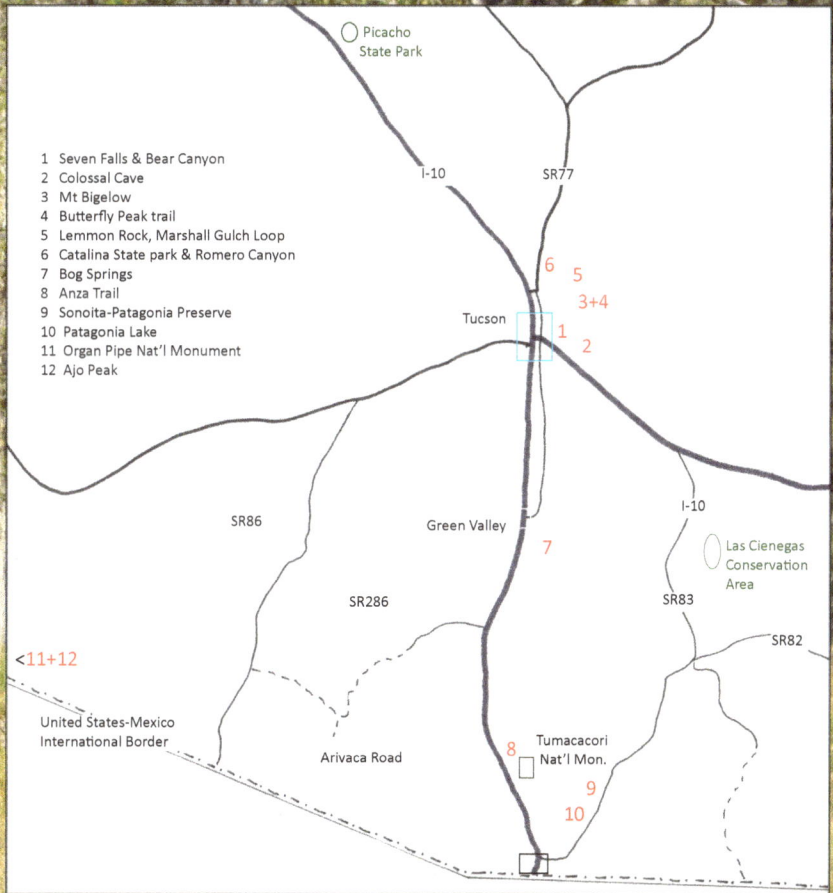

1 Seven Falls & Bear Canyon
2 Colossal Cave
3 Mt Bigelow
4 Butterfly Peak trail
5 Lemmon Rock, Marshall Gulch Loop
6 Catalina State park & Romero Canyon
7 Bog Springs
8 Anza Trail
9 Sonoita-Patagonia Preserve
10 Patagonia Lake
11 Organ Pipe Nat'l Monument
12 Ajo Peak

Picacho
State Park

I-10

SR77

6
5
3+4

Tucson
1
2

Green Valley

7

Las Cienegas
Conservation
Area

I-10

SR86

SR83

SR286

SR82

<11+12

United States-Mexico
International Border

Arivaca Road

8 Tumacacori
Nat'l Mon.

9

10

Seven Falls & Bear Canyon

Towering over the northeastern edge of Tucson, the Santa Catalina Mountains have become the playground of both Tucson's residents and out-of-town visitors. As the trails are so popular, some hikers may look for a more pristine experience. Yet, it would be a shame to ignore Seven Falls. So, brush up on those social skills and join the trek into the Santa Catalinas!

Sabino Canyon

There are two ways to enter Sabino Canyon. Private vehicles are prohibited so visitors hike to the trailhead of choice or board the correct tram. There are two trams, one up Sabino, the other Bear Canyon. Sabino Canyon features several stops including Esperero Trail to Bridal Veil Falls at the last stop and West Fork Canyon to Hutch's Pool.

Seven Falls is spectacular as the water descends through seven pools in Bear Canyon. During the spring runoff, the number of visitors is also astounding. From the intersection with Tanque Verde/Grant Road, follow Sabino Canyon Road to the Visitors Center. Be prepared to pay a parking fee and if you wish to save yourself a three-mile walk to the trailhead, pay a fee for the tram as well.

From the trailhead, the trail drops into a canyon and then begins to ascend along the creek. Over 1.5 miles, the trail crosses Bear Creek 7 times. During the spring when the water is high visitors should be prepared to get their feet wet as they skip from rock to rock. Just past the last crossing, the trail ascends switchbacks up the right or south canyon wall.

From the overlook, the falls are an inspiring sight. Visitors lean out to catch a glimpse of the pool at the bottom of the lowest fall, then look upward to where it all begins. Each waterfall alone would be unique but together they are awesome. Beyond the overlook, the trail descends to the largest pool where sunbathers spread towels across the rocky flats and take a dip in the coffee-colored pools. Be sure to plan your departure carefully so as not to miss the last tram back to the Visitor's Center.

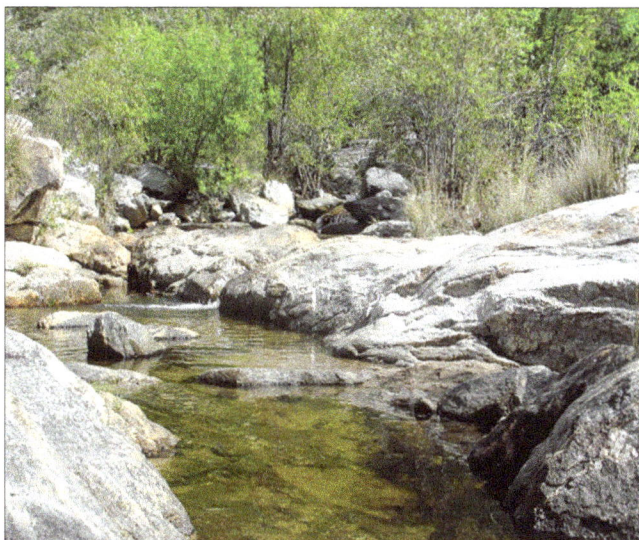

Bear Canyon Creek

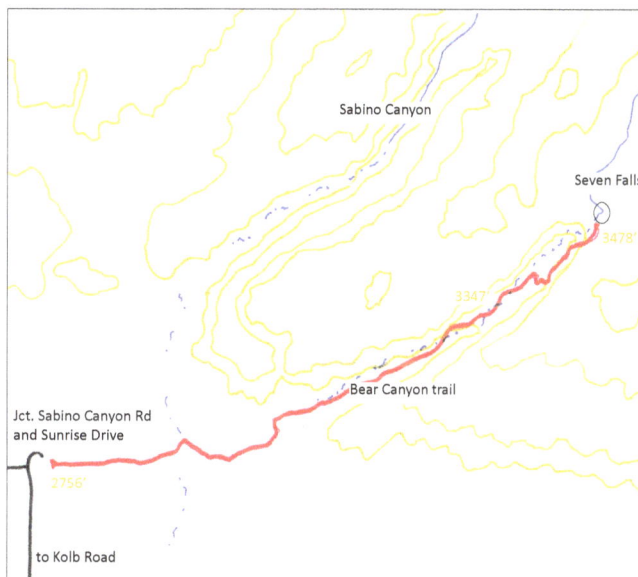

Hiking Distance: 2.5 miles one way
Rating: Moderately easy
Elevation: 2700 - 3000'
Best Season: Spring
Special Features: A beautiful set of waterfalls with swimming holes and hiking along a scenic creek.

Precautions: Rock ledges at falls are extremely slippery in places. Do not trust your feet! High heat in summer. Possible poisonous reptiles and insects.
Maps: Sabino Canyon Recreation Area map
Information: Sabino Canyon Recreation Area (520) 749-8700

Colossal Cave

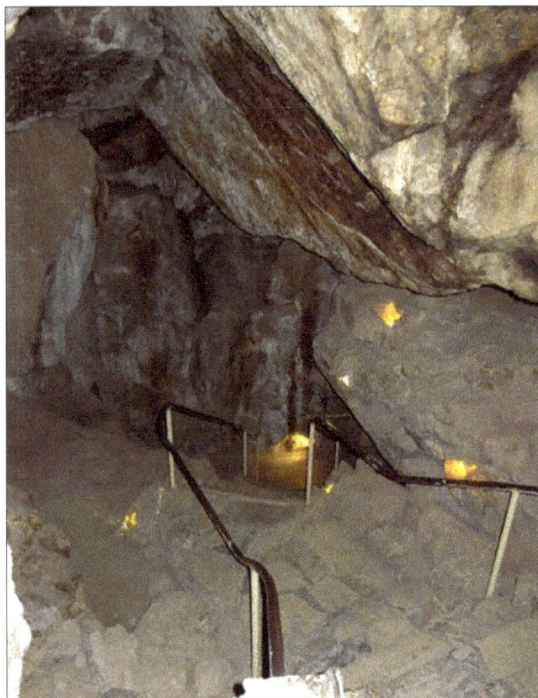

Stepping down into Collossal Cave

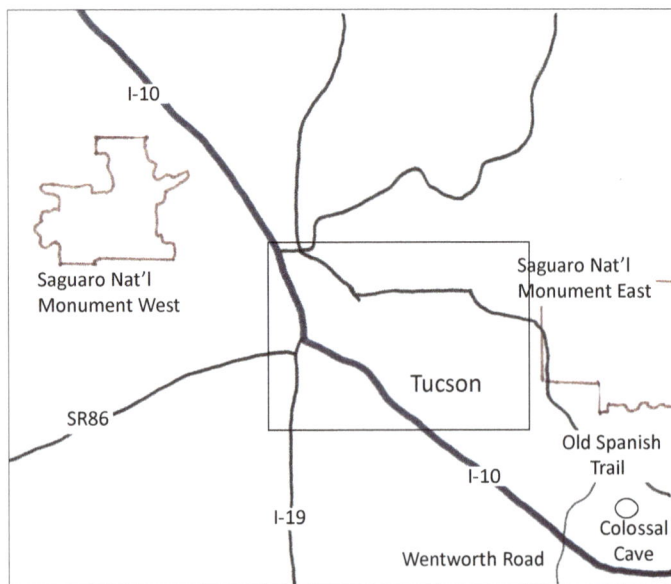

There's nothing like a good cave, providing it has all the essentials, including guides, lights and emergency exits! **Colossal Cave** has all these and more. Not only is it a fascinating place to visit but visitors get some exercise hiking through the narrow passages as they climb through the cave.

The first white man to explore the cave was a bit devious about his tours. For 25 cents he would give customers a length of rope, several candles and a week's supply of food for what was to be a half-day tour. Only after reaching the depths of the cave would he reveal the true length of the tour which took several days. In their time underground, visitors would see some spectacular secrets hidden well below the earth's surface.

Today, guides keep their tours around 45 minutes as they detail the history and geology of Colossal Cave. The Visitors Center and walkways were constructed by the CCC in the 1920's. Visitors pass through a locked wrought-iron gate, descending six and a half stories into the dark depths along dimly lit passages, past 'Old Baldy' and other rock formations.

The guides may describe how bank robbers are believed to have hidden their loot in the cave and exited through a back entrance, eluding the attempts of a posse to arrest them. The gold stolen in the robbery was never recovered.

By the time hikers return to the surface, they have great respect for the early visitors who descended by rope with only candles to light their way.

To reach the Visitors Center, drive southeast on I-10 from Tucson to exit #279. Turn north and follow the paved road 5.9 miles through Vail to the turn off to Colossal Cave. The main road continues northwest to Saguaro National Monument in the Rincon

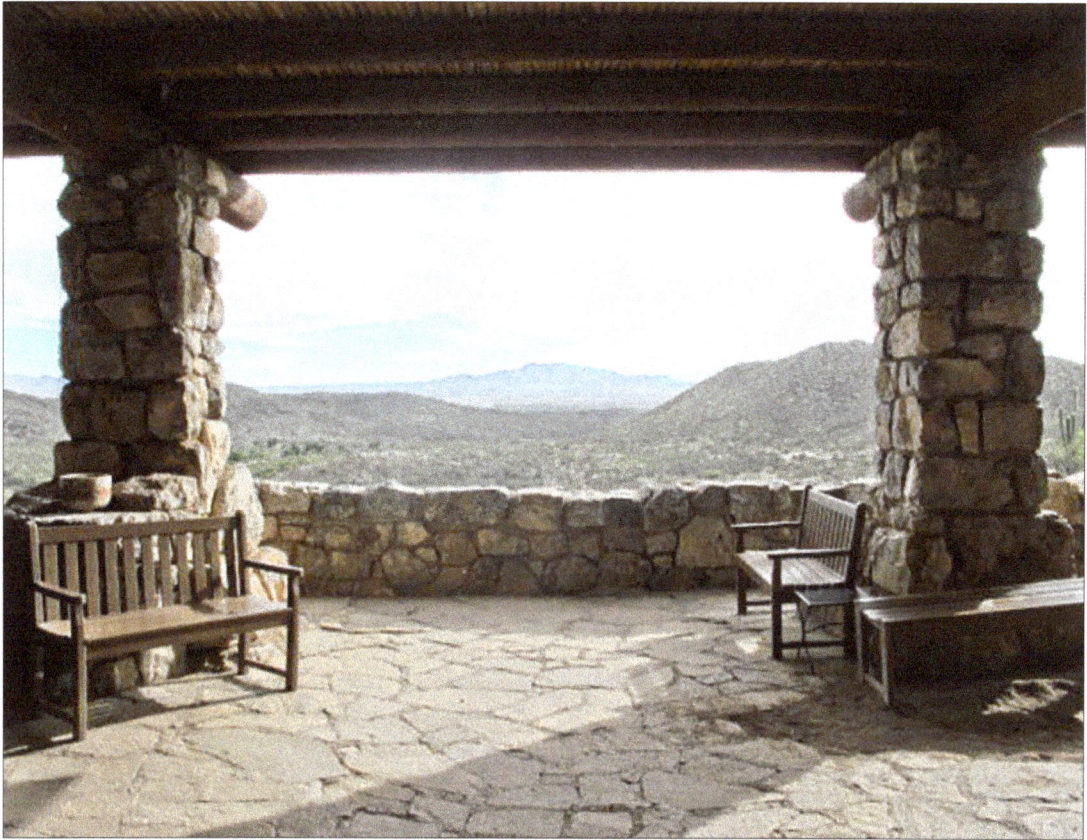

Patio overlooking Posta Quemada Canyon

Mountains. From the turnoff, drive .6 mile to the Visitors Center where tickets are purchased for the next tour.

The Posta Quemada Canyon, below the Visitors Center, stands as a welcome refuge of green in a dry desert. The canyon, just .25 mile from the Center, has day use ramadas and a small trail leading down into the creek. About five miles upstream is Papago Springs which feeds the creek. The stream is a source of water to local wildlife. Watch for tracks and other signs of animal life in the damp earth.

Driving Distance: Via I-10, 25 miles from
    Tucson
Hiking Distance: Through the cave .75 mile.
Rating: Easy
Best Season: All year, hot outside in summer.
Special Features: A live cave with mineralized
    rock formations. Shallow creek with
    signs of wildlife.
Precautions: For those who struggle with
    claustrophobia, passages in cave may
    seem a bit close. Watch for rattlesnakes
    and cactus along creek.
Information: Colossal Cave Mountain Park

Mount Bigelow

The Santa Catalina Highway winds through the foothills of the Santa Catalina Mountains which rise above Tucson. The highway steadily ascends till reaching Summerhaven a small community at the summit. Along the route are several campgrounds with opportunities to hike and explore.

Nineteen miles from Tucson, the **Palisades Ranger Station** is located on the left or south side of the highway. This is a good place to stop and browse the gift shop while asking any questions about the hiking trails.

Across from the Palisades Ranger Station is **Mount Bigelow,** the site of several radio towers as well as a fire lookout tower. A footpath takes hikers up a short ascent from the Ranger Station to the towers - a nice way to stretch our legs after the long drive.

The Mt. Bigelow Lookout tower is seldom used these days. But when lightning starts snapping and thunder rolls over the mountains, the Forest Service may send a staff member to stand watch for a couple of hours.

Only a few years ago, fire swept across the Santa Catalinas, leaving large swathes of hillside blackened with charred pine totems. Summerhaven survived the flames and has come back stronger than ever - a nice place to stop for lunch or maybe a cold drink after a hike on a warm afternoon.

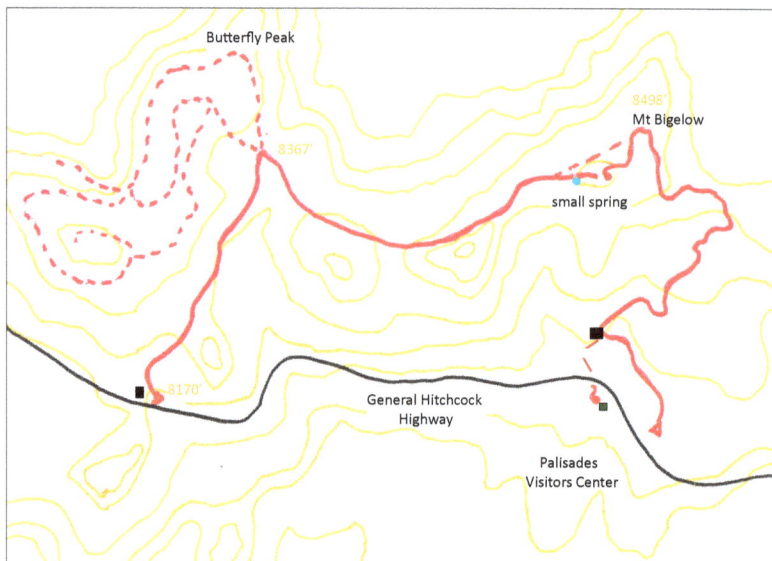

Butterfly Peak · 8498' · Mt Bigelow · 8367' · small spring · 8170' · General Hitchcock Highway · Palisades Visitors Center

Butterfly Peak Trail

A longer alternative to the Sunset Trail is the Butterfly Peak trail. Hikers start at Soldiers Camp, decending in elevation 400 feet to a trail junction. A side trail directs hikers left to the summit while the right branch continues to drop enroute to a small spring and reparian zone. The trail passes the site of a plane crash, frequently visited by hikers.

We found the ascent became a bit confusing as we neared Mt Bigelow. Be careful not to stray onto the Kellogg trail if you intend to end up at Palisades. The route back along the road is 3 miles and a pre-arranged shuttle is wonderful for tired hikers.

> Distance: 4.5 - 5 miles
> Elevation: 8,500' - 8,600'
>   1,500' drop between two points
> Rating: Moderate to Difficult
> Best Season: Summer, shoulder seasons
>   the trail may be icy in spots.
> Map: CFS Santa Catalina District map
> Information: Palisades Ranger Station

Sunset Trail to Mt Bigelow

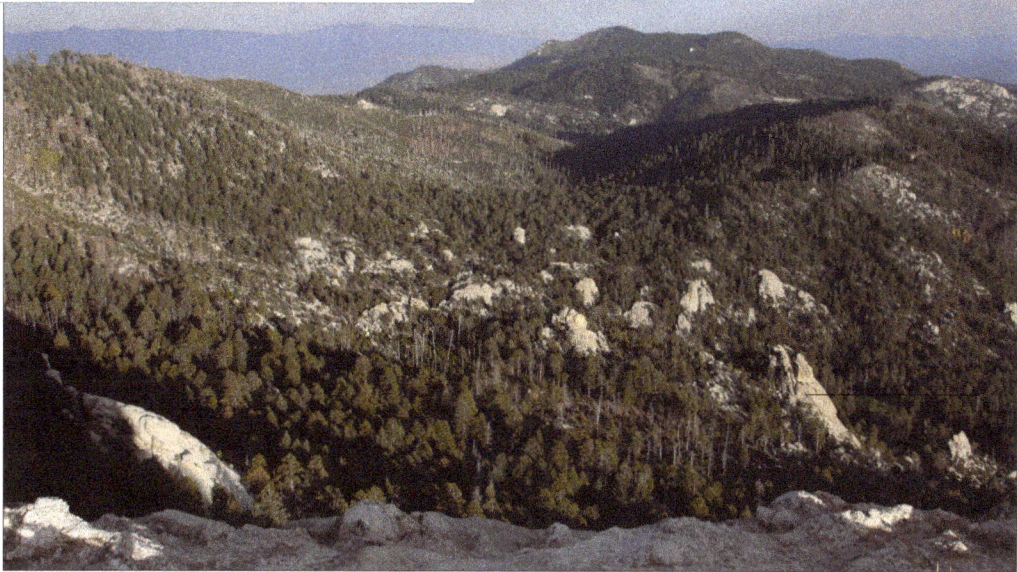

Looking east from the Santa Catalina Mountain Highway, above the Butterfly Peak trail

Nearly 20 years ago, flames swept over the Santa Catalinas, leaving hillsides with blackened poles rather than lush green ponderosa. Two decades later, vegetation has returned and the slopes are beautiful again.

A portion of the **Sunset Trail**, just east of Soldiers Camp is a good choice for day hikers who want a hike with time to explore other areas. The trailhead is east of Soldiers Camp at a wide bend in the highway. Along the route, the trail passes below the Mt Bigelow campground with dispersed camping. A number of trails are woven around this site - stay on course for Mt. Bigelow.

The trail drop 360 feet in elevation before ascending Mt Bigelow to Palisades. From Mount Bigelow, hikers return back to their vehicle or have a shuttle arranged at Palisades.

Sunset Trail to Mt Bigelow & Palisades
Hiking Distance: 2 miles one way.
Driving Distance: 19 miles from
     Tanque Verde Road
Rating: Moderate
Elevation: 8500' - 8600'
Best Season: Summer, fall.
Special features: A beautiful sky island retreat
Precautions: Hopefully trail junctions are signed
     or a bit of route finding may be necessary.
Maps: Coronado NFS map /
     Santa Catalina District
Information: Palisades Ranger Station (walk in)
     CNF Santa Catalina District
     (520) 749-8700

Mt. Bigelow fire tower may be used to keep watch over the northeastern slopes but a second lookout looks over the southwestern slopes and the desert plains surrounding Tucson. **Lemmon Rock** is now off limits to visitors as the lookout is required to keep watch without idle interruption.

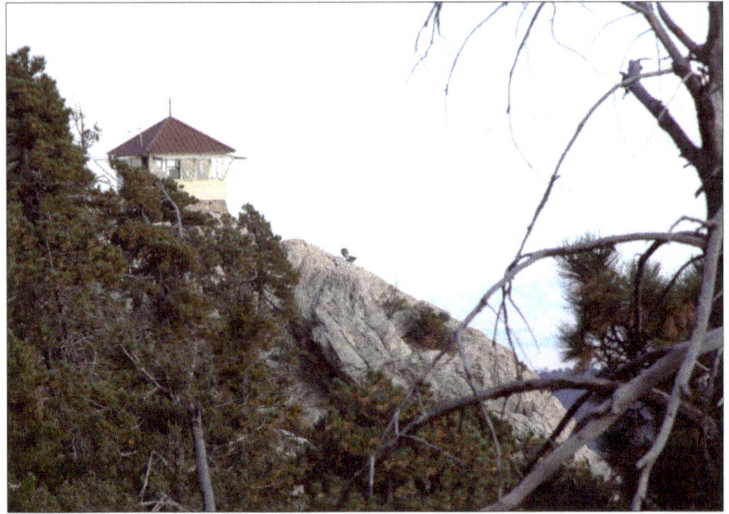

Around Lemmon Rock, a network of trails follows the terrain across the peaks and ravines on either side of the lookout. Hikers may choose to do one, two or three sections of trail as a loop combined with a section of the highway. To reach the summit, hikers drive the Santa Catalina Highway 30 miles, passing the Ski Area to arrive at the gate enclosing the Mt Graham Observatory. From the parking area, walk to the electrical grid station. The path passes behind the chain link fence and drop down the slope, following the terrain. At the first junction, signage points toward either the Marshall Gulch trail or Lemmon Rock. Turning toward Lemmon Rock, at a second fork in the trail, stay left for the cabin. The right fork leads to Quartzite Spring. The water is channeled through a pipe with the overflow released down the hillside to maintain the riparian area.

Top Photo: Lemmon Rock Fire Cabin
Bottom: Along the Marshall Gulch trail

For those wishing to complete the 9.5-mile loop, return to the first junction and turn right. The trail follows the terrain to the Marshall Gulch trail, then climbs to the Aspen-Marshall Gulch trail head. Hopefully, hikers have arranged a shuttle back as it is a long walk to the observatory.

Another option within this network is to drive through Summerhaven to the **Aspen-Marshall Gulch** trailhead. The two trails form a 3.7 mile loop with the right side of the loop called the Aspen Trail, the left side designated as Marshall Gulch. From any combination of trails, hikers have wide-open views of the lower slopes of the Santa Catalinas as well as the Tucson Mountains and the desert plains. If a summer storm moves in, it woud be wise to find shelter or get off the trail completely.

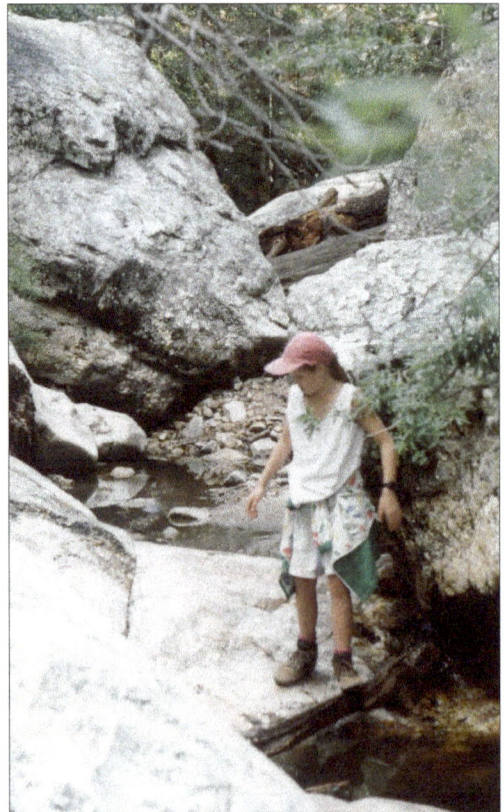

162

Lemmon Rock and Marshall Gulch - Aspen Trail

Driving Distance:

Hiking Distance: Lemmon Rock Lookout   1.5 mile out and back

         Aspen - Marshall Gulch trail   4.2 mile loop

Rating: Moderately

Elevation: Lemmon Rock   9,088 - 8,760'

         Aspen - Marshall Gulch   7,513' - 8,104'

Best Season: Summer, fall.

Special features: Historic fire cabin, natural spring, beautiful
         boulder-choked canyon.

Precautions: Watch your feet along the aspen trail for toe catchers.

Maps: Coronado NFS map / Santa Catalina District

Information: CNF Santa Catalina District (520) 749-8700

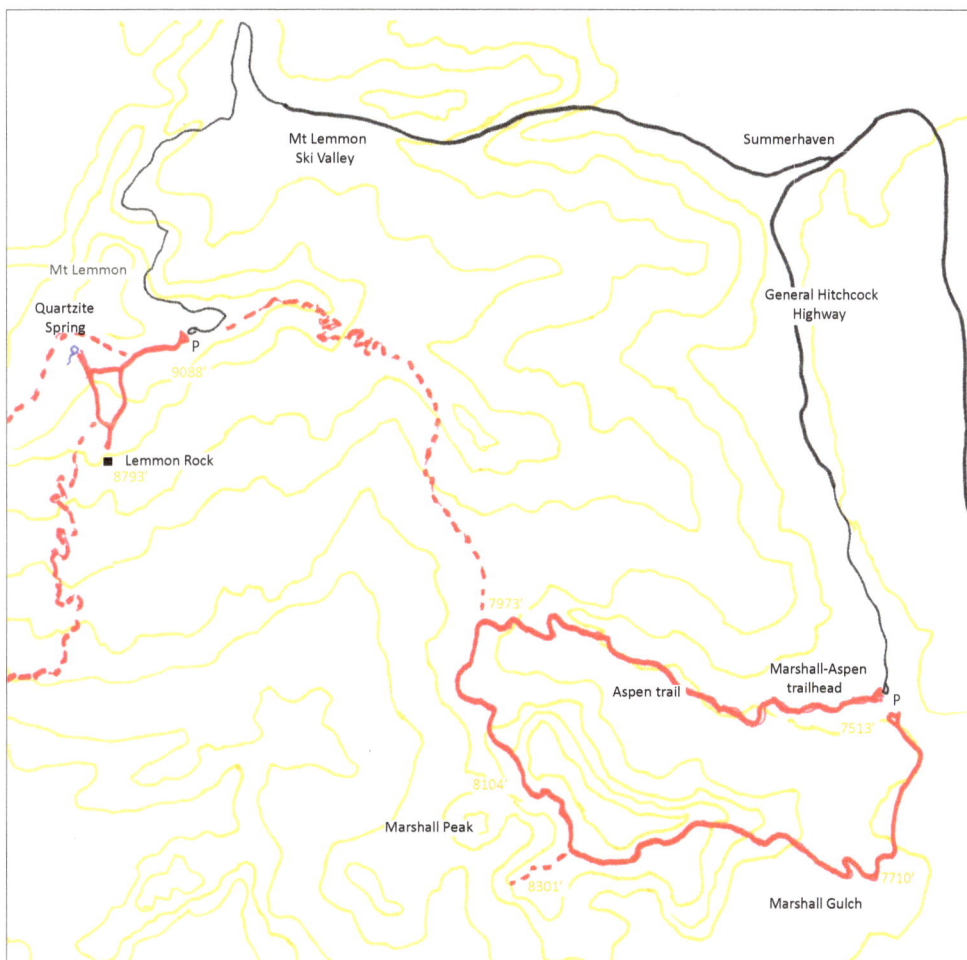

Catalina State Park, Romero Canyon and the Montrose Pools

Catalina State Park lies north of Tucson along Sutherland Wash. Nice campgrounds with several short trails and access to the longer trails of the Santa Catalinas have made this a favored spot for hikers in southern Arizona. The campground fills up quickly on weekends during the cooler months. To reach the park, follow Oracle Road (Hwy 89) north from Tucson. At mp 81.1, turn right into Catalina State Park. The state charges an entrance fee. The main road runs through the park to a day-use parking area for the **Romero Canyon** and **Sutherland** trails.

Romero Canyon Trail

The Romero Pools are a delightful retreat from the heat of early summer, but hiking in high temperatures with the heat reflecting off the rocks can be brutal on a summer day. An alternative to the Romero Pools are the Montrose Pools just a mile from the trailhead.

The trailhead for Romero and Sutherland Canyons is just a few yards away from Sutherland Wash. Notice that there are a couple of other routes, one a nature trail, the other through thick brush favoring bird watchers. With low water,

be prepared to rock hop or even wade across the stream. Do not attempt to cross the wash if flooded. After a short ascent, the trail is an easy walk to the foot of the Catalinas. At the base of the foothills the trail begins to climb through switchbacks to an intersection with the trail down to the **Montrose Pools trail**. If this is your destination, watch your steps over the loose rock.

Continuing on to Romero Pools, stay left at the junction and climb to the wilderness boundary where a sign states that dogs are not permitted. The trail continues up the side of Romero Canyon through cuts in the hillside, switchbacking past large boulders that bake hikers' skin during warm weather. After reaching a false summit, the trail descends, only to climb again. Winding through large boulders and brush, watch the cairns to remain on the trail. There are great views from a steep drop-off on the left side. After topping a small rise, the trail drops past the Romero Pools enroute to ascend Romero Pass and the summit of the Catalinas. Many hikers spend a pleasant afternoon in Romero Pools before returning to the trailhead.

Hiking Distance: (all indicated mileages are one-way)
     Romero-Sutherland loop 2.3 miles
     Romero to Montrose Pools 1.1 miles
     Romero Pools trail 2.8 miles
     Romero Pass 7.2 miles
Rating: Lower elevation - easy, Route to pools, moderate.
Elevation: 2700'-3600' at Romero Pools, 6000' Romero Pass Best Season: Spring, fall
Special Features: Beautiful pools in a mountain canyon. During hot weather, check with the Forest
     Service as to whether there is water in the pools.
Precautions: Watch footing around pools to avoid a dangerous fall.
Maps: Catalina State Park trail map, Coronado NFS map
Information: Catalina State Park   (520) 628-5798

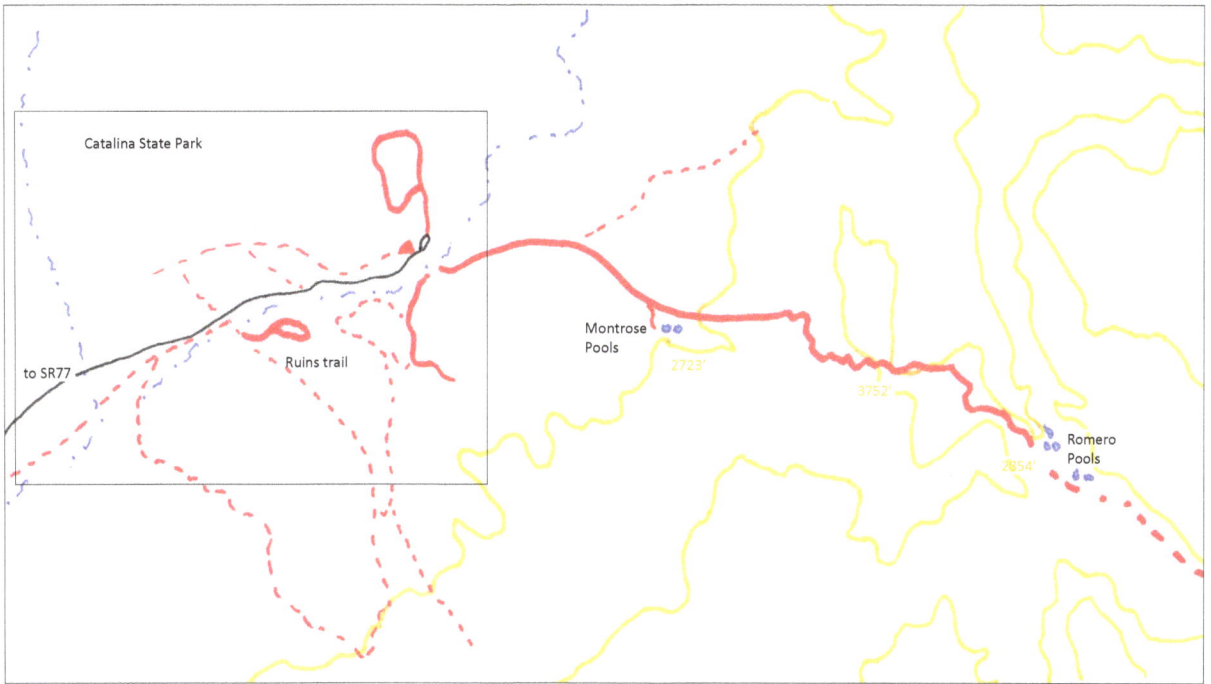

Romero Ruins Trail

These ruins gives us a glimpse of the lives of early residents. From the trailhead at Catalina State Park, the trail crosses Sutherland Wash, then climbs a bluff to visit a prehistoric site with explanatory signs. First, the prehistoric people, then later, the Spanish built their homes using the materials around them. The interpretive signs explore the vital role of water and plants to the Native American people who lived in the area. This mile-long loop brings hikers back to Sutherland Wash and the parking lot. The trail is easily combined with other short trails in the area. The campground makes a good base for exploring the network of trails over a couple of days.

Hiking Distance: approximately .75 mile
Rating: Easy
Elevation: 2700'

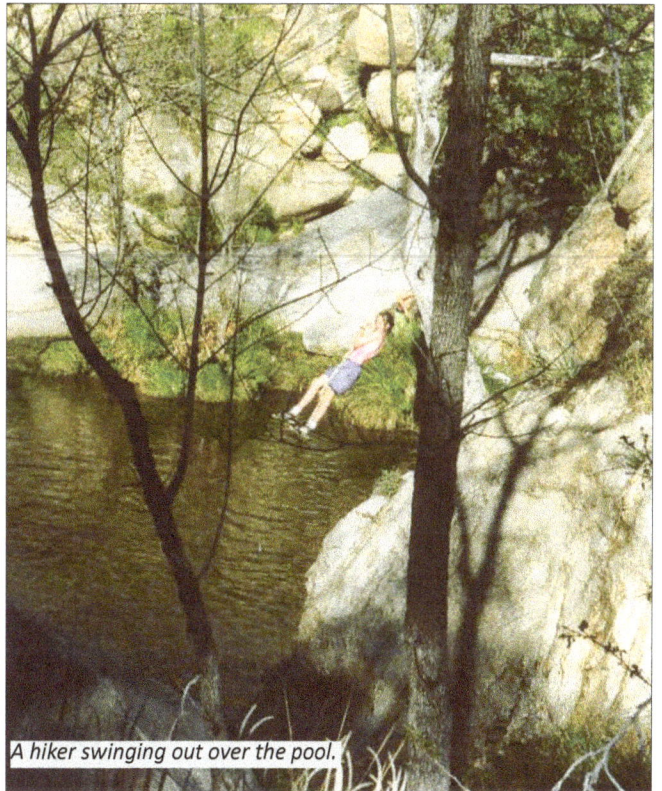

A hiker swinging out over the pool.

Bog Springs/ Santa Rita Mountains

This five-mile trail in Madera Canyon is actually a loop but many hikers proceed as far as Bog Springs and call it a day. I prefer the trail head in Bog Springs Campground. The trail ascends along a hillside before reaching a fenceline and turns left to Bog Springs. A right turn into the loop would take hikers to Kent Spring first.

From the junction, it is .8 miles to Bog Springs with the trail following the contours of the terrain. The spring emerges in a fold on the hillside, sheltered by a rich stand of Arizona walnut trees with sycamores and silver leaf oak.

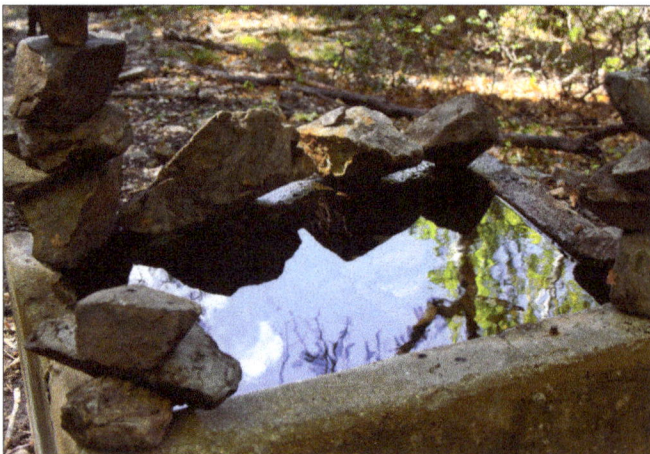

Photo: Bog Spring
Opposite: Sycamore near Bog Spring

One late afternoon when the kids and I hiked up to the spring, a mother bear with two cubs had been actively grazing in the area. We made lots of noise as we approached the spring rather than risk surprising her. As much as we would like to have seen the bear, we were relieved to miss her as she had been rather aggressive toward intruders that week. Watch for the small Coues white tail deer that graze in this area.

From Bog Springs, the trail climbs through switchbacks toward Kent Springs, another 1.2 miles. Beyond Kent, the trail turns east, back toward the campground, passing Sylvester Spring in a half mile. Past Sylvester, the trail climbs out of a ravine and another two miles returns visitors to the campground. Total distance is about 5 miles but with the springs it is a pleasant hike and an opportunity to see some wildlife.

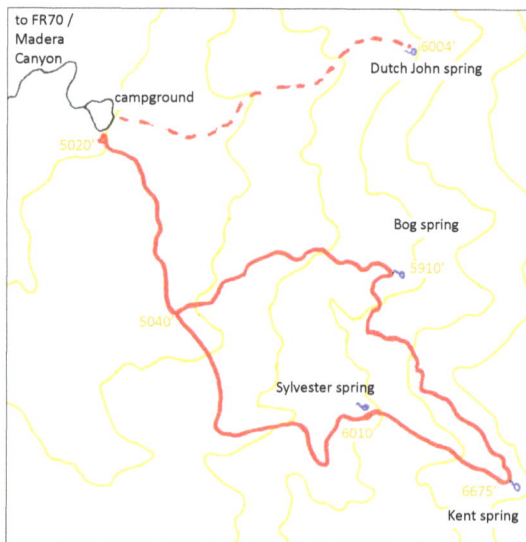

Driving Distance: 11.5 miles from I-19
Hiking Distance: 3 miles Bog Springs, round trip
        5 miles Bog Springs/Kent Springs loop
Rating: Moderate
Elevation: 5040'-6640'
Best Season: Late spring, summer & fall.

Special Features: Lots of wildlife & Arizona walnuts supported by perennial springs.
Precautions: Watch for bears, poisonous reptiles. Great to see, not so great if threatened.
Maps: Coronado NFS map / Nogales District
Information: CNF Santa Catalina District (520) 749-8700

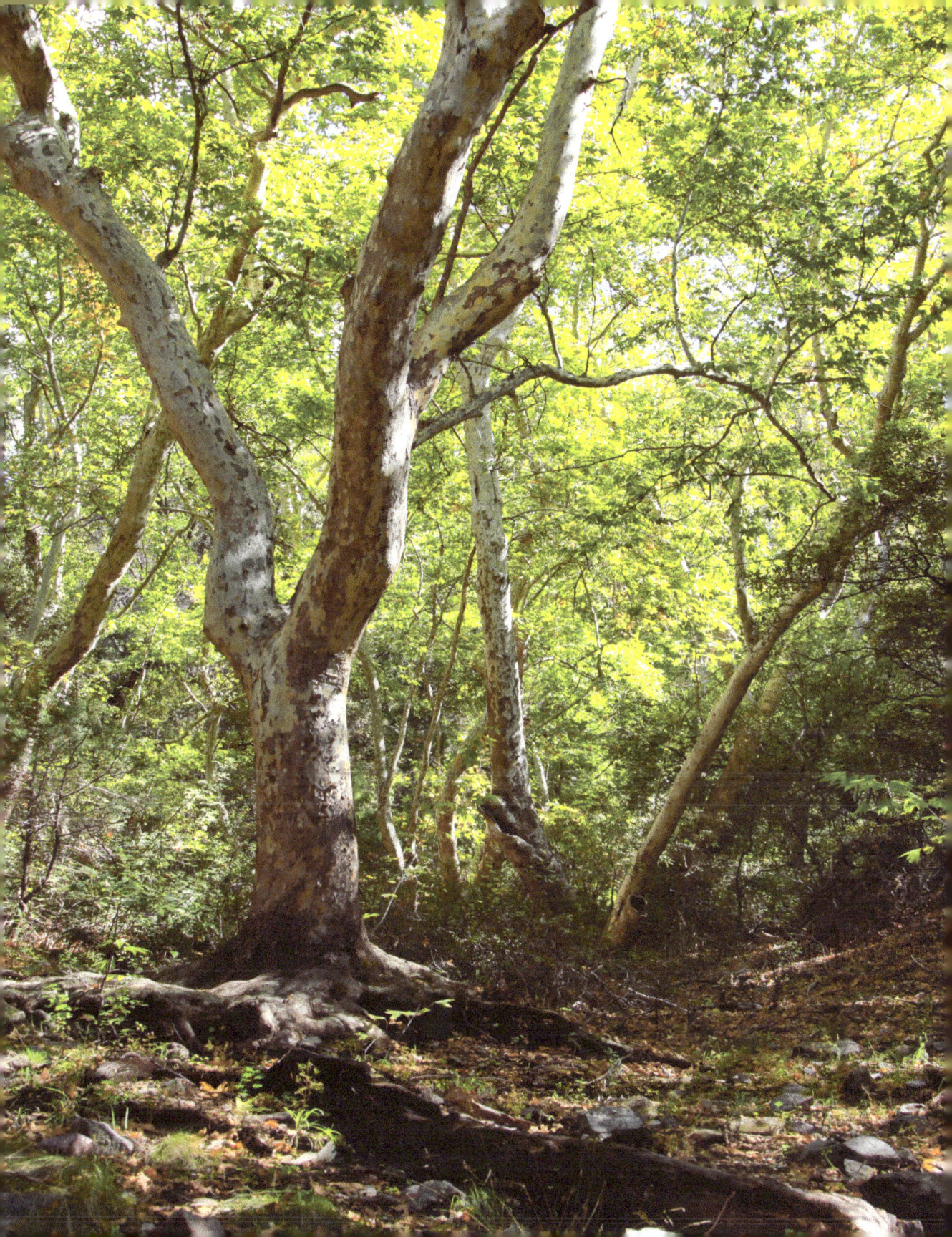

Anza Trail: Tubac Presidio to Tumacacori Mission

In 1776, as 13 colonies along the eastern coastline of North America were celebrating their proclamation of freedom, Captain Juan Baptista de Anza led an expedition north out of New Spain (Mexico) to Monterey, California. Their route? Right through the community of Tubac, north to the Gila River and across to the Colorado River. We can still walk part of this historic route along the Anza trail.

Drive south along I-19 from Tucson toward Nogales. Note that the mileage along the interstate is listed in kilometers. At exit 48, drop under the freeway and drive into the market at Tubac. Park at the historic Presidio. Hikers could take the time to tour the museum and learn more about the Spanish presence in North America.

The trail head is just beyond the Presidio along the Santa Cruz River. The trail follows the bank of the stream, at one point crossing to the opposite bank, for 2.3 miles in length. In places the path is nearly overgrown by vegetation - push through but watch for snakes.

At Tumacacori National Historic Site, visitors pay a fee to tour the grounds. An attempt has been made to restore the Catholic Mission. It gives visitors an idea of the importance of such an outlier of civilization in a raw land in the 1600s. Arrive on a festival day and the effect can be dynamic with vendors and performances.

To return, either arrange a shuttle or walk back on the path, thinking about the men and women who once made their way along the Santa Cruz to a new life.

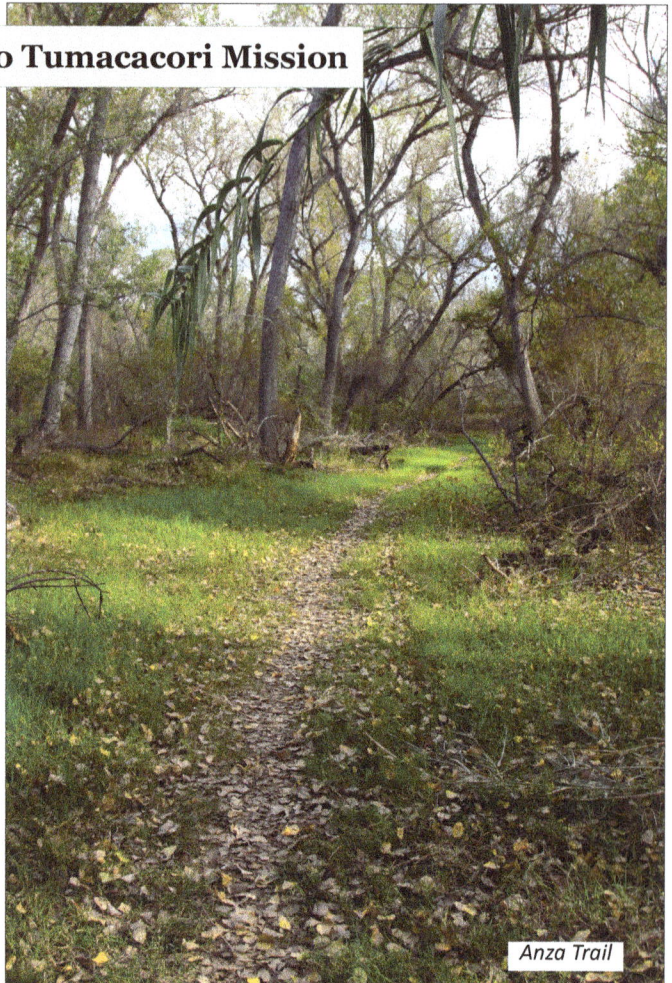

Anza Trail

Driving Distance: 44 miles from Tucson
Hiking Distance: 2.3 miles one-way
Rating: Easy   Elevation: 3857 feet
Best Season: Winter, spring, & fall.
Special Features: Historic Spanish Mission and Presidio.
Precautions: Watch for poisonous reptiles. Use mosquito repellent if mosquitos are present. A pipe at the Nogales dump has repeatedly broken, sending trash downstream toward Tubac. Mosquitos alight on the muddy bank and then on us.
Maps: Area map from either the Presidio or the Mission
Information: Presidio Historic Park (520) 398-2522

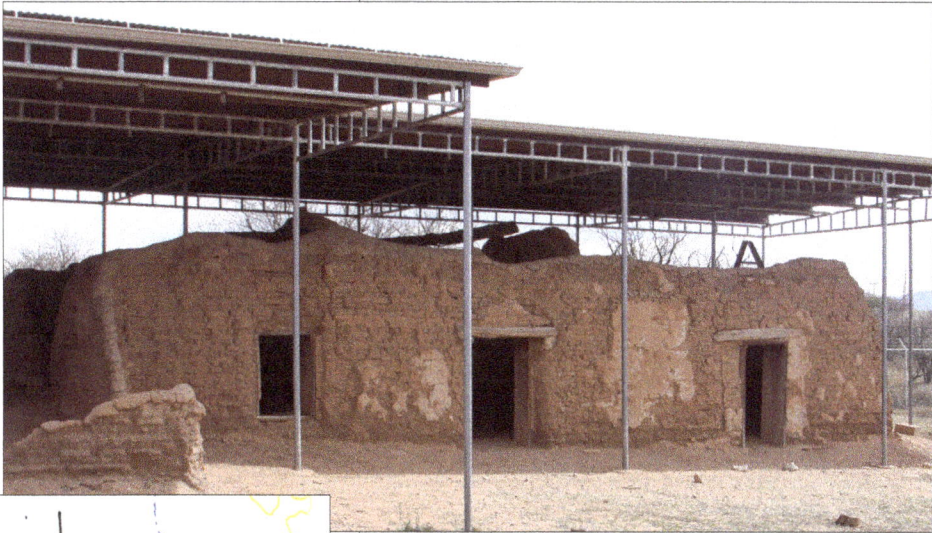

Calabasas Mission Ruins

Visiting the Spanish Missions: Tumacacori, Calabasas & Xavier del Bac

Spanish priests first entered Arizona, following the Conquistadors in their exploration for the Cities of Gold. The Conquistadors were disappointed in the poor brush shelters of the native tribes and returned to New Spain. The priests remained, determined to bring the native tribes into the Catholic faith. The Mission at Tumacacori was one of a chain of missions built across southern Arizona and would have been the center of community celebrations. When the territory of southern Arizona became part of the United States, the old missions fell into decline for a period of time until interest grew in restoring them.

San Xavier Del Bac near Tucson has been fully restored and is visited by hundreds of thousands each year. Two mission sites, Guevavi and Calabasas, may be visited by reservation during the cooler months - call Tumacacori Historical Park for information.

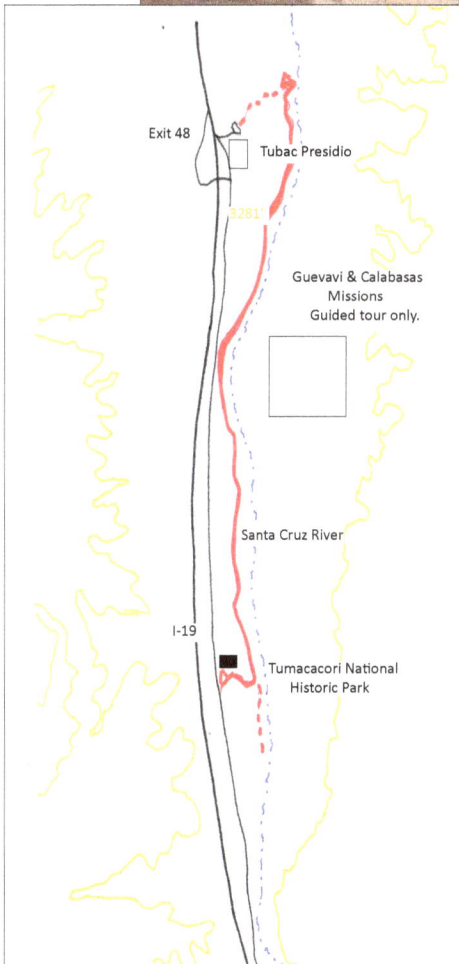

Exit 48

Tubac Presidio

Guevavi & Calabasas Missions Guided tour only.

Santa Cruz River

I-19

Tumacacori National Historic Park

Patagonia-Sonoita Creek Preserve

The little town of Patagonia is located on State Route 82, just 19 miles northeast of Nogales. On the southern edge of the community, a riparian area has been set aside to protect wildlife and preserve fragile wetlands from encroaching development. Sandwiched between the Santa Rita Mountains and the Patagonia Mountains, **Sonoita Creek** provides a welcome refuge to desert wildlife as well as the people of southern Arizona.

Visitors park at the Visitors Center. A trail loops around the Preserve and back to the Visitors Center. There is no established destination - instead visitors watch for wild life and unique species of birds as they move along the creek. Throughout the refuge the meadows and woodlands preserve open space for the species that favor the Preserve. Walk quietly and you may have an opportunity to see raccoons, coatimundi, deer and squirrels.

The bird life is what really draws visitors to the refuge. The director noted that if a rare bird shows up, within days he may see bird watchers arrive from around the world seeking a siting of the species. Binoculars and a good bird book are helpful to identify the small feathered creatures that emit their calls through the woodland.

Hiking Distance: .5+ mile
Rating: Easy
Elevation: 3325'
Maps: Coronado NFS map /
        Nogales District
Information:
        Patagonia Lake State Park
        (520) 287-6965

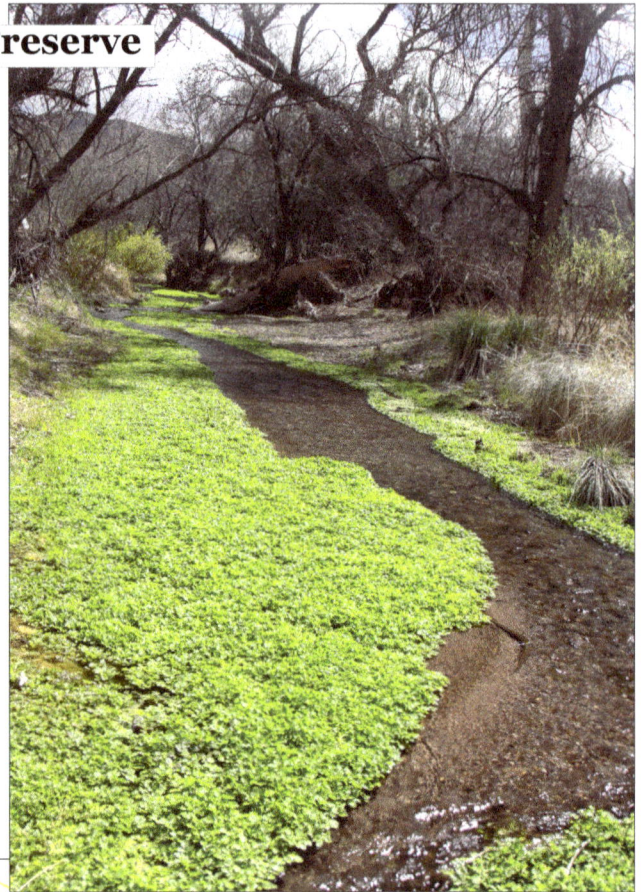

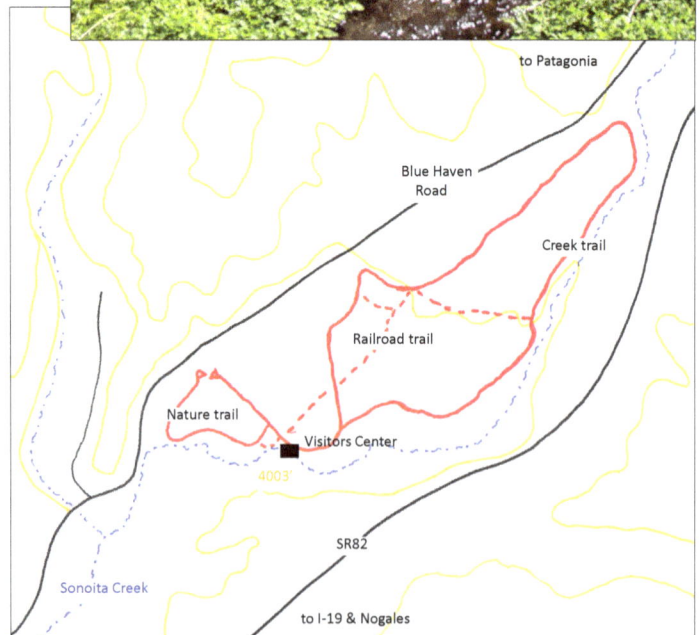

to Patagonia

Blue Haven
Road

Creek trail

Railroad trail

Nature trail

Visitors Center

4003'

SR82

Sonoita Creek

to I-19 & Nogales

Patagonia Lake

Patagonia Lake was created when Game and Fish placed a dam across Sonoita Creek in 1974. The lake has a marina for launching private or rented water craft. A sandy beach offers a shallow area for swimming. Both fishermen and water skiers share the surface area. However, this lake is more than recreation. It offers water and refuge to a variety of wildlife and birds.

To reach the lake, drive 16 miles northeast from Nogales on State Route 82. Turn north onto Patagonia Lake Road. The entrance is open from 8:00 am to 10:00 p.m. daily with a users fee. Drive past the turnoff to the park rangers' residence and turn right, to either the marina or a large parking lot above the beach.

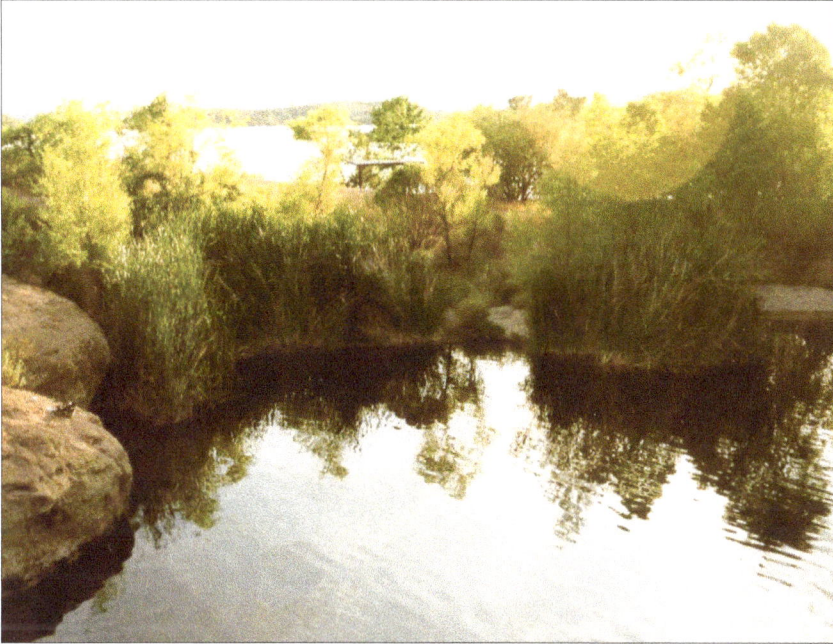

A short trail winds along the shoreline about a half mile to the point where Sonoita Creek enters the lake. As hikers approach the creek, a wide expanse of thick brush and small trees grow close to the shore intersected by a number of cow trails. Choose a trail and navigate through the brush. The creek isn't very deep but it carries a fair amount of water in a dry climate. Keep an eye on the skyline for large raptors sailing the thermal currents as they watch the lake for a meal. Hikers may spot large herons fishing, balanced on one leg along the shoreline.

Historically, this is a unique area. Before the United States acquired Arizona and New Mexico from Mexico, a number of large land grants were awarded to wealthy land owners. When the United States acquired Arizona, some of these land grants were legally honored, including the one known as the Jose de Sonoita Grant. To walk the creek is to walk through history, across the land grant and to remember the Spanish and Indian vaqueros that once herded stock along its shoreline.

For those who don't speak Spanish this area can be a unique experience since so many of its residents come from the Mexican culture with Spanish language and customs.

Organ Pipe Cactus National Monument

Organ Pipe National Monument is a refuge dedicated to preserving the animals and plants of the Sonoran Desert. The monument's namesake is the organ pipe cactus. The Monument offers U.S. citizens a chance to see an environment that covers much of northern Mexico, our neighbor to the south, with a glimpse of the struggle for life in such harsh territory.

It is best to visit Organ Pipe during the winter months when the Park is teeming with activity under moderate temperatures. In the summer, temperatures can reach 115 degrees. This is a popular stop with both retirees in their recreational vehicles and visitors to Rocky Point, Mexico.

Two scenic car routes take visitors through the back country of the Park. The most poular route takes visitors through Arch Canyon past Mount Ajo. The second route starts just north of the Lukeville Border Station and passes the Quitobaquito Spring before turning north through the back country of the Monument.

Three trails start near the Visitors Center. The **Palo Verde Trail** parallels the road from the Visitor Center to a circular path around the campground. The **Desert View Nature Trail** is at the campground. Last and longer is the **Victoria Mine Trail** leading from the campground to the site of an old mine, 4.5 miles round trip. Check with Monument rangers before embarking on this trail. In peak production, the mine produced both silver and gold but is now boarded up for the safety of visitors.

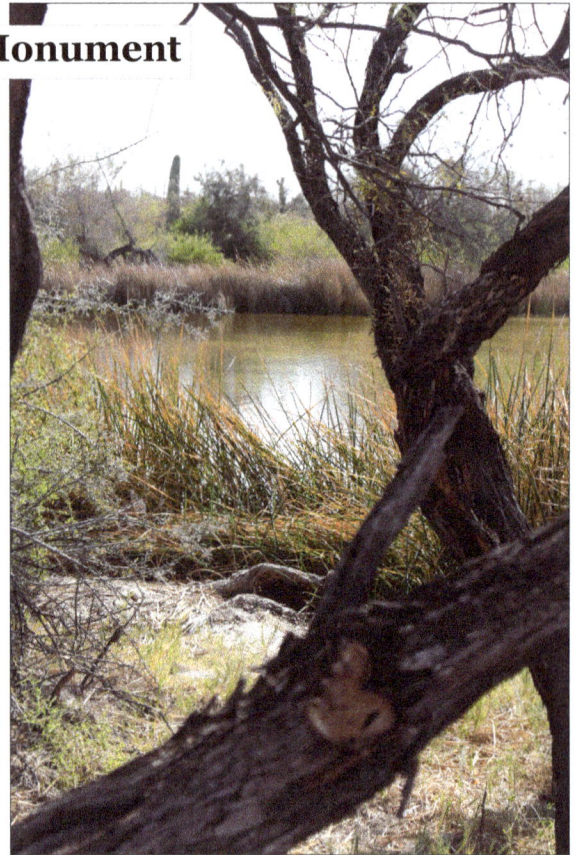

Quitobaquito Spring

Quitobaquito spring has been a vital source of water to people for centuries. Tohono O'odham people still follow an ancient route each year, passing by the spring enroute to collect salt from the Sea of Cortez in Mexico. The pool was created by Spanish settlers and later enlarged by the Park Service. It is a welcome delight after our eyes have grown weary of the glare from the desert.

Hiking Distance: Desert View Nature Trail - 1.2 miles / Victoria Mine Trail - 2.6 miles one way	Precautions: Avoid contact with shin stickers, a native succulent with narrow leaves ending in sharp points!
Rating: Easy	Maps: Organ Pipe National Monument Map
Elevation: 1720'-1840'	Info: Visitors Center, Organ Pipe National Monument (520) 387-6849
Best Season: Winter	
Special Features: Introduction to use of native plants	

The **Ajo Mountain Drive** take visitors along the base of the Ajo Range. Two trails ascend the peak, **Arch Canyon** climbs toward a small arch high on a ridge. The **Bull Pasture trail** climbs to an overlook of a basin at the foot of the range. At one time the trail led to a fire lookout at the summit of Mount Ajo but the cabin was removed after it was no longer needed. On either of these trails, pay close attention to the rock cairns marking the path to avoid losing the trail in the loose sand and rock boulders.

The trail to Bull Pasture ascends a low ridge speckled by small caves and depressions, inviting discovery. About half way into the ascent, the trail begins to switchback up the ridge. There is one confusing spot where the trail appears to cut through heavy brush, forcing hikers to scramble upward on hands and knees. Wrong way, go back and look for the cairns.

At a junction, high on a rocky ledge overlooking the valley, hikers turn left, walking to a viewpoint overlooking Bull Pasture. The wind-swept overlook of Bull Pasture is a popular destination for day hikers.

Beyond the viewpoint, the lure of the trail beckons. Be aware this trail climbs cross-country to the summit of Ajo Peak, 3.5 miles one way from the parking lot. Hikers should check with rangers in advance for directions and the condition of the trail.

Returning along the ridge to the junction, hikers continue straight rather than turning right. The loop trail descends past rock hoodoos on the back side of the ridge to the parking lot.

Driving Distance: 21 miles one-way loop, about two hours.
Hiking Distance: 4.1 miles loop trip
Rating: Moderate
Elevation: 2400' - 3000'
Best Season: Winter, early spring
Special Features: Desert land with educational exhibits.
Precautions: Carry sufficient water. Watch for poisonous reptiles and insects.
Maps: OPC National Monument Trail Guide
Information: Organ Pipe Cactus Nat'l Mon. (520) 387-6849

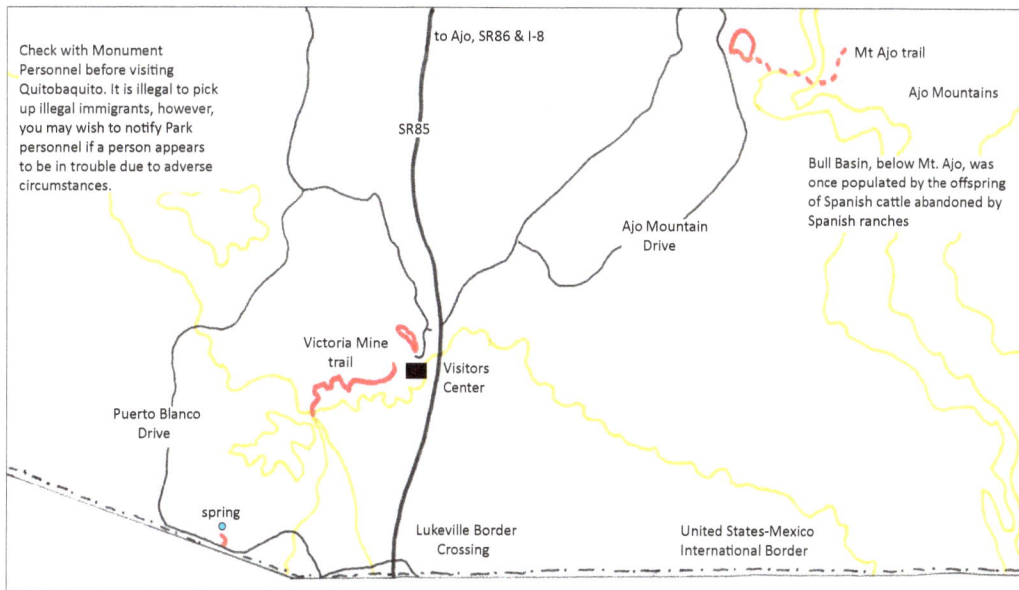

Check with Monument Personnel before visiting Quitobaquito. It is illegal to pick up illegal immigrants, however, you may wish to notify Park personnel if a person appears to be in trouble due to adverse circumstances.

to Ajo, SR86 & I-8

Mt Ajo trail

Ajo Mountains

SR85

Bull Basin, below Mt. Ajo, was once populated by the offspring of Spanish cattle abandoned by Spanish ranches

Ajo Mountain Drive

Victoria Mine trail

Visitors Center

Puerto Blanco Drive

spring

Lukeville Border Crossing

United States-Mexico International Border

Southeastern Arizona

Southeastern Arizona is the background for legends of the old west as told in countless books and movies. The vast plains caught between the sky islands are carpeted with sage brush and grass that turn golden in the late summer afternoon.

The spectacular Karchner Caverns have drawn many visitors to explore further into this quiet corner of the state. There is so much more to explore in Cochise County. The sky islands promise adventure for those willing to explore the back roads and hidden niches of southern Arizona. The lure of the hoodoos in Chiricahua National Monument draws visitors from across the country. An exhibit at the Visitor's Center educates those who come about the tremendous contribution of the Civilian Conservation Corps to the western United States.

We can't forget the allure of the old west, found in the play-acting of the gunfights in Tombstone or the mining history along the winding steps of Bisbee, an old mining town. The somber old Cavalry Forts of Bowie and Rucker remind us that this land was bought, not just in dollars, but with the blood of those who sacrificed to retain their stake among the grasslands of southeastern Arizona.

Again, we are reminded that Arizona shares part of our southern border with Mexico and many people from other countries seek a route into the state - Be safe.

1 Reef Townsite & Comfort Spring
2 Ramsey Canyon
3 San Pedro House & River
4 Coronado Nat'l Monument &
5 Montezuma Peak
6 Slaughter's Ranch
7 Rucker Dam & Camp
8 Rustler Park & Fly Peak
9 Cottonwood Canyon
10 Echo Canyon
      & Chricahua Nat'l Monument
11 Fort Bowie
12 Webb Peak & Heliograph Peaks
13 Dragoon Mountains
      & Cochise Stronghold

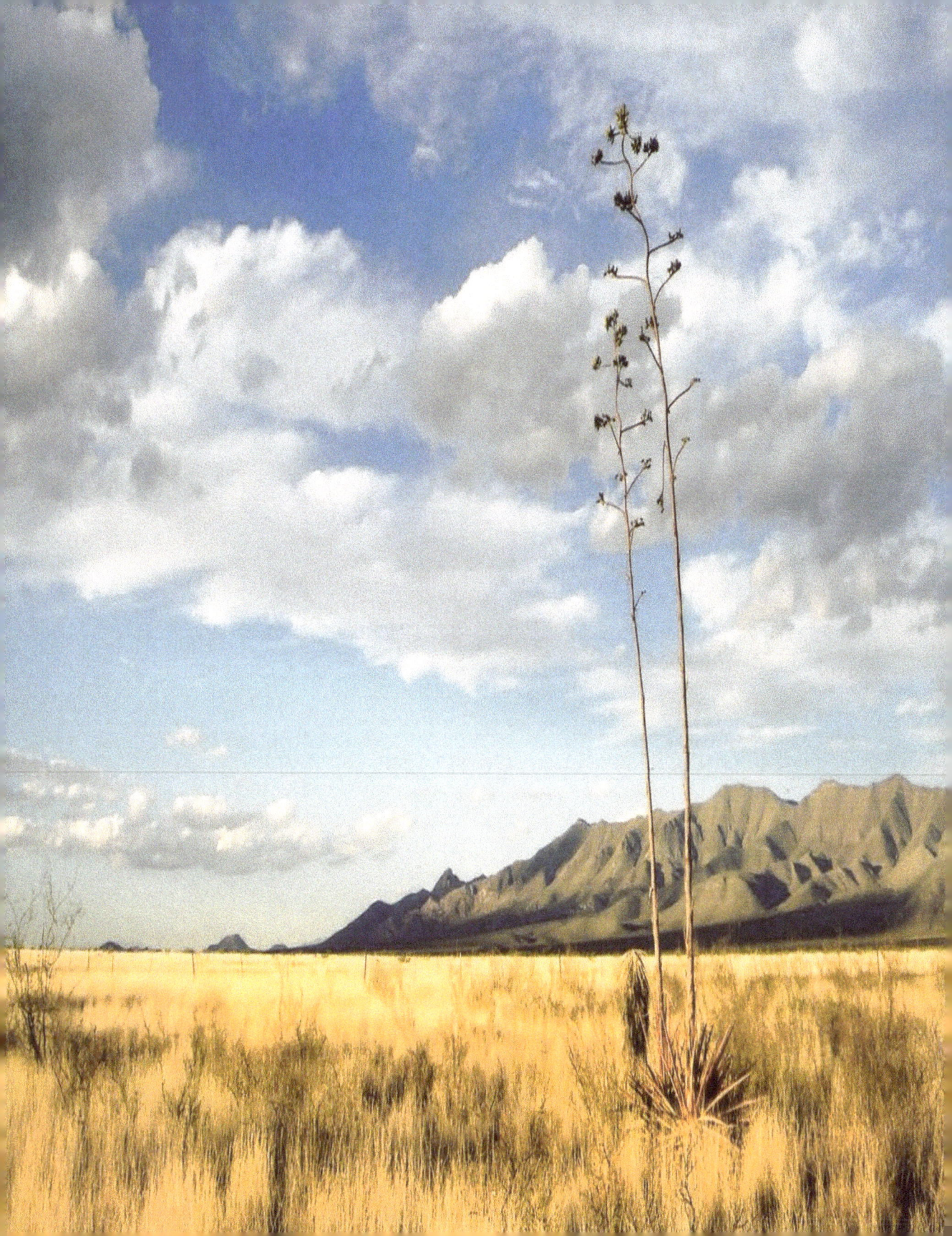

Reef Townsite Trail

The sheer cliffs of the Huachuca Mountain Range, as seen from Sierra Vista, are a bit intimidating. Years ago, prospectors climbed the peaks seeking valuable minerals. Their detritus remains but now, hikers and campers climb the peaks. To open the upper heights of the Huachucas, the Forest Service built a road through Carr Canyon and up over the cliffs. From Sierra Vista, drive south on SR 92. Turn west at mp 327.9 onto Carr Canyon Road. In 1.5 miles, the road takes a sharp left turn, passing a side canyon, once the site of an old moonshine still. Within two miles the asphalt turns to dirt and ascends steeply along the contours of the mountain. The dirt road is passable for passenger cars but drivers will want to ease over the rocky areas, noting the absence of guard rails.

Reef Townsite Campground is 6.5 miles and Ramsey Vista Campground 8 miles from SR 92. Four trails begin from these two campgrounds. The historic Reef Townsite trailhead is located at the first campground. The one-mile long trail passes several sign-boards discussing the area history and and the abandoned mine as it drops into a steep-sided canyon. The climb out will leave some breathless but remember, the miners did it first!

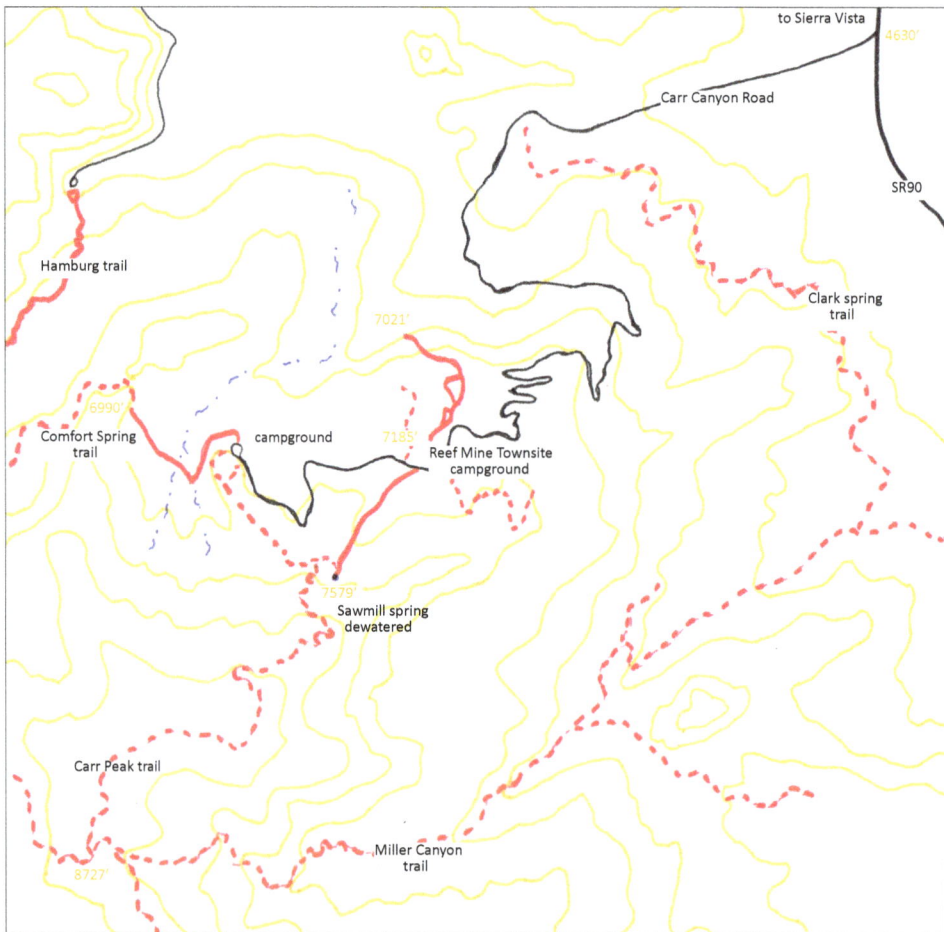

Miners removed tons of ore containing gold and silver, copper ore, tungsten and quartz from the Reef mine. Each of these was mined in turn to supply the demand from industry at the time of operation.

An old road leads to the mine ruins but visitors are discouraged from exploring the site due to unstable rock on the steep slope. It is possible to see the rusting hulk of abandoned machinery. As visitors turn to leave, they could take a moment to look back. Did the last miner stop to look back a final time as he left? What did he think about as he rattled down the steep hillside one last time?

Across the road from the townsite, a trail climbs Carr Peak to dewatered Sawmill spring which once supplied the campground with drinking water. Two other popular trails depart from the Ramsey Vista Campground, one climbing Carr Peak, the other dropping down to Comfort Spring.

The northern section of the Huachucas is set aside for military use at Fort Huachuca. Visitors must obtain permission from the military installation to hike in this area.

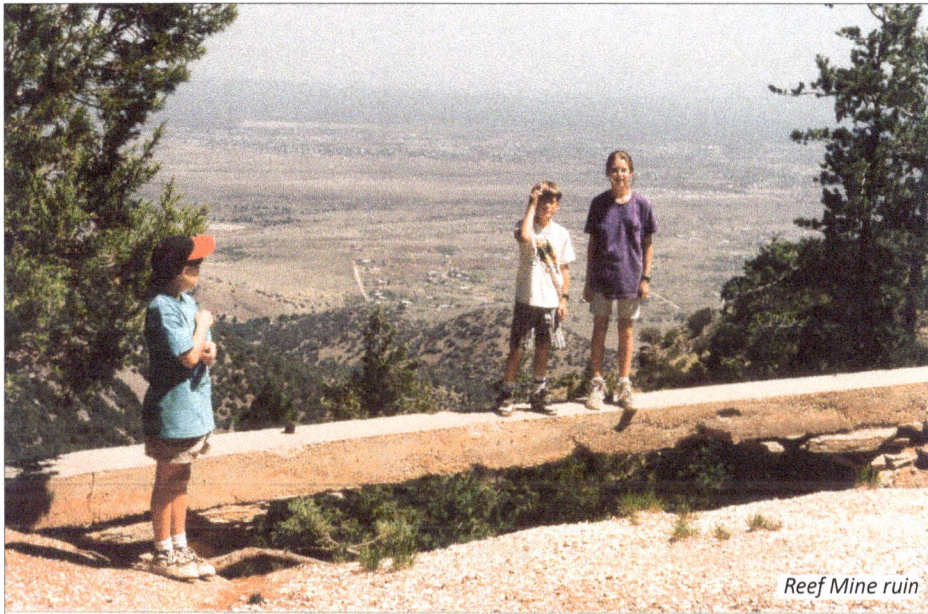

Reef Mine ruin

Reef Townsite
Driving Distance: 7.5 miles one way from SR 92
Hiking Distance: .75 mile loop   Rating: Easy
Best Season: Spring, summer & fall
Special Features: Historic mine site
Precautions: Watch for black bear and reptiles.
        Off trail, rock may be loose underfoot,
        causing a rock slide.
Maps: Coronado NFS map

Comfort Springs
Hiking Distance: .75 mile one way
Rating: Moderate
Best Season: Summer & fall
Special Features: Riparian retreat with wildlife
Precautions: Watch for bears and poisonous
                snakes.
Information: Sierra Vista Ranger District
        (520) 378-0311

Ramsey Canyon

Ramsey Canyon has an international reputation for hummingbirds! The canyon is a refuge for many animal species and a treat for human visitors who seek to quietly observe the world around them.

In 1975, Dr. Nelson C. Bledsoe donated 280 acres in Ramsey Canyon to the Nature Conservancy in order to preserve this beautiful riparian domain. Visitors are welcome from 8-5 daily, except Christmas and New Years.

From SR92, turn west on Ramsey Canyon Road and drive four miles to the Nature Conservancy Preserve. Parking is very limited. On busy days, visitors may be forced to park some distance from the entrance. As Ramsey Canyon has become so popular, reservations may be necessary.

A hiking pass can be obtained at the Visitors Center. The **Nature Trail** is a .75 mile loop with sign-boards describing the plants and history of the area. An old cabin remains from one of the first settlers in the canyon. The trail reaches a junction; the left branch ascending along the **Hamburg Trail**. The right branch loops right back to the Visitors Center.

Visitors see a great number of birds, squirrels, maybe a snake. I've caught glimpses of a deer and a coatimundi scurrying up the hillside. The frogs remain submerged in their little pond. As with most of the sky islands of southeastern Arizona, Ramsey Canyon sits on the border between the Rocky Mountains to the north and the Sierra Madre Mountains, the Sonora and Chihuahua Deserts to the south, meaning species from diverse habitats cross paths in the canyon.

Meet the Hummers!

Hummingbirds are the race drivers of the bird world. These fantastic aerial acrobats beat their wings at over 40 count per second to stay airborne as they spread their trail feathers for high speed turns. All that energy burns a lot of calories. Hummers metabolic rate, meaning how fast they turn their food into energy, is 300 times the human rate. There are over 340 species of hummingbirds with 16 species found in Arizona. The most common hummers in Arizona are Anna's, the Black Chinned, the Broad Billed, the Broad Tailed, the Costa's and the Rufous.

The **Chiricahua Leopard frogs** are a protected species. The Nature Conservancy has designed a habitat favorable to the little frogs, hoping to increase their population. The trail passes the ponds where the frogs submerge in the mud, leaving their nostrils just above water level.

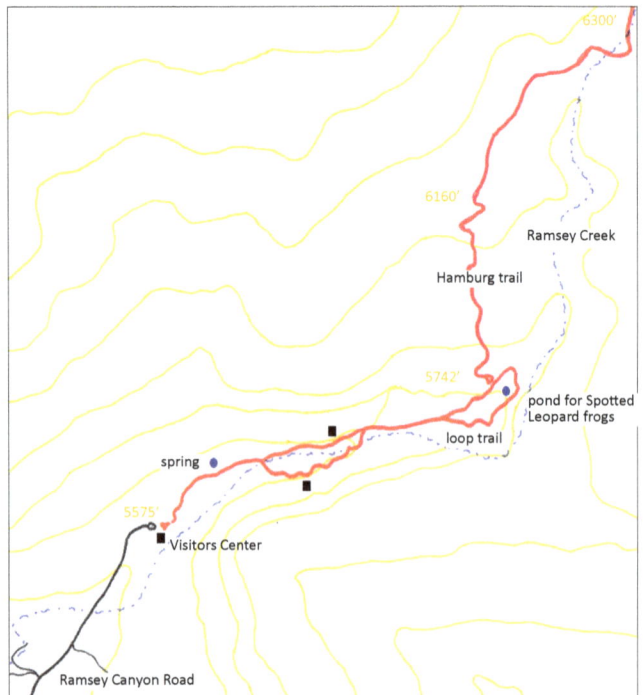

The **Hamberg Trail** climbs to a saddle above Ramswey Canyon. Prospectors first came to the canyons above Ramsey in the 1870s. In 1900, a claim was filed for the Hamberg mine and a 200-foot tunnel developed with several drifts for discarded material. The mine is no longer in operation. Today, hikers drop past the mine, over the saddle, to explore the Pat Scott and Wisconsin canyons.

Hiking Distance: 2.8 miles one way
Rating: Moderately difficult
Elevation: 5,700 - 8,075 feet
Special Features: Nature Preserve,
      historic mine,
Information: Ramsey Canyon
      520-378-2785

Nature Trail
Driving Distance: 4 miles from SR 92
Hiking Distance: 1.5 miles out and back
Rating: Easy   Best Season: Spring, summer & fall.
Special Features: Wildlife preserve with hummingbirds
Information: Ramsey Canyon Preserve   (520) 378-2785

San Pedro River Nat'l Conservation Area / San Pedro House

Forty miles of land bordering the upper San Pedro River was set aside as a National Conservation area by Congress in 1988 to protect and preserve this important riparian ecosystem. The San Pedro River, stretching between St. David in the north and Palominas in the south, is a life line to the wild inhabitants of southern Arizona.

It is easily accessed by two-legged adventurers from SR 92, SR 90, SR 80 or the Charleston Road. First-time visitors and long-time residents visit the San Pedro House and its network of trails extending along the banks of the stream. The House is located on SR 90, 7 miles east of Sierra Vista.

A footpath extends from the San Pedro House down to the river where visitors hike, fish and bird-watch. Tall cottonwoods shade the river banks. Throughout the seasons, over three hundred species of birds including a number of raptors, take up residence along the San Pedro. Reptiles hidden in the brush along the river banks include Gila Monsters and a variety of rattlesnakes including the Mohave Green. Human eyes may easily find jack rabbits and prairie dogs. Deer or javelina lurk in the late afternoon shadows. The Sonoran Box Turtle and a variety of bats and rodents are also drawn to the area.

For the residents of nearby Sierra Vista, the San Pedro is a refreshing break from the dry desert. Unfortunately, as the town has grown, the demands on the water table have expanded, endangering the San Pedro. Conservations are working to maintain the rio from further encroachment.

> *For those who love history and ghost towns, Fairbanks, a ghost town, is an interesting place to explore off SR82, between SR90 & SR80, north of the San Pedro House.*

Opposite page:
Along San Pedro River

Driving Distance: 7 miles from Sierra Vista, 42 miles
    from I-10
Hiking Distance: .5-3 miles
Rating: Easy
Elevation: 4068'
Precautions: Poisonous snakes and insects. Watch where you put your feet and hands. If wading, quicksand may be present.
Information:
    San Pedro Riparian Nat'l Conservation Area
    (520) 508-4445

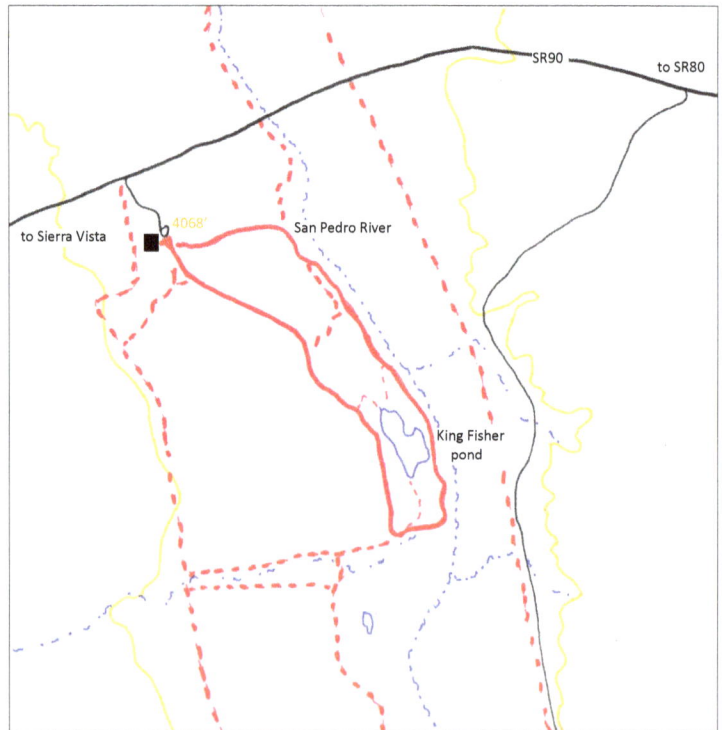

The water in the San Pedro is not potable. Bring your own!

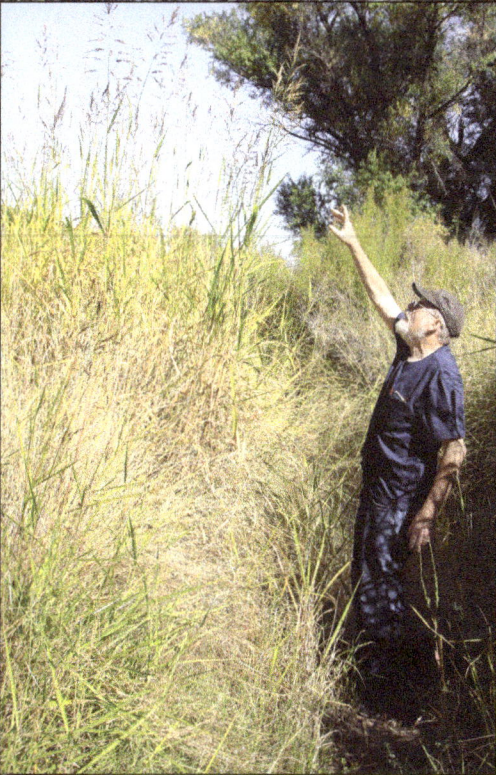

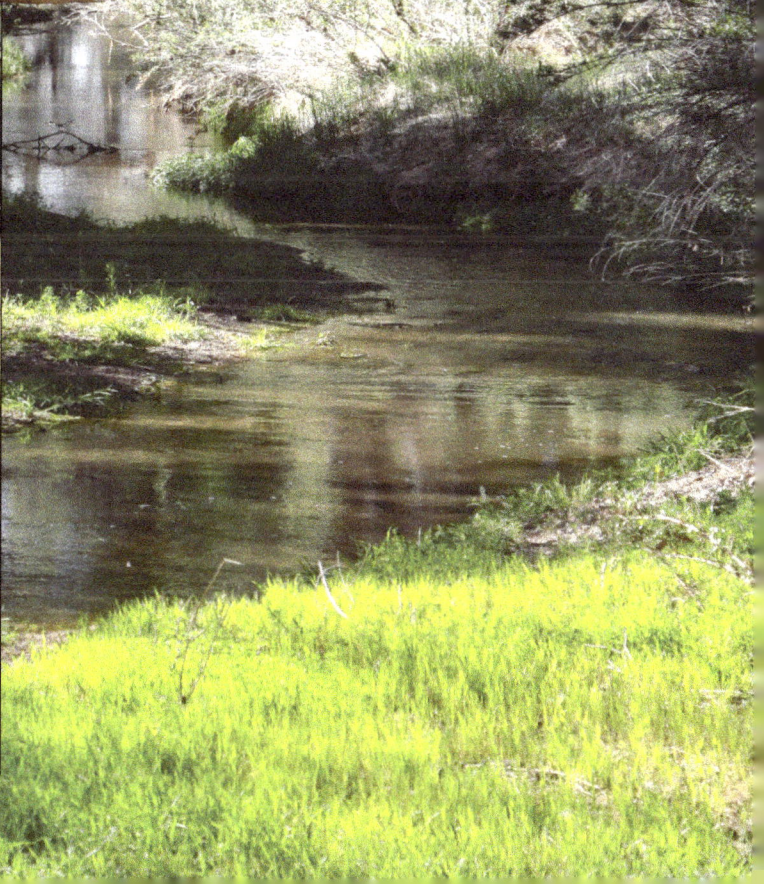

Coronado National Memorial

The southern part of our state is rich in Spanish history. This small monument on the border with Mexico commemorates the historical role Spanish explorers, primarily Don Francisco Vazquez de Coronado, played in exploring the Southwest. But this is not a dry, boring lecture. There is chain mail armor to examine and an oxhide garment to try on with a sword to brandish at imaginary foes. A video and a short walk under a blazing sun give us insight into what these men faced as they toiled through the heat and desert of southern Arizona chasing an elusive promise of golden cities.

To reach the Coronado National Memorial drive south from Sierra Vista on SR 92 about 13 miles. Turn south at the sign for the Memorial onto FR 61. This road leads directly past the Memorial before climbing to Montezuma Pass enroute to Parker Canyon Lake.

At the Coronado National Memorial, the video details the background to Coronado's expedition and the journey through the southwest into the great plains of the U. S. The expedition's diary shows the men entered Arizona, most likely in the Sulphur Spring Valley, at the beginning of summer as temperatures routinely rose to 100 degrees.

The Spanish treated the pueblo tribes of the southwest poorly and eventually native residents told Coronado that the cities he sought were further east. Coronado was quick to follow this erroneous information and the Pueblo people rejoiced in ridding themselves of the Spanish. The expedition eventually returned to Mexico with Coronado's health broken and his fortune gone.

The expedition was a forerunner of what would descend on the pueblo people. Eventually, the Pueblo tribes would lose their land and freedom to Spanish settlers. The Spanish influence in Arizona remains an integral part of Arizona's culture.

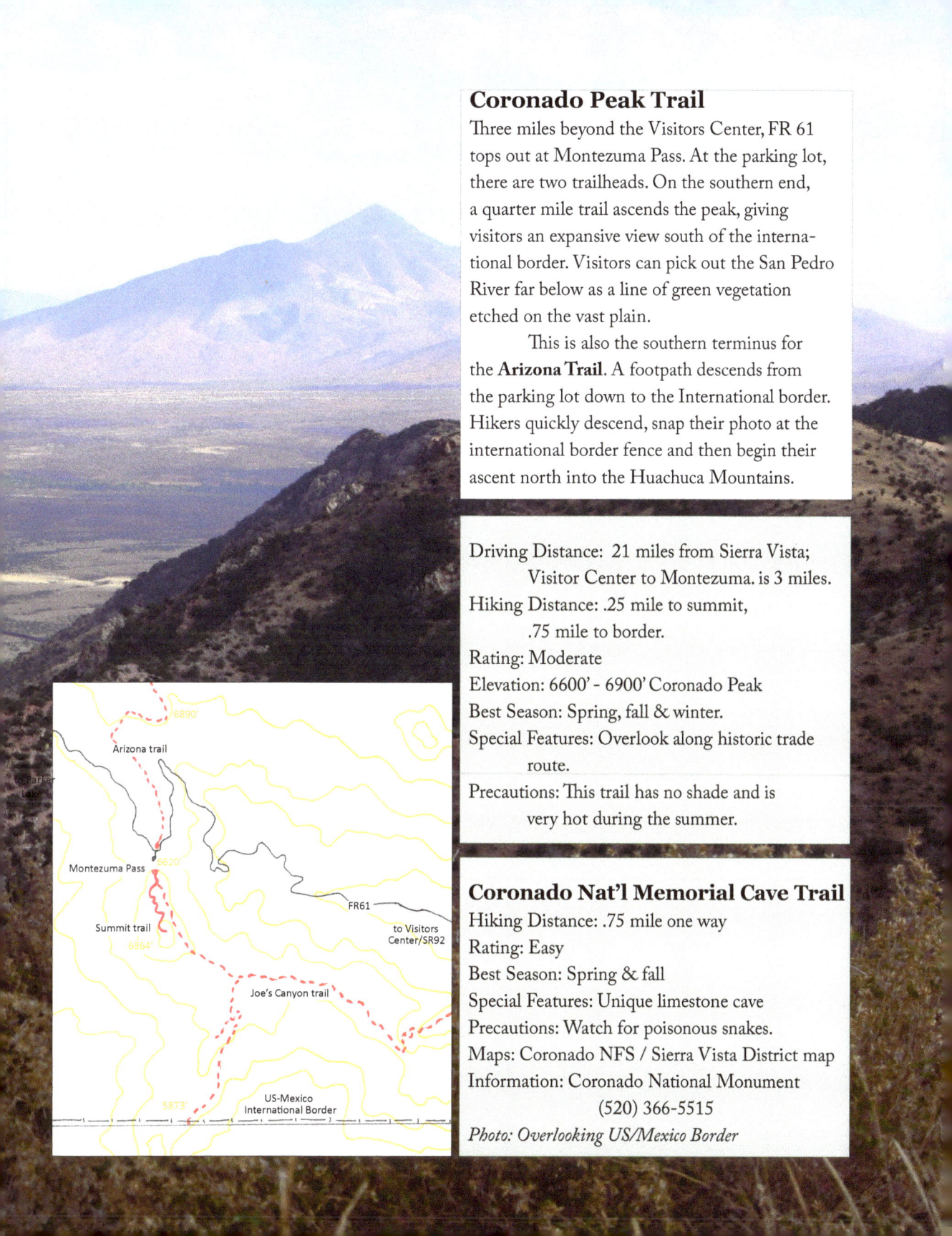

Coronado Peak Trail

Three miles beyond the Visitors Center, FR 61 tops out at Montezuma Pass. At the parking lot, there are two trailheads. On the southern end, a quarter mile trail ascends the peak, giving visitors an expansive view south of the international border. Visitors can pick out the San Pedro River far below as a line of green vegetation etched on the vast plain.

This is also the southern terminus for the **Arizona Trail**. A footpath descends from the parking lot down to the International border. Hikers quickly descend, snap their photo at the international border fence and then begin their ascent north into the Huachuca Mountains.

Driving Distance: 21 miles from Sierra Vista; Visitor Center to Montezuma. is 3 miles.
Hiking Distance: .25 mile to summit, .75 mile to border.
Rating: Moderate
Elevation: 6600' - 6900' Coronado Peak
Best Season: Spring, fall & winter.
Special Features: Overlook along historic trade route.
Precautions: This trail has no shade and is very hot during the summer.

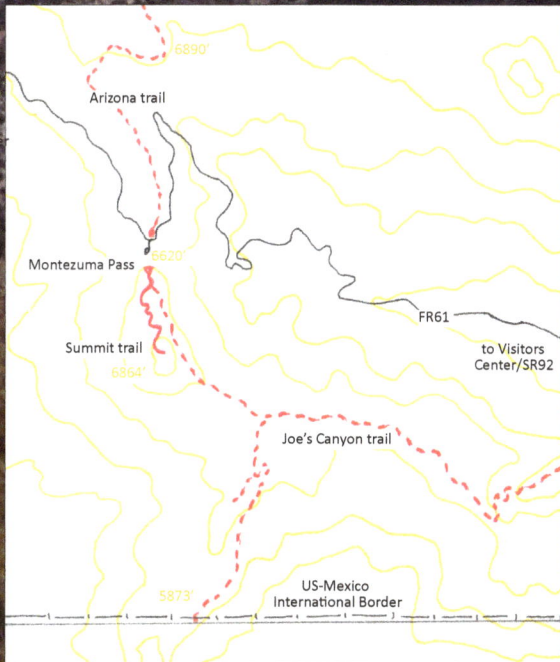

Coronado Nat'l Memorial Cave Trail

Hiking Distance: .75 mile one way
Rating: Easy
Best Season: Spring & fall
Special Features: Unique limestone cave
Precautions: Watch for poisonous snakes.
Maps: Coronado NFS / Sierra Vista District map
Information: Coronado National Monument
(520) 366-5515
Photo: Overlooking US/Mexico Border

Arizona trail

6890'

to Parker Lake

Montezuma Pass

6620'

FR61

to Visitors Center/SR92

Summit trail

6864'

Joe's Canyon trail

5873'

US-Mexico International Border

Slaughter's Ranch & the San Bernardino Wildlife Refuge

Driving Distance: 17 miles from Douglas
Hiking Distance: up to 3 miles
Rating: Easy   Elevation: Just over 4,000'
Special Features: Natural springs, historic site
Precautions: Ranch is open Wednesday - Sunday, 9:30-3:30,
          $5.00 donation for adults. No service after leaving town.
Maps: Arizona Highway map

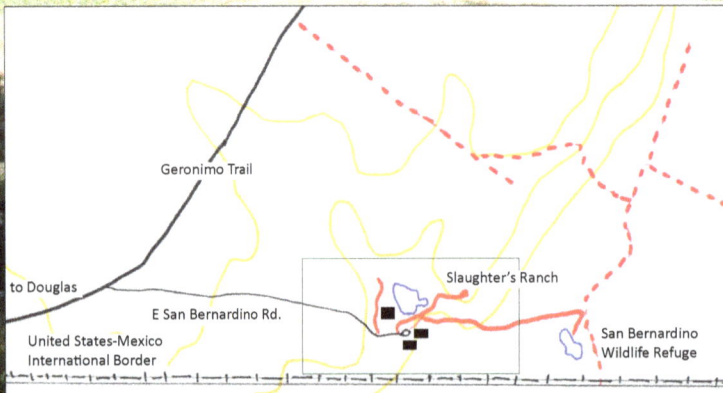

Geronimo Trail

to Douglas

E San Bernardino Rd.

United States-Mexico
International Border

Slaughter's Ranch

San Bernardino
Wildlife Refuge

Slaughter's Ranch is a great place to visit and explore but hiking could become an adventure if visitors choose to explore the **San Bernardino Wildlife Refuge.** The springs at Slaughter's Ranch are a historic site going back to prehistoric time. Living in such an arid climate, ancient people valued the perennial water source. The Spanish, as they moved north, settled at the springs. In the late 1800's, John Slaughter bought the ranch and drove cattle from Texas to his property. After serving a term as Sheriff, John and Violetta Slaughter built an adobe ranch house with outbuildings. John placed a pipe in the springs that released the artesian pressure with the water shooting skyward out of the pipe. He developed two ponds on the ranch, one near the ranchhouse.

During the Mexican Revolution, the Army stationed troops at the ranch, overlooking the border. The footprint of the outpost remains today and visitors follow a short path to the outline of the barracks looking over the international border with Mexico.

Today, the ranch is an oasis in the dry Sonoran desert. Huge cottonwoods and green pasture greet visitors to the ranch. Livestock bleat from the pens. A stroll around the homestead gives visitors a glimpse of the lives of the former occupants.

Hikers may choose to venture beyond the ranch down to the pools in the Buena Aires Wildlife Refuge where local residents at one time pulled large catfish out of the ponds. Today, the United States Wildlife Service raises several strains of native fish. To reach the ranch, follow 15th Street out of Douglas for 16 miles - the pavement turns to dirt and is now listed as the Geronimo Trail. Turn right onto the San Bernardino Road and drive .06 mile through the headgate of the ranch to the parking area below the ranchhouse.

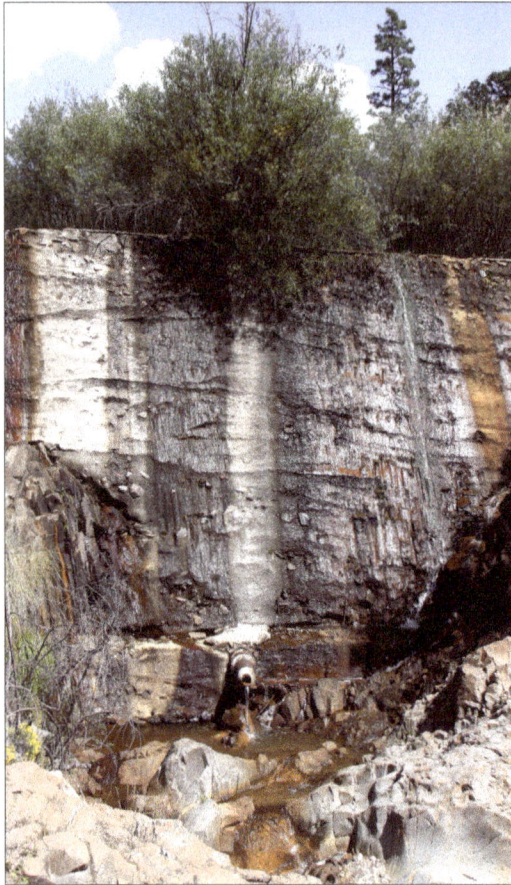
Rucker Dam

Rucker Lake was once a sparkling body of water with good fishing. In 1992 the Rattlesnake Fire swept over the southern Chricahua Range. As the monsoons arrived the following July, flash floods filled the lake bed with silt. The lake has not been dredged leaving a gravel plain with a small stream trickling over the dam.

To reach Camp Rucker, follow SR 191 south from the junction with I-10. About five miles north of Elfrida, turn east onto Rucker Canyon Road. Follow FR 74, into Rucker Canyon and the turnoff to the camp. Rucker Canyon Road has a well maintained surface as the cross-over road between US 191 and State Route 80.

Camp Rucker, a former Cavalry Camp was named for Lt. John Rucker who rode his horse into a flash flood trying to save Lt. Austin Henely. Both men perished in the torrent crashing down the canyon Many of the buildings remain with paths leading through the camp. Small signs identify each building. The old barn that once housed cavalry horses still contains wisps of hay. An old water tower stands on its cement foundation. Visitors can enter most of the buildings. A small tank on the grounds provides water for wildlife.

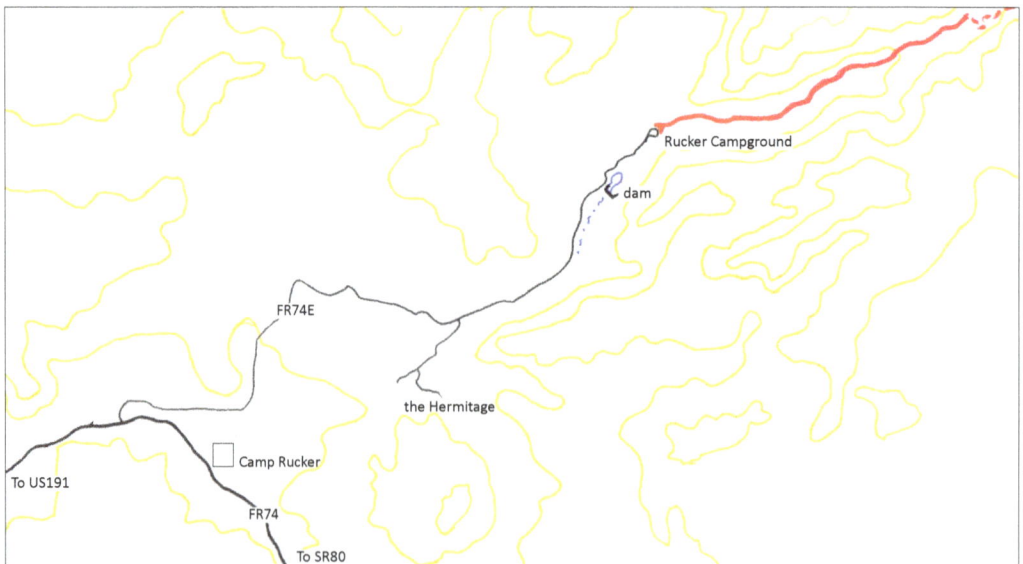

186

Camp Rucker and the Lake that Disappeared

The area around the camp is good for hiking though the rock formations lack the dramatic appeal of the hoodoos in the northern part of the range. The foothills around the lake support a wide diversity of birds as do many of the southeastern sky islands. FR 74E comes to a dead end in the campground above the dam.

Before the Rattlesnake fire this was one of the prettiest lakes in Arizona. One long-time resident recalls the rain starting to fall during a fishing trip. They hurriedly gathered their equipment and his father rapidly drove along the narrow road in an old pickup to cross the creek before a flash flood could cut off their access. It is still a lovely area for camping. In the fall, the maples turn a brilliant red, contrasting with the dark pines.

Several trails ascend the Chiricahuas from a trailhead near the lake, climbing toward Monte Vista, Raspberry and Chiricahua Peaks - all for overnight back packing trip. For more information, check a map for the Coronado National Forest.

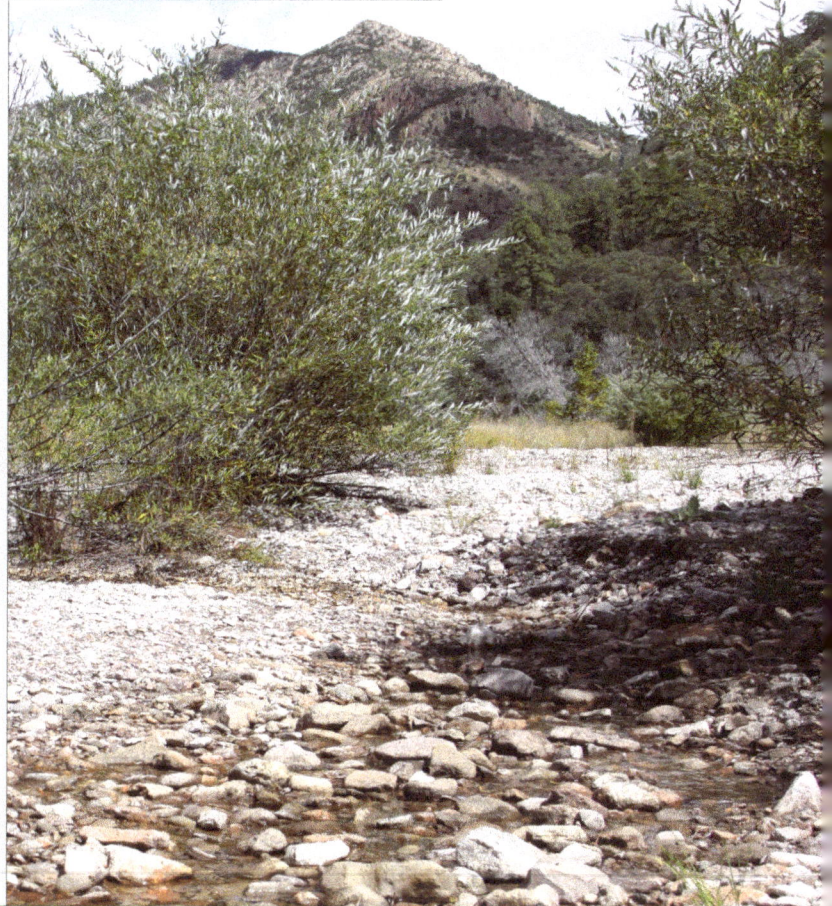

Driving Distance: 25 miles from SR 191.

Hiking Distance: .50 mile loop

Rating: Easy   Elevation: 3300'

Best Season: Late Spring, summer & fall.

Special Features: Explore an old army camp and learn about life with the US Cavalry in southern Arizona. During the summer rains, do not attempt to cross flooded washes water more than 3-4 inches deep.

Precautions: Do not cross flooded washes. Be careful for soft spot walking across the dry lake bed.

Information: Douglas Ranger Station   (520) 364-3468

Photo: Infilled Rucker Lake

Rustler Park - Climbing to Fly Peak and the Crest Trail

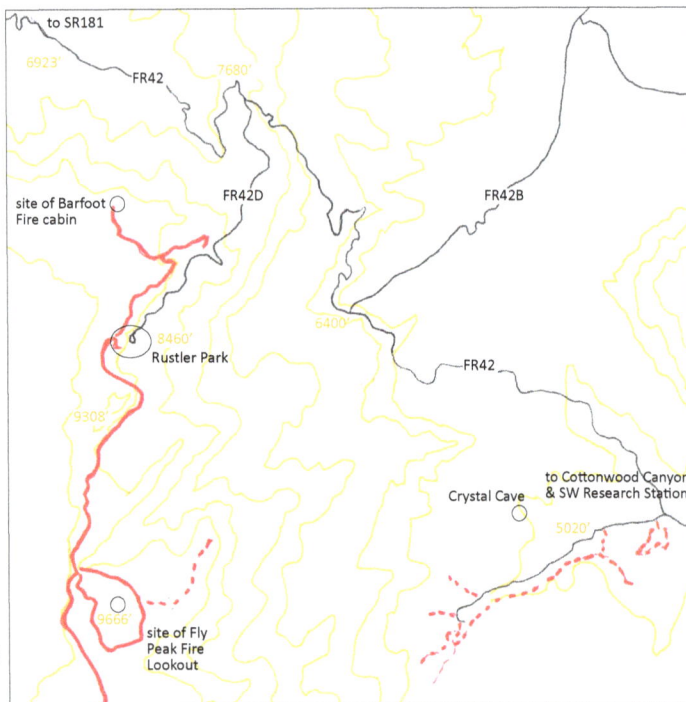

Pinery Canyon Road /FR42 crosses the Chiricahuas Range from Chiricahua National Monument to Cottonwood Canyon on the eastern slopes. Visitors exiting Chiricahua National Monument may turn up Pinery Canyon to seek out **Rustler Park** with a beautiful meadow, rock cliffs and the trailhead for the Crest Line trail that follows the spine of the Chiricahua Range. While the Crest Line trail is a multi-day backpack, hikers can ascend Fly Peak, the first stretch of the Crest Line, as a day hike. The trailhead is located on the north end of Rustler Park. A side trail will take visitors to the site of Barfoot Lookout, a fire cabin that burned several years ago.

To reach Rustler Park, drive SR186 south from I-10 to SR181, the access road into Chiricahua National Monument. Just before reaching the entrance to the Monument, turn right onto Pinery Canyon Road and ascend the steep slopes of the Chiricahuas to Onion Saddle. At the saddle, turn right onto FR42D and drive south into Rustler Park.

Rustler Park is a work site for the Forest Service with only one road into the Park. Returning to FR42, visitors can choose to return to SR186 or to proceed down the eastern side of the Chiricahua Range into Cottonnwood Canyon. Years ago, a fire swept through the canyon and heavy summer rains destroyed much of the infrastructure in the campgrounds. Flooding silted in the ponds behind the small dams built to retain run-off. The Forest Service has worked to restore the campgrounds but the canyon has a ways to go before it will resemble the lush, shaded environment that once lured visitors to wile away their time in the shade.

Driving Distance: 18 miles from Jct. of SR 181 & SR 186.
Hiking Distance: 3.5 miles one way
Rating: Moderate
Elevation: 8500 - 9666'
Best Season: Late spring, summer, fall.
Special Features: Beautiful Rustler Park, fewer visitors than the monument!
Precautions: Loose rock on the trails. The campground has 'bear boxes to protect campers food - be aware of your surroundings!
Maps: Coronado NFS map / Chiricahua District
Information: Douglas Ranger Station (520) 364-3468

Cottonwood Canyon

(from previous page)

Streamside trails are available for hiking along sections of the stream as well as trails to Silver Peak and Cathedral Rock.

A research station is located in the canyon, hosting scientists from around the world. Signs are posted warning visitors that this is private property.

Fire As a Tool

In driving up to Rustler Park, visitors may notice the black trunks and open areas left by a forest fire that once blazed through the area. In the early 1990's, firefighters battled to save beautiful Rustler Park and the Forest Service Administrative site during one wildfire. As the fire crowned in the tree tops threatening the park, Buck Wickham and his crew made one last stand. He set a crescent-shaped burn against the rim of the hill. As the flames of the wildfire surged up the hill, they reached the crescent burn and ran out of fuel. Without fuel, the fire slowed and firefighters gained the upper hand, turning back the flames. Rustler Park was saved for future generations to enjoy. Rustler Park is a former CCC camp and favored by birders from around the world.

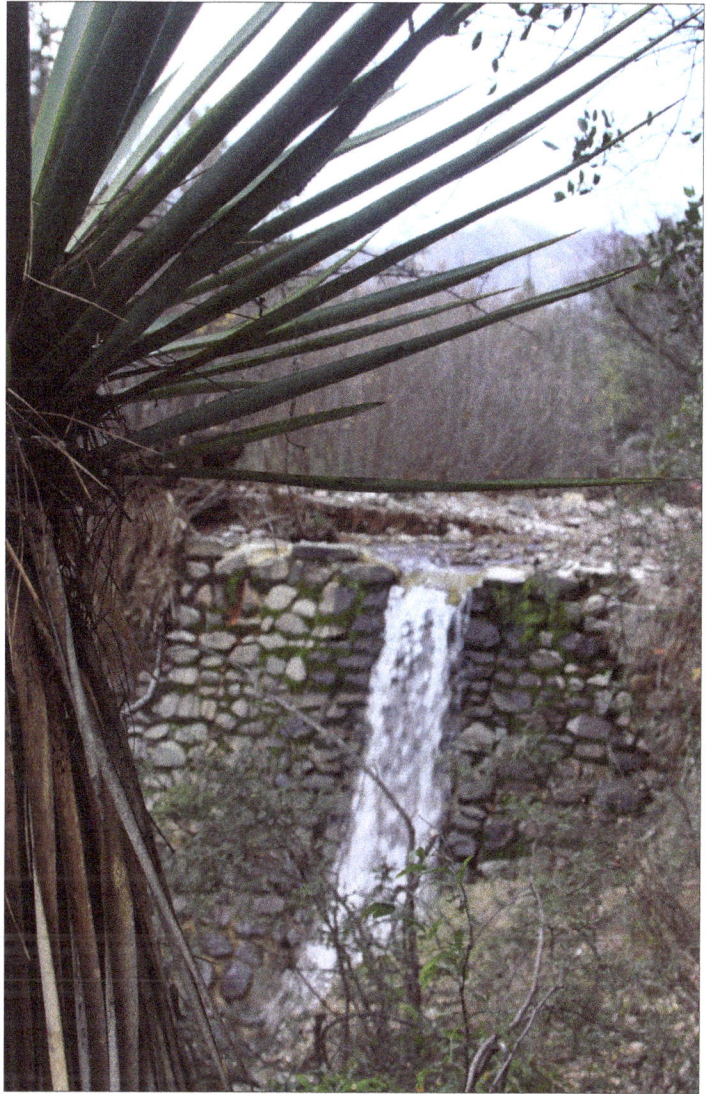

Dam along Cottonwood Canyon Creek

Driving Distance: 18 miles from
     Jct. of SR 181 & SR 186.
Hiking Distance: 3.5 miles one way
Rating: Moderate
Elevation: 8500 - 9666'
Best Season: Late spring, summer, fall.
Special Features: Beautiful Rustler Park,
     fewer visitors than the monument!

Chiricahua National Monument & the Wonderland of Rocks

The campgrounds and trails of this national monument are the work of the Civilian Conservation Corps as part of the federal Works Progress Adminstration instituted by President Franklin Roosevelt. Young men were put to work, following a strict daily regimen on public work projects throughout our nation as part of a program to alleviate unemployment during the Great Depression.

Masai Point, Echo Canyon and the Hailstone Trail

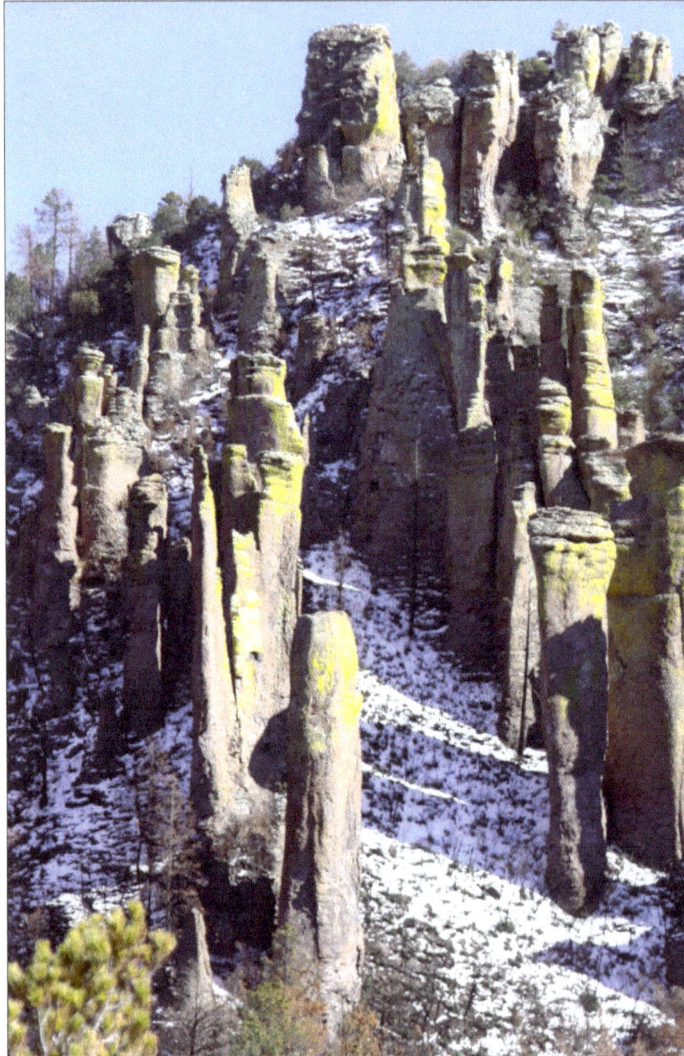

Hoodoos of Chiricahua National Monument, along the Echo Canyon trail
Opposite: Rock grotto along Echo Canyon trail

A 3.9 mile hike loops through a canyon filled with eye-popping rock formations. It is truly one of the highlights of Arizona, allowing hikers to see the Wilderness of Rocks up close.

As visitors begin to descend into Echo Canyon, the hum of traffic remains just a few feet above the path. As the trail moves away from the highway, quiet creeps in. Visitors descend past giant boulders balanced on small pedestals and under a small rock grotto arching over the trail.

After descending 1.6 miles, hikers leave behind the rock hoodoos and enter the shadowy green glens of Echo Canyon. Small swallows dart and glide through tall pines coming to rest in mud nests on the side of cliffs. The silence is pierced by their calls and the voices of other hikers. The trail crosses a small creek, then climbs the opposing ridge to an intersection with the Rhyolite Canyon Trail. At the junction, hikers can turn west (right) toward the Heart of Rocks Trail, an additonal 1.8 miles, and the Visitors Center in 3.3 miles. Turning left at the junction hikers follow the Hailstone Trail as it climbs 2.1 miles out of Echo Canyon. The trail is aptly named as it follows the terrain, exposed to the elements and lacking the shelter of the tall pines in

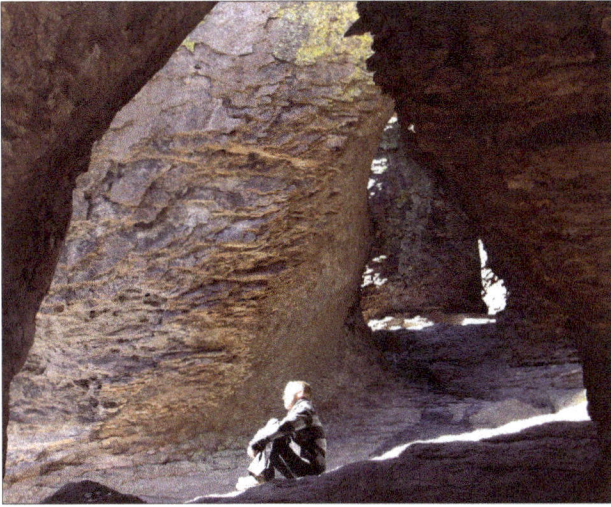

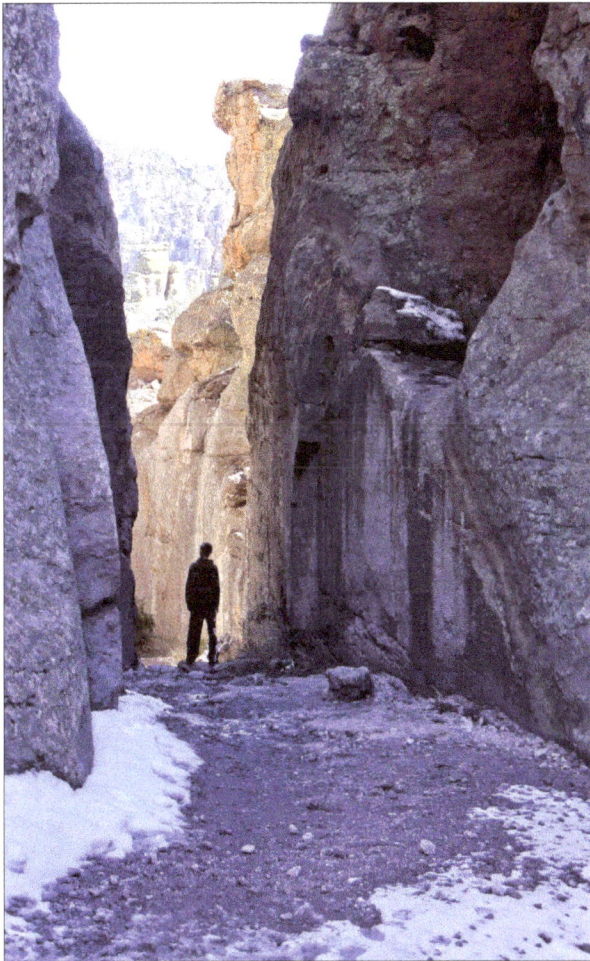

Echo Canyon. On the ascent, at a second junction, a trail splits off to Inspiration Point.

Those who take the time to hike down through Echo Canyon will see more of the monument than the vast majority of visitors who return to the Visitors Center without exploring beyond the edge of the rim overlooking the forest of rock hoodoos. It is well worth the effort.

To reach the Chiricahua National Monument, turn south from I-10 at the Wilcox exit onto SR 186. Drive 31 miles south and turn east onto SR 181, driving toward the Monument. After clearing the entrance booth, follow the main road to the Visitors Center. I would suggest their exhibit on the CCC is worthwhile. Drive 7 miles up the winding road to Massai Point. At the last junction, the right branch takes visitors to Sugarloaf Mountain and the Echo Canyon trailhead. The left branch enters the parking area at Massai Point and is often congested. A trail connects Echo Canyon to Massai Point.

Driving Distance: 8 miles from park
    entrance
Hiking Distance: 3.3 mile loop
Rating: Moderate
Elevation: 6780' - 6330'
Best Season: Late spring, summer and fall.
Precautions: Late snows may leave the trails
    slushy. Keep an eye on the weather,
    especially during summer thunder
    storms. Stay on the trail during
    access to and from canyon.
Maps: Chiricahua Nat'l. Monument map
Information: Chiricahua National Mon.
        (520) 824-3560

Other Trails at Chiricahua National Monument

Rising above the surrounding desert, the Chiricahuas are a cool, green retreat with striking rock formations and shady canyons. The range was once the home of the Chiricahua Apaches. They called this range the "Land of the Standing Up Rock."

Scientists theorize that thousands of years ago a giant volcano began a series of eruptions near what is now Turkey Creek. The volcanic caldera blew ash high into the atmosphere. The ash settled into the crevices and depressions, covering the cooled lava flows. Over the centuries water and wind eroded the rocky crust, leaving pillars of fused lava and ash. The awesome results are the creased and sculptured rocky spires and columns of the northern Chiricahuas. From above, the columns massed together appear as soldiers standing in formation. Massive rocks appear balanced on pedestals. Hiker approach with caution, assessing the chance of a boulder rolling off as they pass along the trail. Around each corner is another great photo waiting to be captured by photographers.

In the 1940's, the Civilian Conservation Corps built roads, retaining walls and a Visitor's Center in this unique sky island. A trail map is available at the entrance booth.

(**Echo Canyon/Hailstone trail** on previous page)

Trails within the Monument at a Glance:

Faraway Meadow Trail   1.2 miles
This easy trail, located near the park entrance, provides access to the cabin of early settlers, Ed and Lillian Riggs. The site is a 'hands-on' place for visitors to explore and get an idea of what home meant to early settlers in the Chiricahuas.

Natural Bridge Trail   2.4 miles
The trailhead is located about 1.5 miles from the Visitors Center on the main road through the Park. Hikers start up Northern Bonita Canyon, then turn into Picket Canyon before turning south toward the natural bridge.

Rhyolite Canyon Trail   1.5 miles
This trail begins just beyond the Visitors Center, climbing 1.5 miles through the Heart of Rocks. Many visitors prefer to hike down from Massai Point, combining either the Hailstone Trail or the Echo Canyon Trail with the Rhyolite Canyon Trail to the Visitors Center. Return by two car shuttle or hike 5 miles back to the top.

Heart of Rocks Trail   3.8 miles (outer loop)
This double loop trail explores the heart of the park away from main roads. The .9 mile inner loop passes around the area known as the Heart of Rocks, featuring several prominent rock formations. Inspiration Point off the Hailstone trail is a worthwhile side trip, .8 mile one way. To access the loops, use either the Hailstone trail, .7 mile, or the Echo Canyon/Rhyolite Canyon Trail for an additional 2.7 miles.

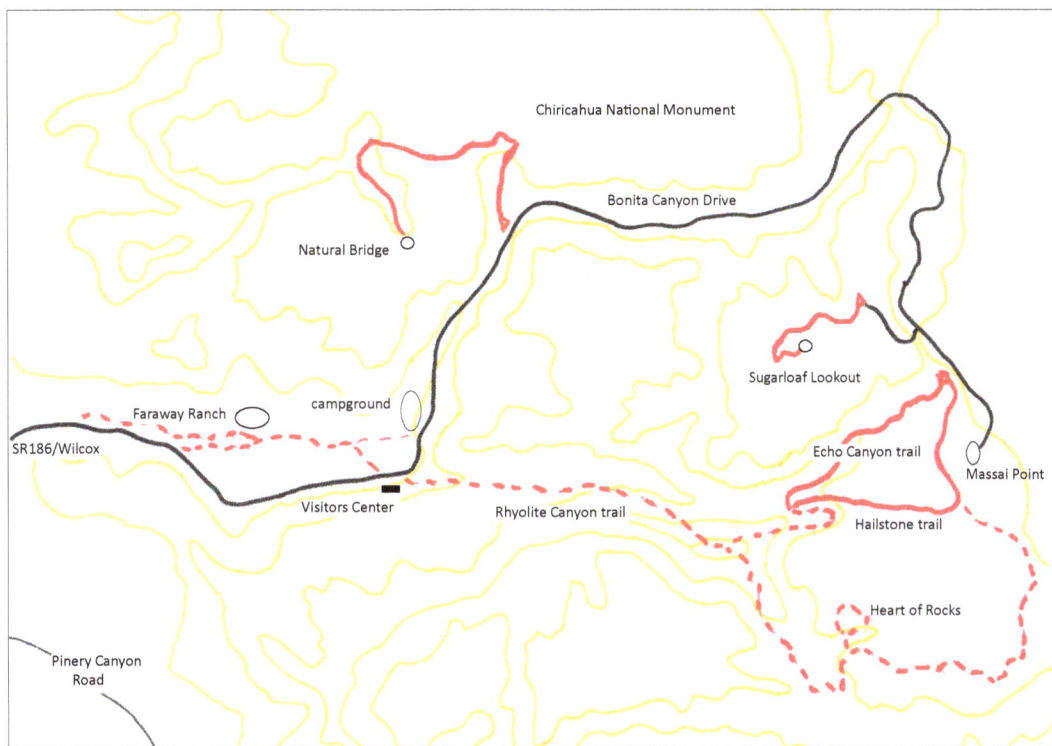

Map labels: Chiricahua National Monument, Bonita Canyon Drive, Natural Bridge, Sugarloaf Lookout, Echo Canyon trail, Massai Point, Faraway Ranch, campground, SR186/Wilcox, Visitors Center, Rhyolite Canyon trail, Hailstone trail, Heart of Rocks, Pinery Canyon Road

Sugarloaf Fire Lookout

In the effort to protect our forest against wildfire, men and women are stationed in fire towers or cabins in remote locations overlooking the valleys and mountains of Arizona. Sugarloaf Mountain, in the Chiricahua National Monument is one such location, accessed by driving 8 miles from the Visitor's Center to Massai Point. Just before reaching the summit, a signed fork directs visitors to the trailhead.

Within .25 mile of the trailhead, hikers pass through a rocky tunnel. The trail circles the peak toward the summit with good views of the rock hoodoos in the canyon's below. The simple one-room cabin at the summit was once a live-in location, offering a bunk and counter along with the Osborne Fire Finder. The 12 x 12 foot cabin offered panoramic views in all directions as the lookout scanned the horizon for a trickle of smoke.

This lookout cabin is similar to the cabins at Lemmon Rock and those destroyed by fire on Atascosa Peak, west of I-19, and Barfoot Peak above Rustler Park. Sugarloaf is rarely used now. A ranger may be sent up for a couple of hours during particularly violent storms to watch for lightning strikes.

Driving Distance: 8 miles from park entrance
Hiking Distance: .9 miles one way
Rating: Moderate
Elevation: 6840' - 7310'
Best Season: Spring, summer (hot) and fall.
Precautions: Wide trail but watch your footing.
Maps: Chiricahua National. Monument map
Information: Chiricahua National Monument
(520) 824-3560

Fort Bowie National Historic Site

Fort Bowie is a page out of Arizona history from a time when the U.S. Cavalry and the Apaches fought over the use of land and water. Visitors gain a better understanding of how history played out in southeastern Arizona where the high ground was an advantage and water could mean life to the victor.

From I-10, exit at mp 340. Drive southeast from Wilcox along SR 186 toward the Chiricahua Mountains. After 22 miles, turn left or north onto Apache Pass Road, an important trade route for both the Apaches and the white settlers. Six miles from SR 186, turn into the small parking area. A footpath leads east 1.5 miles toward the Fort Bowie National Historic Site.

The trail passes an old stage stop on the Butterfield Overland Trail. Beyond the stage stop, a fenced cemetery is a reminder of the risk to those who traveled the route and who settled the western lands. The next stop on the trail is the foundation for the Chiricahua Indian Agency. Tom Jeffords settled here when he was first appointed Indian agent for the newly formed Chiricahua Apache Reservation in 1872. He had earned the respect of officials in Washington and the Apaches for his decisions. However, local ranchers convinced officials to later remove him.

The trail climbs to Apache Spring, the site of a battle between the Cavalry and the Apaches. Due to a misunderstanding on the part of Major Bascom, the Apaches declared the spring off limits for all but their tribe. The Union Cavalry, in pursuit of an expedition force aligned with the southern states, desperately needed water. The Apache warriors ambushed the Cavalry as they approached the spring. Due to the presence of mountain howitzers, the Cavalry did prevail but not without

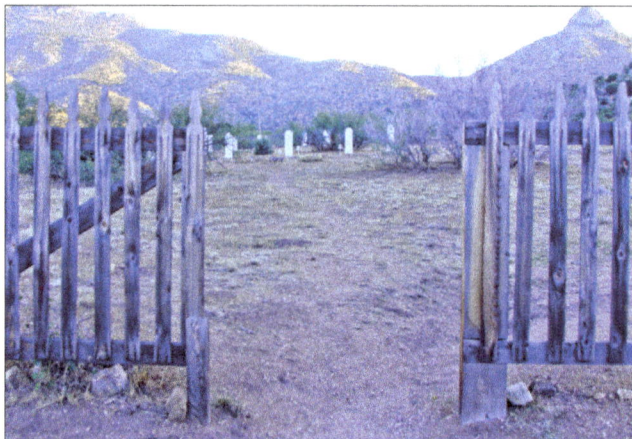

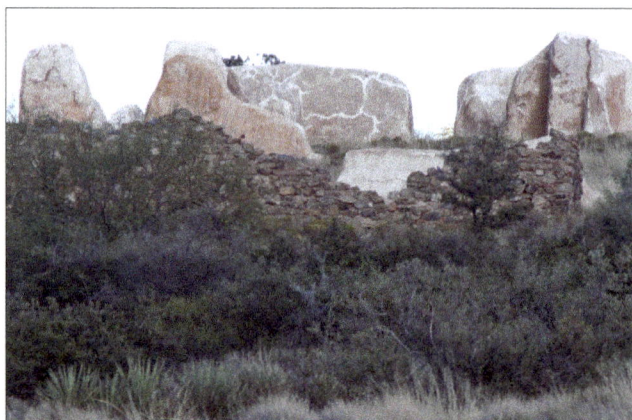

Cemetery & ruin walls

Driving Distance: 28 miles from
    Wilcox/I-10
Hiking Distance: 2+ miles
Rating: Easy   Elevation: 5325'
Best Season: Winter, spring & fall
Special Features: Historic Army Post
Precautions: Take lots of water in warmer
    months. Spring water is not potable.
Maps: Arizona Highways map, Park trail
    guide.
Information: Fort Bowie Visitors Center
    (520) 847-2500

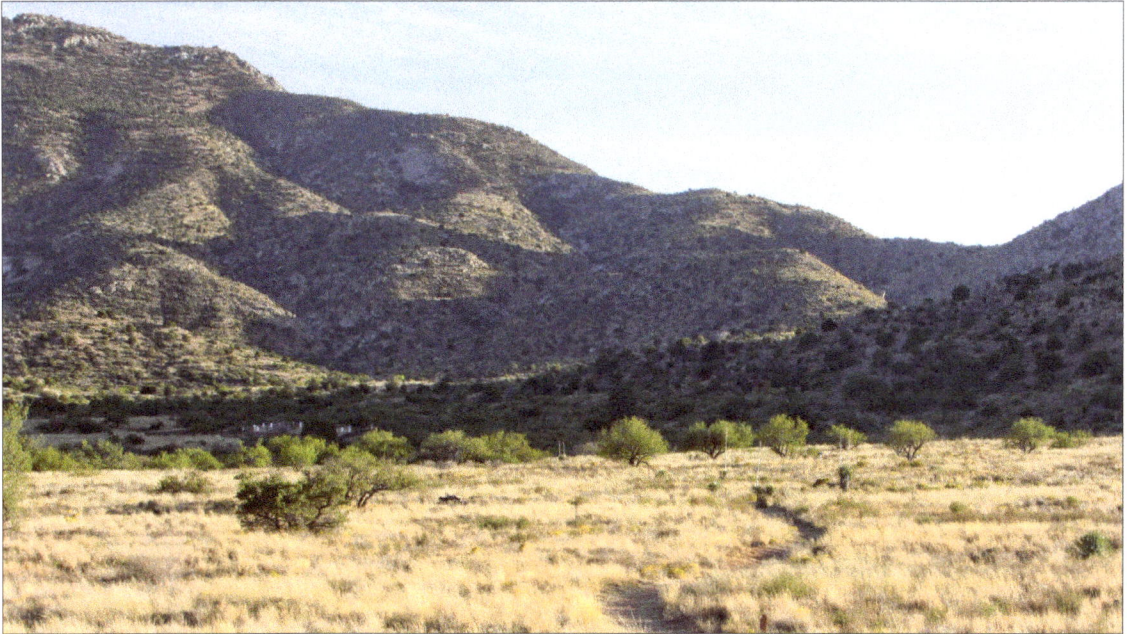

Looking up Apache Pass toward Fort Rucker

significant fatalities on both sides. Without the howitzers, the result might have been decided differently.

From the spring, visitors climb up to the old fort. Today, only scattered adobe walls remain on the quiet hillside. Fort Bowie was constructed in 1862, to defend the settlers throughout the area and to protect the route through the Pass. The last of the Apaches surrendered in 1886. The fort was decommissioned and abandoned after 27 years of service.

Visitors may examine old photos and displays at the Visitors Center. The fort wasn't a comfortable place to live, conditions were rough. In the quiet of the high desert, take a moment to imagine the squeak of leather cavalry saddles and clop of horses' hooves as they returned from patrol or the sound of a bugle playing taps at sunset as the flag is lowered over the Fort. Imagine sitting in the rocks high on the ridge above the fort as an Apache Indian observing life below, wondering what it would

take to send the white men back east so that your tribe might once again live a nomadic lifestyle.

Visitors either return the way they came or follow the trail up the ridge above the fort before descending along switchbacks toward the trail they first hiked from the parking area.

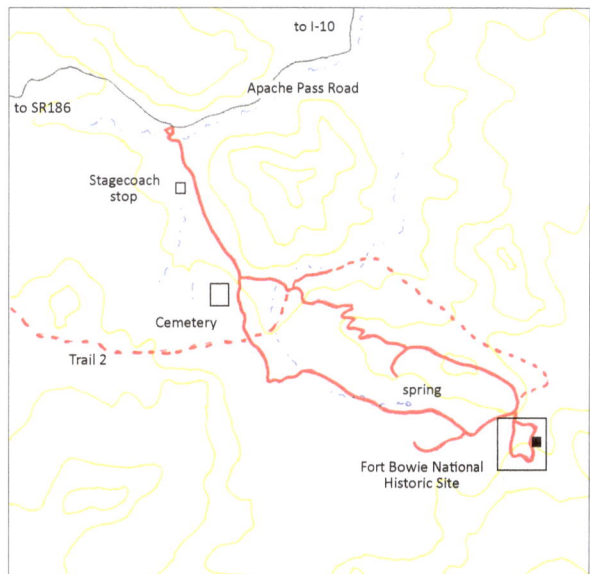

195

Heliograph Peak

No telephones! No cars! And certainly no radio or TV! So how could the US Army Cavalry receive the news of an Indian attack?

In the 1800's, as white settlers first moved into the Southwest, communication was limited to word carried by horseback or on foot. The US Army Cavalry built forts across the frontier and used a heliograph system with light and mirrors to flash messages in Morse Code between stations located on tall peaks. Heliograph Peak was the location of one such station.

Decades later, the Forest Service built a fire tower on the same summit. Around a hundred feet tall, this tower is one of the tallest in the Southwest. Heliograph Peak is located in the Pinoleno Mountains, along SR 366, one of only three state highways with a dirt surface in Arizona. Turn west onto the Swift Highway / SR366 from US Highway 191, south of Safford. Drive about thirty miles to the turnoff for Shannon Campground.

The trailhead is located at the far end of the campground. The trail starts as a gentle incline through tall pines, then switchbacks up the peak. After climbing about a mile, hikers break into the open on top of a rocky knob with a great view of the valley below. Beyond the knob, the trail hugs the hillside, a steep climb over loose rock. Much of the slope below was burned over in 2003 but vegetation has recovered, though not the majestic pines that once provided some nice shade.

From the summit, visitors look out beyond the Piñalenos, across the deserts into New Mexico and central Arizona. The tower also has an access road but it may not be open to visitors.

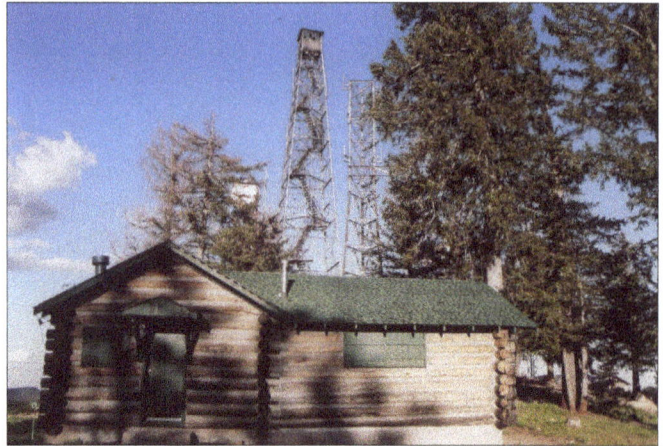

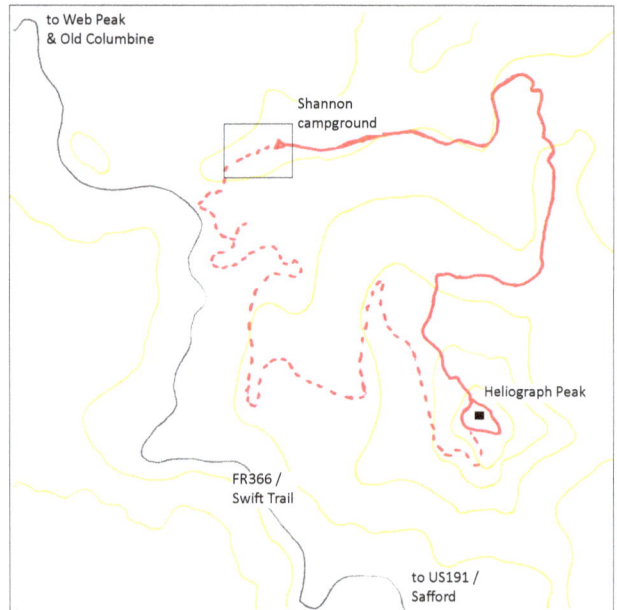

Driving Distance: Approx. 20 miles from Safford
Hiking Distance: 2 miles one way
Rating: Moderately difficult
Elevation: Heliograph Peak 10,028'
Best Season: Summer and early fall.
Special Features: One of tallest fire lookouts in the Southwest, site of an early heliograph station.
Precautions: Bear country. Watch footing over loose rock.

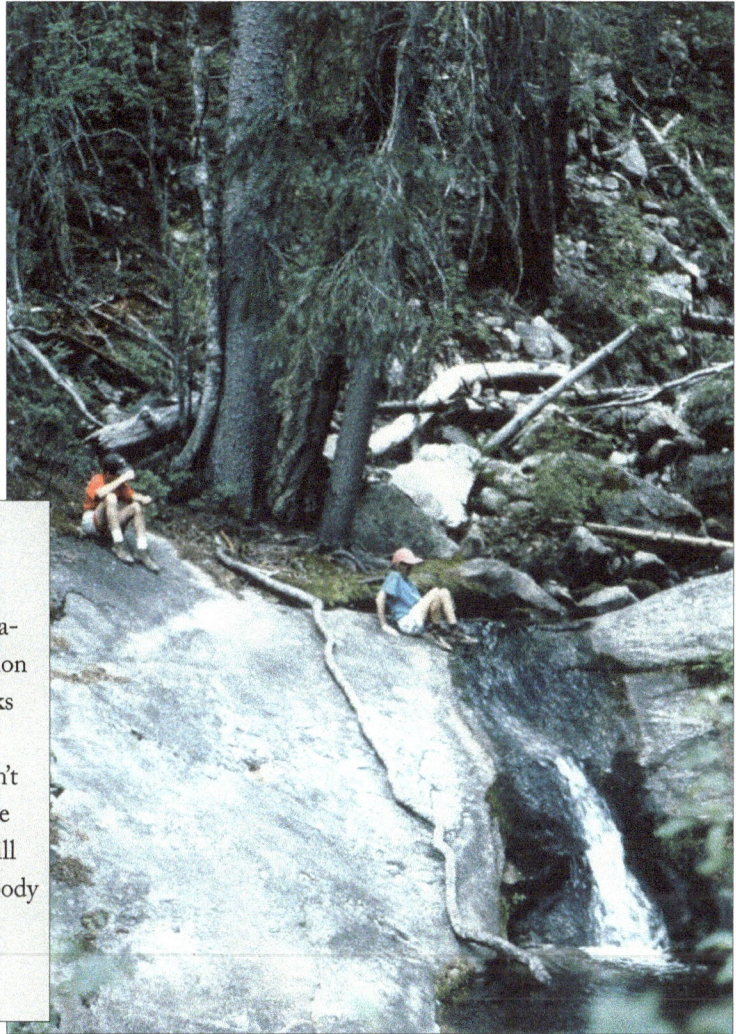

Along Ash Canyon Trail

Rhubarb?

Shannon Campground has a special niche set aside to protect the Chirica-huadock. This wild relative of common rhubarb flourishes in the moist banks along streams in eastern Arizona, including Ash Creek. The stalks aren't red like rhubarb but the showy white flowers towering above the leaves will catch your eye. The next time somebody offers you rhubarb think of 'rumex', rhubarb's wild relative.

Webb Peak and Old Columbine

An alternative hike to Heliograph Peak is a visit to Old Columbine Ranger Station and the Webb Peak Fire Tower. These structures are located at the end of the Swift Highway, just beyond the turnoff to the Mount Graham Observatory. A short hike take visitors from the road up to the fire tower.

Before fires swept the range, this was one of my favorite places to visit in Arizona. The Ash Creek trail is located across from Old Columbine. Before the fire in 2003, the canyon was a lush wilderness of wildflowers, tall fir and spruce with

a sparkling mountain stream. Plan on a full day to make this drive as it is a mountain road laden with twists and turns.

Driving Distance: 36 miles from Safford.
Hiking Distance: 2.2 miles one way to Slick Rock.
Rating: Moderate
Elevation: 9500' - about 9,000'
Maps: Coronado NFS map / Safford District
Info: Safford Ranger Station   (928)428-4150

Dragoon Mountains

The Dragoon Mountains resemble a pile of jumbled rocks dumped by a giant hand. The idea that anyone could find a passage into the mountains or a secluded valley with shade trees and pools of water seems far fetched. The early settlers thought so and failed to recognize the Dragoons as a refuge for the Apaches.

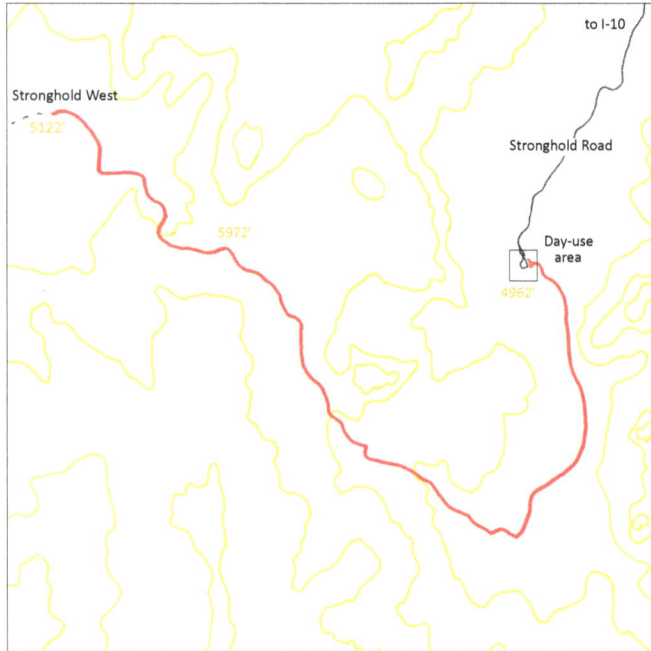

To reach the trailhead, turn south from I-10 at either exit 318 or 331. From exit 318, drive east 11 miles, skirting the north end of the Dragoons. Turn south onto US 191. Or from exit 331, drive south 15 miles on US 191 to the turnoff just north of Sunsites. Turning right onto Stronghold Road, drive 9 miles west into the Dragoons over a good dirt road. The Visitors Center includes a day use area with ramadas and restrooms, a nature walk and the trailhead. Campgrounds are nearby.

The nature trail, just under a half mile, crosses a bridge over a rock-studded swale and leads through desert vegetation at the base of the Dragoons. Plant identification placards explain their use by native peoples. These plants were used by the Apaches as they made their summer camps in the Dragoons.

The trail that most visitors seek out winds upward through the boulders to a pass on the ridge above. In the summer, these rock reflect the intense summer heat. The cooler months are a better choice for making the trek. Be sure to take lots of water.

The trail traverses the range, from Cochise's Stronghold to Stonghold West with a secondary trail turning south from Cochise's Stronghold to Middle March. Check with the Forest Service for additional information and trail conditions.

Driving Distance: 20 miles from I-10.
Hiking Distance: Nature Trail .4 mile, easy
    Stronghold Trail 5 miles one way, difficult
Best Season: Spring or fall
Special Features: Historical site
Precautions: Come prepared for rugged area far from emergency services.
    Watch for rattlesnakes.
Maps: Coronado NFS map / Dragoons
Information:
Douglas Ranger Station   (520) 364-3468
or Safford Ranger Station (928) 428-4150

The Arizona Trail: Footwork from the border with Utah to Mexico

One last trail, stretching from the border with Utah to the southern tip of Arizona at its border with Mexico. Dale Shewalter is credited as the 'father of the Arizona Trail.' In 1985, he began scouting a route that would cross the state from north to south. Through years of avocacy, he lived to see his dream completed though in the early years the route was pretty rough.

Today, a well-trod footpath, complete with trail signs, a web site along with a number of books and maps lay out the route. The 819 mile trail scales mountain ranges reaching its highest elevation at 9, 148 feet, dropping to the lowest elevation at 1,700 feet. The AzT was designated a National Scenic Trail in 2009, joining the ranks of other state transects like the Pacific Crest.

With the passage of time, this route has become ever more popular, whether covered one passage at a time or in one long stretch over several months. Volunteers now maintain a watch over each passage and are available online for those who have questions or a concern to report about the trail's condition.

So, when you're out hiking, somewhere toward the center line of the state and you come across a wooden sign proclaiming that this is the Arizona Trail, take a moment to appreciate the long hours that volunteers expended to create this route. Maybe plan a hike along one of the passages and invite a few friends to learn more of our beautiful state one step at a time.

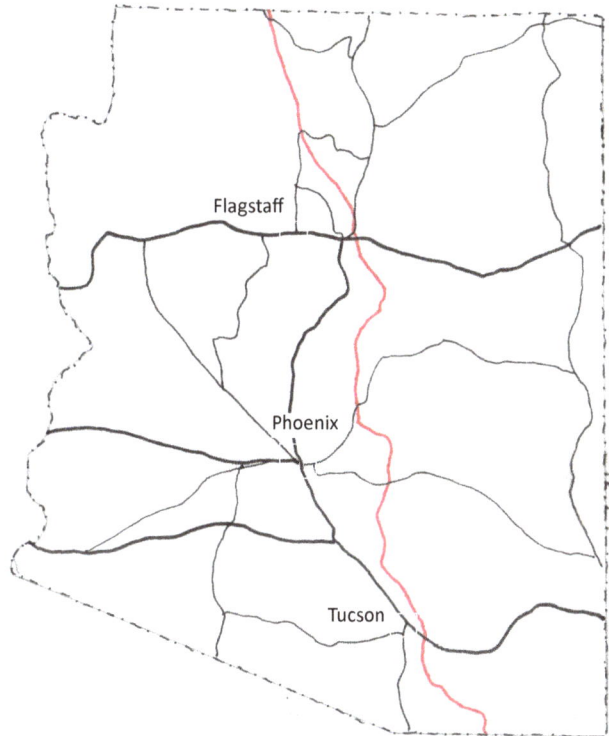

The Arizona Trail winds south from the Utah border through 43 'passages' to the southern terminus at the International border with Mexico.

Index

www.ingramcontent.com/pod-product-compliance
Lightning Source LLC
Chambersburg PA
CBHW042357030426
42337CB00030B/5132